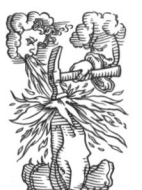

Basler Beiträge
zur Geschichtswissenschaft

Band 186

Begründet von
E. Bonjour, W. Kaegi und F. Staehelin

Weitergeführt von
F. Graus, K. v. Greyerz, H. R. Guggisberg, H. Haumann,
G. Kreis, H. Lüthy, M. Mattmüller, W. Meyer, J. Mooser,
A. v. Müller, M. Schaffner und R. Wecker

Herausgegeben von
C. Arni, S. Burghartz, L. Burkart, M. Lengwiler,
C. Opitz-Belakhal und F. B. Schenk

Lukas Meier

Swiss Science, African Decolonization and the Rise of Global Health, 1940–2010

Schwabe Verlag Basel

Published with the support of the Swiss National Science Foundation

Cover illustration: General Tropical Course,
Archive Swiss Tropical and Public Health Institute, 1947/51

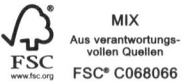

Editorial work: Jeff Acheson
Produced by: Schwabe AG, Muttenz/Basel
Printed in Switzerland
ISSN 1661-5026
ISBN 978-3-7965-3347-1

rights@schwabe.ch
www.schwabeverlag.ch

Contents

Foreword by Thierry A. Freyvogel and Marcel Tanner   7

Acknowledgments   9

Abbreviations 10

Introduction
Science, Medicine and Decolonization 13

Chapter 1
Decolonization, Development and Geographies of Knowledge 35
Refashioning Science: Science for Development 36
Establishment of the IDERT at Adiopodoumé 39
Science and Expertise in Mahenge (Ulanga) District, Tanganyika 42
Science and Decolonization 57

Chapter 2
Switzerland in the World 59
Science and the Postwar Economic Order 60
Shifting towards Colonialism? 98

Chapter 3
Scientists in the Field 101
The Discovery of Côte d'Ivoire 102
The Permanent Expedition: Tanganyika 1954–1961 114
Inventorizing and Improving Africa: Swiss Science in the Field 130

Chapter 4
The Charitable Impulse: Development and Nutritional Research
in Switzerland and Africa 131
"A New Ethic of Giving" 132
Développement Manqué: The Case of Côte d'Ivoire 154
The Nestlé Foundation and the Construction of Moderate
Protein-Calorie Malnutrition in Côte d'Ivoire 164
Variations of Development and the Power of Phenomenotechnique 178

Chapter 5
The Empire Retreats: Medical Research, Development
and the Rise of Social Medicine 181
Dismantling the Rural Aid Center – The Road to Preventive Medicine 184
The Medical Assistants Training Center 1973–1978................... 186
The Rise of Social Medicine in Switzerland.......................... 191
Decolonizing Swiss Medical Research in Tanzania.................... 199
Bringing Science Back in: The Emergence of a New Dispositive 214

Chapter 6
The Transformation of Swiss Science in the Era of Structural Adjustment .. 217
Development's Hangover and the Failure of Primary Health Care 220
*Integrating the Swiss Tropical Institute Field Laboratory
into Tanzanian Health Structures*................................... 223
*The End of the "Pacte Colonial": Scientific Disconnects
and the Africanization of the* CSRS *in Côte d'Ivoire* 237
Towards a New World Order 248

Chapter 7
The Governance of Malaria Research in Tanzania 251
SPf66 – A Vaccine Candidate from the South 254
*Intermittent Preventive Treatment of Malaria in Infants –
History in the Making* 269
*The Forgotten Southern Zone: Implementation Research
in Mtwara and Lindi Regions 2004–2009*........................... 271
Beyond the Laboratory 284

Epilogue
Science and Decolonization Revisited.............................. 285
Colonial Science 285
Development 288
Switzerland's Late Decolonization................................. 291
Writing a Swiss History of Science in Africa........................ 293

References
Archives, Sources, Publications................................... 295

Foreword

History has to be rewritten time and again, for each generation has its own viewpoint. Some historians adhere strictly to scientific methods; others pass judgment on the behavior of historical actors, sometimes disregarding the context in which they acted. To avoid this pitfall, Lukas Meier combined archive work with oral history.

His extensive archive research took him to Abidjan, Basel, Bern, Dar es Salaam and Paris. He gathered oral evidence by interviewing numerous (retired or still active) members of the Swiss and African scientific communities, as well as collaborators and villagers in Côte d'Ivoire and Tanzania.

This book, based on a PhD thesis in history, provides an impressive account of how Switzerland and Swiss science "discovered Africa" and sought to reconcile the tensions between undertaking science and contributing to development – particularly in the postindependence era when Tanzania and Côte d'Ivoire began to develop their own science capacity. It is interesting to note that the notion of achieving good science through equal research partnerships prevailed from the outset, though viewed with a certain skepticism by the former colonial powers. The Swiss founders of the Ifakara Health Institute (IHI, known until 1996 as the Swiss Tropical Institute Field Laboratory) and the Centre Suisse de Recherches Scientifiques en Côte d'Ivoire (CSRS) were keen to pursue their own strategy of becoming a major partner in the host countries' scientific and technological development, partly linked to the economic interests of the partnering private sector.

Reading Lukas Meier's careful analyses and well-documented case studies, it becomes clear that the Swiss Tropical Institute (known since 2010 as the Swiss Tropical and Public Health Institute) – like many other Swiss institutions engaged in action-oriented research – would not be what it is today without having had the opportunity to collaborate with Africa, and in particular with the IHI and CSRS. This important experience has also – albeit belatedly – contributed to the recognition of Swiss science in North-South partnership and its translation into development policy, as reflected in a wide variety of bi- and multilateral activities. The present study provides the first comprehensive basis for understanding the roots, determinants and dynamics of the Swiss North-South scientific collaboration and development partnership, with particular reference to the health sector.

The study guides us through successive periods, starting with the time when science was seen as aid, then moving towards the notion of cooperation, and finally leading to the current approach whereby "mutual learning for change" is used to address global problems. The wealth and depth of information unearthed by the book is especially valuable when we consider – against a backdrop of overrated economic considerations – how bi- and multilateral commitments should be evidence-based, and how much scientific partnership and technical cooperation is still required in jointly addressing diseases of poverty (such as HIV, tuberculosis and malaria) and neglected tropical diseases. Moreover, since the case studies also examine more recent large, community-based projects and clinical trials as part of the overall aim of understanding the decolonization process, Lukas Meier's findings should have a direct impact – not only in the context of individual and public health ethics – on improving the design and implementation of key intervention studies and public health interventions for the benefit of the populations concerned.

This work reveals the fundamental change in the attitude of Europeans to Africans, from sheer scientific curiosity to sound assistance, which occurred after the end of World War II. The analysis also illustrates what it means to see the multidisciplinary nature of questions and problems encountered in the field and the need for interdisciplinary approaches so as to achieve transdisciplinary solutions. Finally, it is gratifying to observe how a country as small as Switzerland can successfully contribute to international development.

It has been a privilege to work with Lukas Meier. The co-authors of this foreword – both former students of Rudolf Geigy, the founder of the Swiss Tropical Institute – have themselves witnessed the transition from colonial rule to independence, and the struggle for good governance and partnership. Much to their surprise – and indeed to their advantage – they have now, in their own lifetime, become objects of historical research and critical questioning.

Finally, we are indebted to the venerable Basel publisher Schwabe Verlag – founded by Johannes Petri in 1488 – for producing this edition of Lukas Meier's thesis.

Thierry A. Freyvogel   Marcel Tanner
Director of Swiss Tropical Institute   Director of Swiss TPH
1972–1987   since 1997

Acknowledgments

This book could not have been written without the help of many people. First, I want to thank Marcel Tanner, Director of the Swiss Tropical and Public Health Institute (Swiss TPH), who initiated the project and has supported it over the years, and the staff of the Swiss TPH. I am grateful to the R. Geigy Foundation, the Freiwillige Akademische Gesellschaft (Basel), the Commission for Research Partnerships with Developing Countries (KFPE), the Dr. H. A. Vögelin-Bienz-Stiftung (Staatsarchiv Basel-Stadt), the Josef und Olga Tomcsik-Stiftung (Basel) and the Swiss National Science Foundation for their generous financial support. In Tanzania, I would like to thank the Commission for Science and Technology (COSTECH) for research clearance, as well as Frederick Kaijage and Bertram Mapunda (Department of History, University of Dar es Salaam) for their hospitality. Special thanks go to the staff of the Ifakara Health Institute (IHI) in Dar es Salaam, Ifakara and Mtwara, who did everything possible to facilitate research at the various field sites. Likewise, in Côte d'Ivoire, I am indebted to the Ministère de l'Enseignement Supérieur et de la Recherche Scientifique (Direction Générale de la Recherche Scientifique et de l'Innovation Technologique) and to the staff of the Centre Suisse de Recherches Scientifiques (CSRS) for all their generous support. In Switzerland, this study benefited from the inputs of my supervisors – Martin Lengwiler, Patrick Harries, Guillaume Lachenal and Marcel Tanner – who carefully guided me over the years. Invaluable support came from the members of my thesis advisory board (Howard Phillips, Catherine Burns, Julie Parle, Vanessa Noble, Harriet Deacon, Lizy Hall, Helen Sweet, Anne Digby, Shula Marks, Walter Bruchhausen, Brigit Obrist, Piet van Eeuwijk, Elisio Macamo, Paul Jenkins, Socrates Litsios, Hines Mabika and Jean-Paul Bado). The intellectual generosity of all those who commented on draft chapters of the manuscript cannot be overestimated. Apart from my colleagues Marcel Dreier, Pascal Schmid, Rita Kesselring and Nanina Guyer, this applies to Marcel Tanner, Thierry Freyvogel, Kurt Schopfer, André Aeschlimann and Bernhard Schär. Sincere thanks are also due to Tony Clarke and Jeff Acheson, who spent countless hours helping to resolve English language issues. Thanks goes to Schwabe Verlag Basel and the editors of the Basler Beiträge zur Geschichtswissenschaft series for their decision to publish the manuscript and for carefully guiding the publication process. I am also grateful to my family for their constant encouragement and support. My deepest gratitude is owed to Anna Schorner, who has provided assistance and support for several years.   Lukas Meier

Abbreviations

A-OF	Afrique-Occidentale française
BMGF	Bill & Melinda Gates Foundation
CHMT	Council Health Medical Team
COSTECH	Tanzania Commission for Science and Technology
CSRS	Centre Suisse de Recherches Scientifiques en Côte d'Ivoire
DftZ	Dienst für technische Zusammenarbeit
DHMT	District Health Management Team
DMO	District Medical Officer
ENHR	Essential National Health Research
EPI	Expanded Program on Immunization
FAO	Food and Agriculture Organization
FDA	Food and Drug Administration
FIDES	Fonds d'Investissement pour le Développement Economique et Social des territoires d'outre-mer
HSR	Health Systems Research
IC	Ifakara Center
IDERT	Institut d'Enseignement et de Recherches Tropicales
IHI	Ifakara Health Institute
IHRDC	Ifakara Health Research and Development Center
IIRSDA	Institut International de Recherche Scientifique pour le Développement en Afrique, Adiopodoumé
IMF	International Monetary Fund
IPTi	Intermittent preventive treatment of malaria in infants
KDHS	Kilombero District Health Support
KIHERE	Kilombero Health and Research Project
KMP	Kilombero Malaria Project
LSHTM	London School of Hygiene & Tropical Medicine
MATC	Medical Assistants Training Center
MMS	Medicus Mundi Schweiz
MOH	Ministry of Health
MRC	Medical Research Council
NA	Native Administration
NIMR	National Institute for Medical Research
NMCP	National Malaria Control Program
OCP	Onchocerciasis Control Program
ORSTOM	Office de la Recherche Scientifique et Technique Outre-Mer
PCM	Protein-calorie malnutrition
PDCI	Parti Démocratique de Côte d'Ivoire
PHC	Primary health care
RAC	Rural Aid Center
RMO	Regional Medical Officer
SAP	Structural Adjustment Program
SCOA	Société Commerciale de l'Ouest Africain
SDC	Swiss Agency for Development and Cooperation

SNG	Schweizerische Naturforschende Gesellschaft
SNSF	Swiss National Science Foundation
SP	Sulfadoxine-pyrimethamine
STI	Swiss Tropical Institute
STIFL	Swiss Tropical Institute Field Laboratory
TANU	Tanganyika African National Union
TAZARA	Tanzania-Zambia Railway Authority
TPHA	Tanzania Public Health Association
UDEC	Union d'Entreprises Coloniales
UNICEF	United Nations Children's Fund
URDS	Ulanga Rural Development Scheme
UTC	Union Trading Company
VHW	Village health worker
WGH	Working Group Health
WHO	World Health Organization

History isn't the lies of the victors, as I once glibly assured
Old Joe Hunt; I know that now. It's more the memories of the survivors,
most of whom are neither victorious nor defeated.

Julian Barnes, The Sense of an Ending

Introduction
Science, Medicine and Decolonization

The scene is the Thai-Vietnamese border, sometime in the 1950s. It is one of those tropical nights when the temperature never falls to a tolerable level. Two Swiss malariologists are sitting in front of their basic field lab, recovering from an exhausting day studying anopheles mosquitoes, when they notice a figure emerging from the dark surrounding bushes. It is obvious that the man approaching their table has come a long way. His shirt and trousers are in rags, and the Chinese dialect he speaks is barely comprehensible to the two researchers. The stranger has been sent on a secret mission. He pulls out a sealed envelope and asks the two scientists to safely transmit the confidential information to a Swiss diplomat in Bern.

As often in tales of this kind, things rapidly go awry. Russian and British protagonists appear on the scene, with a keen interest in the secret information. The envelope changes hands quickly and soon ends up on the African continent, coming into the possession of Swiss scientists in Tanzania, where the Basel-based Swiss Tropical Institute (STI) operates a small research station in the rural Ulanga District – the Swiss Tropical Institute Field Laboratory (STIFL). Next, it travels in the suitcase of an unsuspecting scientist to Côte d'Ivoire, where another Swiss-run research station is located – the Centre Suisse de Recherches Scientifiques (CSRS) at Adiopodoumé, near Abidjan.

The detective story[1] by Rudolf Geigy – the first director of the STI – paints a striking portrait of Switzerland as a secret power in Africa in the aftermath of World War II. Swiss scientists are present all over the continent and, back home, éminences grises are pulling the political strings. Geigy's account is a suitable point of entry to the major themes discussed below. This book is about Swiss science and development in the context of African decolonization. I will argue that Switzerland – as a noncolonial power – had an important role to play in the context of empire.[2] Swiss sci-

1   Rudolf Geigy, *Siri, top secret*, Basel 1977.
2   Richard Behrendt, *Die Schweiz und der Imperialismus: Die Volkswirtschaft des hochkapitalistischen Kleinstaates im Zeitalter des politischen und ökonomischen Nationalismus*, Zurich 1932; Thomas David, Bouda Etemad, *Gibt es einen schweizerischen Im-*

entific organizations, pharmaceutical corporations and charities were able to take advantage of a period of transition where empires as political entities began to fall apart. Swiss scientific initiatives were well received by French and British colonial governments, and later also by independent African states. While, for the former, collaboration with a country presumed to be neutral was a clear demonstration of incremental changes in colonial policy, for the new African nations it represented a radical break with the colonial past.

However, the following story is as much about Africa as it is about Switzerland. Africa should be given center stage in the twentieth-century history of Swiss science: in remote corners of the African continent, Swiss scientific institutions emerged and researchers worked in the field, collecting specimens, exchanging ideas and developing new forms of collaboration. Looking at the impact of the "periphery" on scientific fields such as botany, zoology and medicine provides a valuable corrective to the Eurocentric approaches that have tended to focus on the "big sciences" in Switzerland.[3] The history of the STI and the two field laboratories in East and West Africa offers a lens through which Switzerland's role in a postcolo-

perialismus?, in: Traverse, Schweiz-Dritte Welt. Von der Expansion zur Dominanz, No. 2, 1998, pp. 17–27; Lyonel Kaufmann, *Guillaume Tell au Congo. L'expansion Suisse au Congo Belge, 1930–1960*, in: Etemad and David (eds.), Les Annuelles. La Suisse sur la ligne bleue de l'Outre-mer, Vol. 5, 1994, pp. 43–94; Niklaus Stettler, Peter Haenger, Robert Labhardt, *Baumwolle, Sklaven und Kredite. Die Basler Welthandelsfirma Christoph Burckhardt & Cie. in revolutionärer Zeit, 1789–1815*, Basel 2004; Andrea Franc, *Wie die Schweiz zur Schokolade kam. Der Kakaohandel der Basler Handelsgesellschaft mit der Kolonie Goldküste, 1893–1960*, Basel 2008; Serge Reubi, *Gentlemen, prolétaires et primitifs. Institutionalisation, pratiques de collection et choix muséographiques dans l'ethnographie suisse, 1880–1950*, Thèse Université de Neuchâtel 2008; Patrick Minder, *La Suisse coloniale? Les représentations de l'Afrique et des Africains en Suisse au temps des colonies, 1880–1939*, Bern 2011; Patrick Harries, *Butterflies and Barbarians. Swiss Missionaries and Systems of Knowledge in South-East Africa*, Oxford 2007; Andreas Zangger, *Koloniale Schweiz. Ein Stück Globalgeschichte zwischen Europa und Südostasien, 1860–1930*, Bielefeld 2011; Bernhard Schär, *Tropenliebe. Basler Naturforscher, holländische Imperialisten und die "Entdeckung" von Celebes um 1900*, Dissertation Universität Bern 2013 (forthcoming); Patricia Purtschert, Barbara Lüthi, Francesca Falk (eds.), *Postkoloniale Schweiz. Formen und Folgen eines Kolonialismus ohne Kolonien*, Bielefeld 2012.

3   Bruno J. Strasser, *The Coproduction of Neutral Science and Neutral State in Cold War Europe. Switzerland and International Scientific Cooperation, 1951–1969*, in: Osiris, Vol. 24, 2009, pp. 165–187; Strasser, *La fabrique d'une nouvelle science. La biologie moléculaire à l'âge atomique*, Florence 2006; Stephan Zellmeyer, *A Place in Space. The History of Swiss Participation in European Space Programmes, 1960–1987*, Basel 2007.

nial world order can be assessed. This book thus stands at the crossroads of two intellectual endeavors – the history of science and biomedicine in Africa and an analysis of the relationship between science and decolonization.

Science and Biomedicine in Africa

Colonial science has been widely discussed in scholarly accounts of Africa. It has been assumed that, if colonizing states differed from noncolonizing states in their ways of mobilizing resources or exerting power over their colonial subjects, then there must also be a specific notion of colonial science. Many authors claimed that science and technology was colonial in its strong preference for certain topics, such as race and eugenics; it focused on Europeans (i.e., the military) rather than the colonized, and consequently on urban centers rather than rural areas.[4] In short, science was a tool of empire and Africa a laboratory where new practices and technologies could be tested before being applied at home.[5] However, as the volume of empirical material and theoretical reasoning increased, the reading of colonial science took a new turn. Scholars inspired by postcolonial thinking and cultural history increasingly began to portray science in the periphery as being influenced by local intermediaries, contested and prone

---

4   Shula Marks, *What is Colonial about Colonial Medicine? And What has Happened to Imperialism and Health?*, in: Social History and Medicine, Vol. 10, No. 2, 1997, pp. 205–219, here: p. 211; David Arnold, *Medicine and Colonialism*, in: William F. Bynum and Roy Porter (eds.), Companion Encyclopedia of the History of Medicine, Vol. 2, London, New York 1993, pp. 1393–1416, here: p. 1398; Patricia M. E. Lorcin, *Imperialism, Colonial Identity, and Race in Algeria, 1830–1870. The Role of the French Medical Corps*, in: Isis, Vol. 90, No. 4, 1999, pp. 653–679; Meredeth Turshen, *The Impact of Colonialism on Health and Health Services in Tanzania*, in: International Journal of Health Services, Vol. 7, No. 1, 1977, pp. 7–35.

5   Daniel R. Headrick, *The Tools of Empire. Technology and European Imperialism in the Nineteenth Century*, New York 1981; Maynard W. Swanson, *The Sanitation Syndrome. Bubonic Plague and Urban Native Policy in the Cape Colony, 1900–1909*, in: Journal of African History, Vol. 18, No. 3, 1977, pp. 387–410; for critical accounts of the laboratory metaphor see: Dirk van Laak, *Kolonien as "Laboratorien der Moderne?"*, in: Sebastian Conrad and Jürgen Osterhammel (eds.), Das Kaiserreich transnational. Deutschland in der Welt, 1871–1914, Göttingen 2004, pp. 257–279; Guillaume Lachenal, *Le médecin qui voulut être roi. Médecine coloniale et utopie au Cameroun*, in: Annales HSS, Vol. 1, 2010, pp. 121–156.

to failure.[6] In a recent book, historian Helen Tilley refused to accept any notion of colonial science whatsoever. Knowledge, she contends, might be generated locally, but it is constantly on the move: "There is too much circulation between metropole and colony, across colonies and between colonies and nation-states to warrant the designation colonial science."[7] Aside from the close interconnection between colonial and metropolitan science, can the study of a noncolonial power yield new insights into the problems of colonial and postcolonial science? Perhaps. As I will argue, there was little difference between Swiss science as practiced in Switzerland and in the tropics. Swiss researchers deployed the same methodologies and similar technical equipment when studying parasites in the Bernese Alps or in the French and British colonies. Rather than describing science as merely "local" and thus "colonial", it will be important to analyze the power structures inherent in scientific projects – irrespective of whether such activities took place during colonial times or in the context of today's global health research. Swiss actors differed from those of other nations in their ability to undertake research projects in Africa, to seek vital collaborations, to control the scientific process and to obtain significant results. Time and place play an important role in explaining these differences. Generally speaking, Swiss science became more powerful in the period after African independence, when the influence of the former colonial powers declined

6   Megan Vaughan, *Curing their Ills. Colonial Power and African Illness*, Stanford 1991; Nancy Rose Hunt, *A Colonial Lexicon: Of Birth Ritual, Medicalization, and Mobility in the Congo*, Durham, London 1999; Luise White, *Speaking With Vampires. Rumor and History in Colonial Africa*, Berkeley, Los Angeles, London 2000; Walter Bruchhausen, *Medizin zwischen den Welten. Geschichte und Gegenwart des medizinischen Pluralismus im südöstlichen Tansania*, Bonn 2006; Lyn Schumaker, *Africanizing Anthropology. Fieldworks, Networks and the Making of Cultural Knowledge in Central Africa*, Durham, N. C., London 2001; Nancy Jacobs, *The Intimate Politics of Ornithology in Colonial Africa*, in: Comparative Studies in Society and History, Vol. 48, 2006, pp. 564–603; Patrick Harries, *Field Sciences in Scientific Fields. Entomology, Botany and the Early Ethnographic Monograph in the Work of H. A. Junod*, in: Saul Dubow (ed.), Science and Society in Southern Africa, Manchester, New York 2000, pp. 11–41; Helen Tilley, *Global Histories, Vernacular Science, and African Genealogies; or, Is the History of Science Ready for the World?*, in: Isis, Vol. 101, No. 1, 2010, pp. 110–119; Peter Redfield, *Space in the Tropics. From Convicts to Rockets in French Guiana*, Berkeley, Los Angeles, London 2000; Peter Redfield, *The Half-Life of Empire in Outer Space*, in: Social Studies of Science, Vol. 32, No. 5–6, 2002, pp. 791–825; David Arnold, *Colonizing the Body. State Medicine and Epidemic Disease in Nineteenth-Century India*, Berkeley, Los Angeles 1993.
7   Helen Tilley, *Africa as a Living Laboratory. Empire, Development, and the Problem of Scientific Knowledge, 1870–1950*, Chicago 2011, p. 10.

and new global health paradigms emerged. Furthermore, Tanzania offered more opportunities for Swiss science to get off the ground than did Côte d'Ivoire, where – even after independence – France controlled much of the economy and foreign policy. Thus, the development of Swiss science appears to have been closely related to the process of African decolonization.

Science and Decolonization

In what follows, I will seek to show how Swiss science relates to the political and cultural processes of African decolonization. The main argument is that science and decolonization are not only closely interrelated, but mutually co-productive.[8] The term "decolonization" has many connotations, and it will be necessary to define clearly what is meant when it is used throughout the study.

Firstly, I use the term "decolonization" in probably the most conventional sense, to indicate a historical process roughly covering the period from 1930 to the wave of independence which many African countries were drawn into at the end of the 1950s and the beginning of the 1960s. This process can be understood neither as the result of nationalist struggle nor as a deliberate transfer of power to the former colonial "subjects", controlled by their colonial "masters". As recent scholarship has suggested, decolonization was fraught with contingencies, and its outcome could never be taken for granted.[9] The period under discussion coincides with major advances in the sciences, and with the development of an international health regime that had its roots in the nineteenth and early twentieth centuries, culminating in the foundation of the WHO in 1948.[10] Emblematic of these

---

8   Guillaume Lachenal, *Biomédicine et décolonisation au Cameroun, 1944–1994. Technologies, figures et institutions médicales à l'épreuve.* Thèse de doctorat, Université Paris 7 – Denis Diderot, Paris 2006, p. 15.

9   Tony Chafer, *The End of Empire in French West Africa. France's Successful Decolonization?*, Oxford 2002, p. 5; Frederick Cooper, *Decolonization and African Society. The Labor Question in French and British Africa*, Cambridge 2005, p. 8.

10 Theodore M. Brown, Marcos Cueto, Elizabeth Fee, *The World Health Organization and the Transition from "International" to "Global" Public Health*, in: American Journal of Public Health, Vol. 96, No. 1, 2006, pp. 62–72; Milton I. Roemer, *Internationalism in Medicine and Public Health*, in: William F. Bynum and Roy Porter (eds.), Companion Encyclopedia of the History of Medicine, Vol. 2, 1993, pp. 1417–1435; Paul Weindling (ed.), *International Health Organizations and Movements, 1918–1939*, Cambridge 1995.

scientific advances was the antibiotic penicillin which, in the 1940s, revolutionized the treatment of various infectious diseases, some of which had previously been lethal.[11] Faith in scientific progress was also boosted by the insecticide DDT, which proved to be a life-saving tool – notably for military personnel in malaria-infested areas – and which revolutionized the agricultural and public health sectors in what later came to be called the Third World. Widely applied, the new scientific developments played an important role within the larger context of empire. While World War II was instrumental in reframing the relationship between the imperial powers and the populations living in the colonies, the concept of empire itself did not falter. On the contrary, this idea reached its zenith after the war, sustained by the conviction that colonial subjects should also benefit from scientific progress and social welfare, which was gaining ground in postwar European societies.[12] As historian Frederick Cooper concluded, "Postwar imperialism was the imperialism of knowledge."[13] As will be shown later, Switzerland had a stake in the scientific recolonization of Africa in the 1940s. The period after World War II not only witnessed attempts to create a federal scientific system but saw the rise of scientific institutions such as the STI and its expanding network in East and West Africa.

Secondly, decolonization involves a phenomenon for which scientific knowledge was essential – development.[14] Here, the term is used, not to denote a specifically Western way of thinking and acting, typical of a his-

---

11 Mark Harrison, *Disease and the Modern World. 1500 to the Present Day*, Cambridge 2004, p. 168.

12 Andreas Eckert, *Regulating the Social. Social Security, Social Welfare, and the State in Late Colonial Tanzania*, in: Journal of African History, Vol. 45, 2004, pp. 467–489.

13 Frederick Cooper, *Modernizing Bureaucrats, Backward Africans, and the Development Concept*, in: Frederick Cooper and Randall Packard (eds.), International Development and the Social Sciences. Essays on the History and Politics of Knowledge, Berkeley 1997, pp. 64–92, here: p. 64.

14 Andreas Eckert, *Kolonialismus*, Frankfurt am Main 2006, p. 90; in general, the historiography of Swiss development aid is still in its infancy. Substantial works include: Peter Hug, Beatrix Mesmer (eds.), *Von der Entwicklungshilfe zur Entwicklungspolitik, Studien und Quellen*, Vol. 19, Bern 1993; René Holenstein, *Was kümmert uns die Dritte Welt. Zur Geschichte der internationalen Solidarität in der Schweiz*, Zurich 1998; René Holenstein, *Wer langsam geht, kommt weit. Ein halbes Jahrhundert Schweizer Entwicklungshilfe*, Zurich 2010; Monica Kalt, *Tiersmondismus in der Schweiz der 1960er und 1970er Jahre. Von der Barmherzigkeit zur Solidarität*, Bern 2010; Konrad Kuhn, *Entwicklungspolitische Solidarität. Die Dritte-Welt-Bewegung in der Schweiz zwischen Kritik und Politik, 1975–1992*, Zurich 2011; Lukas Zürcher, *Die Schweiz in Ruanda. Mission, Entwicklungshilfe und nationale Selbstbestätigung*, Zurich 2013 (in press).

torical period, but to study the nature, quality and shifting intensities of entanglements between the various actors engaged in the development project.[15] Development did not "emerge" at the end of the 1940s. During the interwar period, colonial governments were already attracted by the promises of development and modernity, to such an extent that they intervened more systematically in African societies, with the ultimate aim of increasing agricultural yields or sustaining a healthy workforce.[16] These efforts saw the rise of many experts who, as a social group, offered their advice to colonial and postcolonial governments.[17]

Development rhetoric continued to flourish in the new postwar world order. In his 1949 Point Four Program, US President Harry S. Truman famously claimed that, by offering technical assistance (and, one might add, democracy and capitalism), industrial nations could bring underdeveloped countries onto the path of welfare. In the President's view, winning the hearts and minds of the wretched was possible through systematic application of science and technology in impoverished territories. Faith in scientific reason as a means of overcoming abject poverty brought together European and African governments, as well as international organizations such as the UN or the Food and Agriculture Organization (FAO). Often, their initiatives were associated with the hope of containing the spread of communist ideology in the Third World. Moreover, development became the structural principle underlying policy decisions and channeling flows of donor money. The fact that development was not the prerogative of former colonial powers but became the postcolonial question par excellence is shown by the example of countries such as Switzerland, which, from the early 1960s, embraced development as a foreign policy strategy. Swiss government initiatives in this area largely relied on the knowledge and expertise of private actors such as missionary societies, pharmaceutical companies, or groups of natural scientists, whose opinions were valued because of their practical experience in Third World countries. More

15   Hubertus Büschel, Daniel Speich, *Einleitung – Konjunkturen, Probleme und Perspektiven der Globalgeschichte von Entwicklungszusammenarbeit*, in: Büschel and Speich (eds.), Entwicklungswelten. Globalgeschichte der Entwicklungszusammenarbeit, Frankfurt am Main 2009, pp. 7–29, here: p. 20.
16   Christophe Bonneuil, *Development as Experiment. Science and State Building in Late Colonial and Postcolonial Africa, 1930–1970*, in: Roy MacLeod (ed.), Nature and Empire. Science and the Colonial Enterprise, Chicago 2001, pp. 258–281, here: p. 259.
17   Joseph Morgan Hodge, *Triumph of the Expert. Agrarian Doctrines of Development and the Legacies of British Colonialism*, Athens 2007.

importantly, development neither described a mere transfer of technology from the West to African countries, nor was it an "extremely efficient apparatus for producing knowledge about, and the exercise of power over, the Third World".[18] As we will see later, development became, on the one hand, a powerful "claim-making instrument" for Tanzanian actors, who were very much able to influence the path to development taken by the field laboratory during the 1960s and 1970s. On the other hand, Swiss development experts became ardent spokespersons for Nyerere's African socialism in turn.[19] Thus, from the perspective of the complex interactions that took place on the ground, little remains of the favored interpretation of development as a powerful weapon against communist ideology gaining a foothold in Africa. Rather, historical actors could exploit Cold War ideologies, or not, according to their various interests.

Thirdly, "decolonization" is used as an analytical concept throughout the book. Compared to many scientific institutions established by former imperial powers, Switzerland today still exerts a strong influence over the CSRS and the STIFL, which has considerably enhanced their scientific performance over the past twenty years. The stronger impact of these two institutions in their respective countries' scientific and medical spheres dates back to the period of structural adjustment in the 1980s, when Swiss science and medical research underwent a process of decolonization. At this time, the two institutions were more closely integrated into the scientific and medical systems of Côte d'Ivoire and Tanzania, increasing numbers of African researchers were recruited, and research activities were adjusted to local and national priorities. This process of decolonization, however, did not mean making oneself dispensable. Rather, it refers to the strategies employed to remain present, to delegate decision-making to Tanzanian and Ivorian stakeholders, and to position oneself within the constellation now known as a research partnership. The strong role played by Swiss science in these two countries was defended on the grounds that the distorted sociopolitical environment prevailing since the 1980s, and the financial constraints imposed on African governments, posed a threat to the high-quality standards set for the scientific venture. It would,

---

18 Arturo Escobar, *Encountering Development. The Making and Unmaking of the Third World*, Princeton 1995, p. 9; for a similar view, see another classic in the field of development literature, Wolfgang Sachs (ed.), *The Development Dictionary. A Guide to Knowledge as Power*, London 1992.

19 Frederick Cooper, *Writing the History of Development*, in: Journal of Modern European History, Vol. 8, No. 1, 2010, pp. 5–23, here: p. 11.

though, be misleading to see these mechanisms as mere neocolonialism or neopaternalism. During the 1980s and 1990s, Swiss science in Africa was shaped by African actors and institutions, as well as by the vagaries of an international research and donor community. The question of how power relations were reshuffled between Swiss and African actors yields different answers, depending on whether one considers intrainstitutional developments, specific experimental situations, or the interplay between various actors within global scientific networks. From this perspective, decolonization becomes more of a lens allowing one to examine the reconfigurations of social hierarchies or the micropolitics of science as practiced in specific constellations.[20]

Methodologies

The scope of this book is ambitious, as it aims to bring multiple field sites into one analytical framework.[21] Comparison is one of the options proposed here to manage messy historical realities. The book not only focuses on the micropolitics of two formerly Swiss research institutions in Africa. It aims to broaden the picture by comparing different regions, different colonial and postcolonial systems, and the two African countries' different trajectories into a postcolonial world. Without oversimplifying, regions are important objects of comparison in African history. Often, the boundaries of colonial states were drawn randomly, cutting across regions with similar ecological, cultural and economic traits. This is equally true of postcolonial states. Whether one focuses on remote rural areas – where the presence of a district commissioner may be the only symbol of an otherwise absent "colonial state" – or on areas close to administrative and economic centers, makes a huge difference for the deployment of an effective science and health policy. This, of course, is not to say that it is less important to analyze differences and similarities at the level of colonial and postcolonial states. French and British colonial policies were too disparate not to have an effect on Swiss science in the African colonies. Côte d'Ivoire and

---

20 Gabrielle Hecht, *Rupture-Talk in the Nuclear Age. Conjugating Colonial Power in Africa*, in: Social Studies of Science, Vol. 32, No. 5–6, 2002, pp. 691–727.
21 Frederick Cooper, Ann Laura Stoler, *Between Metropole and the Colony. Rethinking a Research Agenda*, in: Cooper and Stoler (eds.), Tensions of Empire. Colonial Cultures in a Bourgeois World, Berkeley, Los Angeles, London 1997, pp. 1–56.

Tanganyika played different roles in the overall imperial structures: while Côte d'Ivoire was France's most valuable colony, whose inhabitants were to be molded into Frenchmen, Tanganyika remained outside the sphere of British interest. Not endowed with natural resources and given the status of a mandated territory by the League of Nations, Tanganyika was a country in which Britain was always reluctant to invest. After independence, modernization was the ultimate goal. However, while Ivorian President Félix Houphouet-Boigny considered a market economy and special trade relations with France as the most promising means to this end, Tanzania's Julius Nyerere advocated an African socialism centered around rural development. It was only in the 1980s that – with the imposition of structural adjustment programs by the World Bank and the International Monetary Fund (IMF) – the two African countries succumbed to economic recession and widespread poverty. These roughly sketched differences all have a part to play in explaining the development of Swiss science in Africa. Analytical separation of the institutional, regional, national and international levels will be one of the foremost aims of this book.

Comparison is, however, not the only methodological instrument adopted. Social history in general and comparative approaches in particular have faced serious criticism in recent years. A set of social, cultural and economic phenomena subsumed under the heading of globalization, together with growing global interconnectedness and exchanges, has led to a reassessment of historical instruments and analytical concepts. French historian Michel Espagne, for instance, mainly focusing on cultural transfers within Europe, argued that comparative approaches – implicitly or explicitly – employ a national perspective and tend to cement differences between the objects of investigation.[22] Given the pitfalls of methodological nationalism inherent in comparative research, and the many entanglements between the objects of analysis, he argued that transfer studies should be at the center of historical inquiry.

However, as many authors have noted, the gulf between comparisons and transfers, between the logic of analytical separation and that of entanglement and connectivity, is not as wide as is commonly assumed. Trans-

---

22   Michel Espagne, *Au-delà du comparatisme*, in: Espagne, Les transferts culturels franco-allemands, Paris 1999, pp. 35–49; Johannes Paulmann, *Internationaler Vergleich und interkultureller Transfer. Zwei Forschungsansätze zur europäischen Geschichte des 18. bis 20. Jahrhunderts*, in: Historische Zeitschrift, Vol. 267, 1998, pp. 649–685, here: p. 668.

fer studies can hardly do without a comparison of the specific situations whence and to which specific items are to be transferred. Moreover, the two approaches meet in their ultimate aim of "transnationalizing" historiography.[23] One concept that combines comparative approaches and transfer studies in unprecedented ways is that of *histoire croisée*, developed by the (German-)French historians Michael Werner and Bénédicte Zimmermann.[24] Werner and Zimmermann share the above-mentioned reservations with regard to comparative history. In their view, comparative approaches are ahistorical and constructed on the basis of a range of untenable abstractions and flawed assumptions. Comparative historians tend to "freeze their objects in time", whereas processes of transformation are at work; they assume parity between objects, whereas these objects are constructed by historical forces; and they proclaim a separation of objects, whereas interactions and reciprocal modifications occur.[25] As if this were not enough,

23   Hartmut Kaelble, *Die Debatte über Vergleich und Transfer und was jetzt?*, in: H-Soz-u-Kult, 08.02.2005, http://hsozkult.geschichte.hu-berlin.de/forum/id=574&type=artikel (accessed, 15.03.2012); Jürgen Osterhammel, *Transkulturell vergleichende Geschichtswissenschaft*, in: Osterhammel, Geschichtswissenschaft jenseits des Nationalstaats. Studien zu Beziehungsgeschichte und Zivilisationsvergleich, Göttingen 2003, pp. 11–45, here: p. 43; Jürgen Kocka, Heinz-Gerhard Haupt, *Comparison and Beyond. Traditions, Scope and Perspectives of Comparative History*, in: Kocka and Haupt (eds.), Comparative and Transnational History. Central European Approaches and New Perspectives, New York 2009, pp. 1–32, here: p. 20; for transnational approaches in historiography, see: Kiran Klaus Patel, *Nach der Nationalfixiertheit. Perspektiven einer transnationalen Geschichte. Öffentliche Antrittsvorlesung an der Humboldt-Universität zu Berlin*, Berlin 2004; Jürgen Osterhammel, *Transnationale Gesellschaftsgeschichte. Erweiterung oder Alternative*, in: Geschichte und Gesellschaft, Vol. 27, No. 3, 2001, pp. 464–479; Albert Wirz, *Für eine transnationale Gesellschaftsgeschichte*, in: Geschichte und Gesellschaft, Vol. 27, No. 2, 2001, pp. 489–498; Sebastian Conrad, Jürgen Osterhammel, *Einleitung*, in: Conrad and Osterhammel (eds.), Das Kaiserreich transnational, pp. 7–27; for a critical appraisal by a social historian, see: Hans-Ulrich Wehler, *Transnationale Geschichte – der neue Königsweg historischer Forschung?*, in: Gunilla Budde, Sebastian Conrad and Oliver Janz (eds.), Transnationale Geschichte. Themen, Tendenzen und Theorien, Göttingen 2006, pp. 161–174.
24   Michael Werner, Bénédicte Zimmermann, *Beyond Comparison. Histoire Croisée and the Challenge of Reflexivity*, in: History and Theory, Vol. 45, 2006, pp. 30–50; Werner, Zimmermann, *Vergleich, Transfer, Verflechtung. Der Ansatz der "Histoire croisée" und die Herausforderung des Transnationalen*, in: Geschichte und Gesellschaft, Vol. 28, 2002, pp. 607–636.
25   Werner, Zimmermann, *Beyond Comparison*, pp. 33–35; Jani Marjanen, *Undermining Methodological Nationalism. Histoire croisée of Concepts as Transnational History*, in: Mathias Albert et al. (eds.), Transnational Political Spaces. Agents – Structures – Encounters, Frankfurt, New York 2009, pp. 239–263, here: p. 245.

comparativists are subject to an "optical illusion". They construct the observer's position as being external to the objects, "while scholars are always ... engaged in the field of observation".[26] Though more sympathetic to transfer studies than to comparative approaches, these authors also find fault with transfer studies: in fact, despite their focus on historical processes and transformations, transfer studies suffer from the same shortfalls as do comparisons. They depart from national frameworks as units of reference, employ often static categories, and largely oversimplify matters in assuming linearity of transfers instead of complex patterns of reciprocity.[27] *Histoire croisée*, the authors maintain, is a reasonable solution because it combines the advantages of the comparative approach with those of transfer studies. *Histoire croisée* is especially appealing because it not only emphasizes the "intercrossings" of the research object on different scales (micro/macro levels), or the historicity of concepts, but reflects on the – often asymmetrical – relations between researchers and their objects.[28]

The study undertaken here draws extensively on the insights provided by *histoire croisée*. On the one hand, the history of the two research laboratories in Côte d'Ivoire and Tanzania is conceptualized as a comparative study of Swiss science in a context of colonial and postcolonial domination. It strives for a "variation-finding comparison",[29] seeking to show that the Third World is not the homogeneous entity commonly depicted in public discourses. Côte d'Ivoire and the Tanganyikan trust territory under British mandate not only provided different "local" research settings for Swiss science to evolve. Unsurprisingly perhaps, the two countries diverged substantially with regard to their status in the wider context of the French and British empires, and in the different trajectories leading into the postcolony. However, the two case studies are not sufficiently differentiated to meet the methodological requirements of "pure" comparisons. Not only did institutional models travel between the two sites themselves – more obvious was (and is) the laboratories' connections with Switzerland

---

26 Werner, Zimmermann, *Beyond Comparison*, pp. 33–34; in this sense, Werner and Zimmermann's approach fits neatly with Ute Daniel's idea of cultural history – see: Ute Daniel, *Einleitung: Kulturgeschichte – und was sie nicht ist*, in: Daniel, Kompendium Kulturgeschichte. Theorien, Praxis, Schlüsselwörter, Frankfurt am Main 2001, pp. 7–25, here: p. 17.

27 Werner, Zimmermann, pp. 35–37.

28 Ibid., p. 41.

29 Charles Tilly, *Big Structures, Large Processes, Huge Comparisons*, New York 1984, chapter 7.

and the STI, from and to which there was a steady flow of experts, scientific specimens and ideas. It is this comparison not just of entanglements but of the underlying power structures, the processes of "de-connection" and the redrawing of boundaries – in short, the nature and shifts in intensity of these entanglements, rather than the entanglements per se – that forms the analytical backbone of this study.[30]

Archives and Sources

The book covers the period extending from colonial science to the anthropology of bioscience in Africa, without losing sight of the late-colonial period, the development decade and the era of structural adjustment.[31] The success or failure of such an endeavor depends largely on raw data processed and stored in archives. Archives are as much sites of circulation as they are indicators of connectivity. The power of historical archives, the accessibility of sources, the innate logic of preservation and exclusion, and the systems of classification determine the dominant perspectives in historical narratives. Archives are not just the laws of what could have been said during a specific epoch – equally, they restrict the possibilities of what can be said about the past. As often remarked, archives, as material and imaginary expressions of state power, are closely related to the logic of governance. They are the products, as well as fostering the development, of states. The very term "archive" refers to the conjugation of knowledge and state power. Deriving from the Greek *arkheia*, the Latin term *archiva* denoted the site where official documents and public records were stored. The archival politics underlying the classification, validation, silencing or destruction of sources has put an end to the understanding of archives as innocent sites of knowledge retrieval. Rather, as Ann Stoler remarked, the

---

30 Ulrike Kirchberger, *German Scientists in the Indian Forest Service. A German Contribution to the Raj?*, in: Journal of Imperial and Commonwealth History, Vol. 29, 2001, pp. 1–26; Stacey Langwick, *Geographies of Medicine. Interrogating the Boundary between "Traditional" and "Modern" Medicine in Colonial Tanganyika*, in: Tracy J. Luedke and Harry G. West (eds.), Borders and Healers. Brokering Therapeutic Resources in Southwest Africa, Bloomington Indianapolis 2006, pp. 143-165; Heather Bell, *Frontiers of Medicine in the Anglo-Egyptian Sudan, 1899–1940*, Oxford 1999.

31 Wenzel Geissler, Catherine Molyneux (eds.), *Evidence, Ethos and Experiment. The Anthropology and History of Medical Research in Africa*, New York, Oxford 2011; Melissa Graboyes, *Surveying the "Pathological Museum." A History of Medical Research Ethics in East Africa, 1940–1965*, PhD Boston University 2010.

"archival turn" has given way to the idea of archives as sites of "knowledge production", as monuments of states as well as sites of state ethnography.[32] As a consequence, historical "facts" have become less of a concern in historical accounts than discussions about the mechanisms of how these facts were produced.

The reciprocal relationship of archives as products of states and state-driving machineries is itself deeply rooted in history. At the risk of oversimplification, colonial states in Africa, as elsewhere, were masters in the "art of lexical governance". As Arjun Appadurai and others have claimed, colonial states trusted in numbers. They compiled statistics covering virtually all areas of domestic and public life, or created new political and administrative categories along racial lines.[33] However, it is likely that the colonial archive is itself a blind spot, indicating the failure, rather than the realization, of the bureaucratic ideal. What tends to be the case for the colonial period is even more true of the postindependence era. According to Andreas Eckert – author of the most detailed account to date of the process of bureaucratization and state power in colonial and postcolonial Tanzania – the documents of the ministries and administrative units have only been filed in a very rudimentary fashion.[34] Consequently, written testimonies on postcolonial Africa are not necessarily to be found in Abidjan, Dar es Salaam or Kinshasa, but instead stored in well-organized archives in France, Britain or Belgium. Here, the power of the postcolony becomes most palpable.[35] This is not, however, to imply that written sources about the colonial or postcolonial past in Africa lead a comfortable life in Europe. As a general rule, the closer one gets to the present, the more dispersed, inaccessible and precarious the written accounts become. My own work on the unclassified papers kept in the basement of the STI in Basel underwent a sudden change when it was decided to relocate the historical records in order to make room for a biobank containing large amounts of health-related information and samples from Swiss donors. A variety of conclusions may be drawn from this incident. Firstly, it is an expression of the dif-

32 Stoler, *Colonial Archives and the Arts of Governance*, in: Archival Science, Vol. 2, No. 1–2, 2002, pp. 87–109, here: p. 90.
33 Arjun Appadurai, *Modernity at Large. Cultural Dimensions of Globalization*, Minneapolis, London 1996, pp. 114–135.
34 Andreas Eckert, *Herrschen und Verwalten. Afrikanische Bürokraten, staatliche Ordnung und Politik in Tansania, 1920–1970*, Munich 2007, p. 26.
35 Stephen Ellis, *Writing Histories of Contemporary Africa*, in: Journal of African History, Vol. 43, 2002, pp. 1–26, here: p. 12.

ferent degrees of importance attached to different sorts of information. Secondly, rather than being placed in the storage rooms of a medical history archive, the bulk of health information today is in the hands of research institutes or private companies, deciphered in high-tech laboratories rather than in outmoded reading rooms. Without going into detail here, these new forms of biopolitical repository are subject to their own rules of economic gains, patients' rights and "benefit-sharing".[36] The third lesson I had to learn about the postcolonial archives of these nonstate organizations was that their documents were assembled haphazardly, their status constantly threatened and their survival due more to considerations of space or the importance attached to their contents at a given time than to the selection procedures whereby government archives transform individual items from historical leftovers to "archivable" sources.[37] In other words, these documents were governed by the disorder of things rather than the classification systems of states, which makes a reading "along the archival grain" difficult.

The sources that organize the narrative of the following account reflect both the seductive order of government archives and the more patchy nature of nongovernmental holdings. In general, sources were unearthed at different sites in Switzerland, France, Tanzania and Côte d'Ivoire. The main archives were located in Switzerland. Apart from the STI archive, the Staatsarchiv Basel-Stadt (StABS) and the Swiss Federal Archives (BAR) housed the most relevant documents on the STI's history. While the Staatsarchiv covers important aspects of the early period of this history, the BAR allows one to place the institution within the wider context of Swiss development work. One of the stated aims was to look at the history of the STI and the CSRS through the lens of a wider scientific and economic network. As far as relations between Swiss and French scientists in Côte d'Ivoire were concerned, the papers held in the Archives nationales at Fontainebleau invited one to grapple with the nature of Swiss-French interactions. Additionally, the largely unexplored archives of Novartis and Nestlé in Basel and Vevey provided further nodes within the vast network of technoscientific exchanges.

36 Cori Hayden, *Taking as Giving. Bioscience, Exchange, and the Politics of Benefit-Sharing*, in: Social Studies of Science, Vol. 37, No. 5, 2007, pp. 729–758.
37 Achille Mbembe, *The Power of the Archive and its Limits*, in: Carolyn Hamilton et al. (eds.), Refiguring the Archive, Dordrecht, Boston, London 2002, pp. 19–26, here: p. 20.

In Tanzania, the holdings of the Tanzania National Archives (TNA), the National Bibliographic Agency (NBA) of the National Central Library and the East Africana Collection of the University of Dar es Salaam Library proved to be fruitful, especially for the colonial period. However, written historical evidence petered out as far as the period after independence was concerned. For the institutional history of the STIFL, the small holdings of the Ifakara branch (kept in a container and in an advanced state of decay) and those of the Mtwara branch served as valuable sources for specific aspects of the institute's recent history. In Côte d'Ivoire, the state of historical record-keeping proved even more unfavorable. Due to the political crisis, the operations of the Archives nationales de Côte d'Ivoire came almost to a standstill. The archive of the Ministry of Scientific Research yielded some insights into French-Ivorian scientific relations, but more on a random basis than guided by a catalogue consulted beforehand.

Historians have employed two different strategies in order to cope with the uneven landscape of historical record-keeping. The first is not to let oneself be too seduced by positivism, but to read between the lines, to explain the silence and the omissions of archives, rather than taking their contents as something naturally given. Reading archival sources has become synonymous with a better understanding of the logic of archives themselves, and that of colonial and postcolonial states. The other strategy is methodological diversification. Oral history, especially, provided by critical anthropology, proved to be essential in capturing as many different voices as possible and creating room for a variety of different interpretations that subvert dominant narratives.

For the recent history of the two laboratories, I was fortunate to be able to obtain personal oral testimonies to make up for the unreliability of postcolonial archives. The people I encountered at these field sites can roughly be divided into two groups: on the one hand, there were those who had been (or were still) affiliated to the institutes, who, by their professional status or specific tasks, had shaped and been shaped by the institute's history. On the other hand, I was also eager to look beyond institutional boundaries and to reach those who in one way or another were affected by the biomedical endeavor – patients enrolled in malaria vaccine trials, mothers who opted for additional malaria treatment at rural dispensaries, or nurses trying – sometimes desperately – to keep these health institutions running. In the first case ("studying up"), I found myself confronted with European and African biomedical experts whose specialist knowledge or knowledge of "what worked and what did not work" in rural Africa largely surpassed my own understanding.[38] Given their position and social status, they were likely to determine the course and outcome of the interviews. The encounters with members of the second group were no less tricky. As is often the case in over-researched places such as Kilombero District, people living around Ifakara today are very much used to social scientists arriving on their doorstep and interviewing them about certain experiences. They are experts in reading social scientists' expectations and would most probably often react accordingly. My use of the interview technique was not inspired by a quest for an "authentic" African voice, or for the unfolding of certain "life histories".[39] Rather, I was interested in respondents' recollections and interpretation of specific events, and in filling in the gaps encountered in the archives.

Organization of the Book

This book has a disjointed structure: rather than presenting one case study after another, followed by a general comparative conclusion, it comprises seven (mostly comparative) chapters, which unfold chronologically. This is demanding for the reader, as it often involves jumping from East to West Africa within one chapter. However, this type of structure is more reflective of science, which also shifts back and forth between different places. To facilitate the reader's task, Chapter 1 delineates the history of Adiopodoumé (Côte d'Ivoire) and the Ulanga (Mahenge) District of Tanzania, which, owing to the new importance attached to imperial science during World War II, became major centers of knowledge production and disease intervention. Whereas France embarked on the project of valorizing its colony from a large scientific institute established on the fringes of Adiopodoumé, the colonial state in Tanganyika took the spread of human trypanosomiasis (sleeping sickness) as an opportunity to intervene in African society and to remold African lifestyles according to its homegrown ideas of modernity and progress. Countries without colonies were not unaffected by these developments. As Chapter 2 shows, the Swiss govern-

---

38   Laura Nader, *Up the Anthropologist – Perspectives Gained from Studying Up*, in: Dell Hymes (ed.), Reinventing Anthropology, New York 1969, pp. 284–311.
39   Luise White, Stephan Miescher, David William Cohen, *Introduction. Voices, Words and African History*, in: White, Miescher and Cohen (eds.), African Words, African Voices. Critical Practices in Oral History, Bloomington, Indianapolis 2001, pp. 1–27.

ment was also increasingly concerned about the control of scientific activities during World War II; tropical medicine was a welcome branch of scientific activity to emerge during the war, as it had the potential to be a decisive vehicle for Switzerland's progress into an international postwar order, and to alleviate labor-market pressures, with young members of the Swiss workforce being assigned to the colonies. The chapter argues that this focus on the nation gave way to a transnational turn, culminating in the establishment of the two research laboratories in Côte d'Ivoire (1951) and Tanganyika (1957). The role and nature of scientific practices are discussed in Chapter 3. Largely inexperienced in colonial matters, Swiss scientists started to discover, describe, order and classify the unknown environment. However, the impact of Swiss science remained narrowly confined, and science in the colonies was more often doomed to failure than crowned with success. It is this weakness of science, rather than its strength, that forms the underlying argument of this chapter. Basic science disappeared altogether when the new discourse and practice of development arose on the horizon. Development was powerful enough to forge new networks between scientists, politicians and private companies. However, the two laboratories were drawn into the development euphoria to different degrees. Whereas in Tanzania, Switzerland launched large-scale irrigation projects and started to train paramedical personnel, the CSRS benefited to a lesser extent from the newly released funds. This situation did not necessarily improve when, in 1967, the Nestlé Foundation decided to establish itself in a wing of the CSRS and to embark on a substantial nutritional research project in Côte d'Ivoire. The detour via the history of Nestlé in Côte d'Ivoire (described in Chapter 4) is important in casting light on an early example of where science and development converged. It must be reiterated, however, that development never meant simply the unilateral application of Western science and technology in Third World countries. As used in this context, the term denotes a complex pattern of interactions and negotiations between different global and local actors. The rise of social medicine – the topic of Chapter 5 – is a case in point. Long before international attention was focused on the principles of primary health care by the Alma-Ata Declaration (1978), the Tanzanian government encouraged STIFL to include public health and community medicine more systematically in its research and teaching agenda. As a consequence, the focus of research shifted away from the study of vectors towards rural communities, whose well-being was conceived as constantly threatened by tropical diseases. As the example of the small village of Kikwawila shows, villagers did not rate public health concerns as highly as the material improvement of local infrastructure. One of the lessons from development-oriented research was that "development became less a matter of benevolent outsiders assisting needy people in backward areas of the world than of citizens claiming entitlements".[40] However, the period when development and health were closely intertwined, offering possibilities for claim-making, was short-lived. Chapter 6 explores the processes which, after conflicts between Swiss development actors, led to the disentanglement of research and development. In the 1980s, foreign-imposed Structural Adjustment Programs (SAP) resulted in an increased dependency of African states on outside donors. It was during this period that the two laboratories entered into closer relationships with their host countries and developed into powerful NGOs, within what James Ferguson and Akhil Gupta have called a "transnational governmentality".[41] Thus, this chapter addresses the paradoxical process of decolonization of Swiss scientific research in Tanzania and Côte d'Ivoire, illustrated by the integration of the institutes into national health systems (as was the case with STIFL), the increased involvement of African experts in decision-making processes, and the deployment of large-scale technologies. These technological developments are especially prominent in malaria research, which, in the 1990s, experienced a high tide of global attention and funding. In contrast to previous episodes in the history of the disease, malaria was (and still is) no longer combated by single "silver bullets", but by a variety of integrated approaches. The "technopolitics" of malaria intervention, embedded in malaria vaccines and treatment regimes, makes up the core of Chapter 7.[42] This involves an attempt to break away from the researcher's perspective, prevalent in the earlier chapters, and to satisfy the claims of writing the history of malaria from the perspective of sufferers themselves.[43] It is here that the different strategies of the "users" of biomedical research come to the fore. However, before we delve into the different usages of Western technology, we should start with the geographical features and historical legacies of those areas where science is conducted.

---

40   Cooper, *Writing the History of Development*, p. 15.
41   James Ferguson, Akhil Gupta, *Spatializing States. Towards an Ethnography of Neoliberal Governmentality*, in: American Ethnologist, Vol. 29, No. 4, 2002, pp. 981–1002.
42   Gabrielle Hecht, *Introduction*, in: Hecht (ed.), Entangled Geographies. Empire and Technopolitics in the Global Cold War, Cambridge, Massachusetts, London 2011, p. 3.
43   Schumaker, *Malaria*, in: Roger Cooter and John Pickstone (eds.), Medicine in the Twentieth Century, Amsterdam 2000, pp. 703–717, here: p. 714.

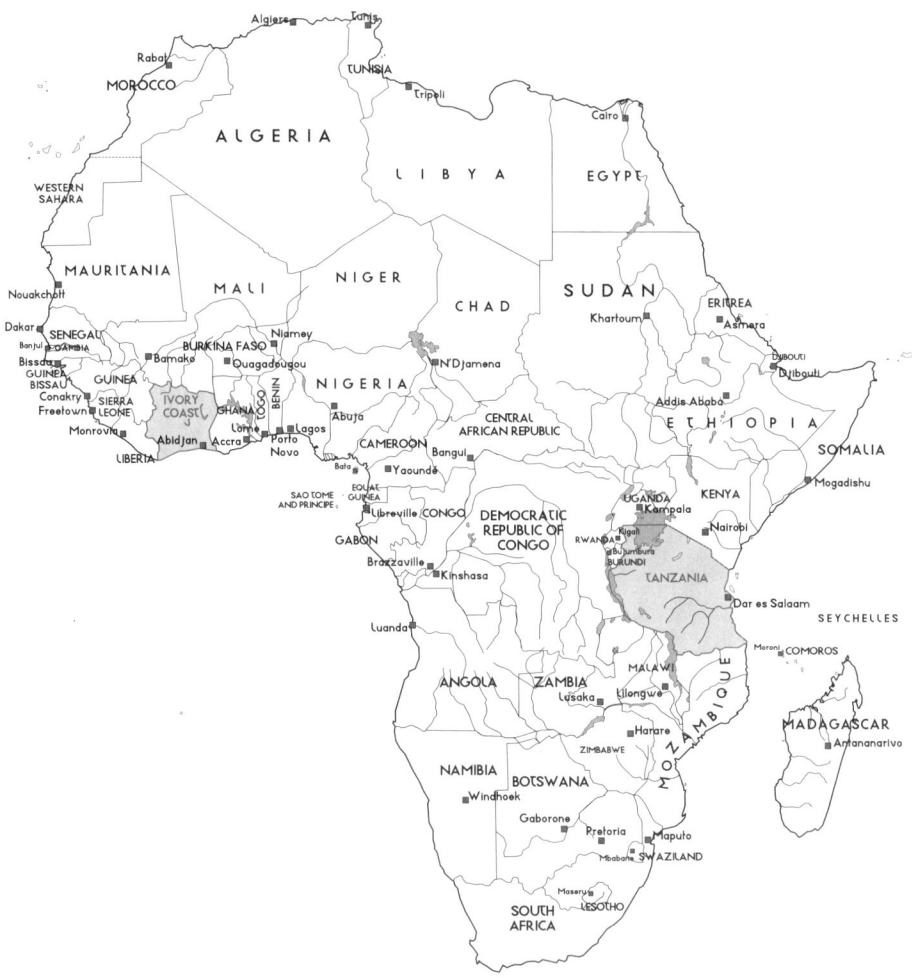

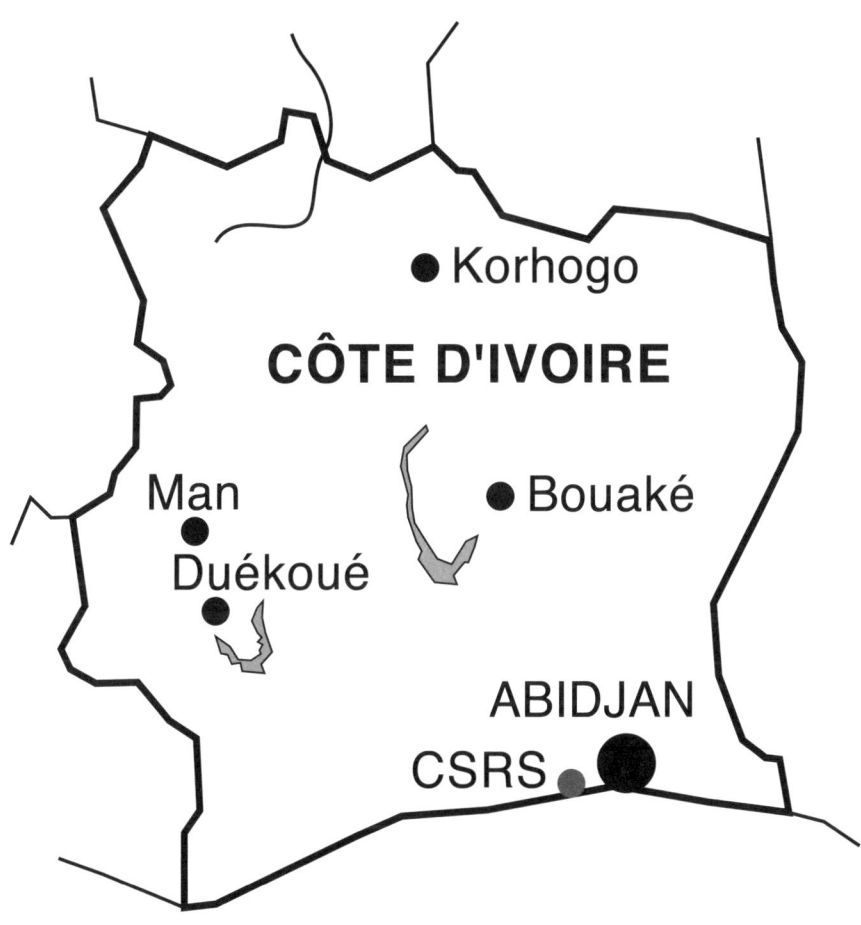

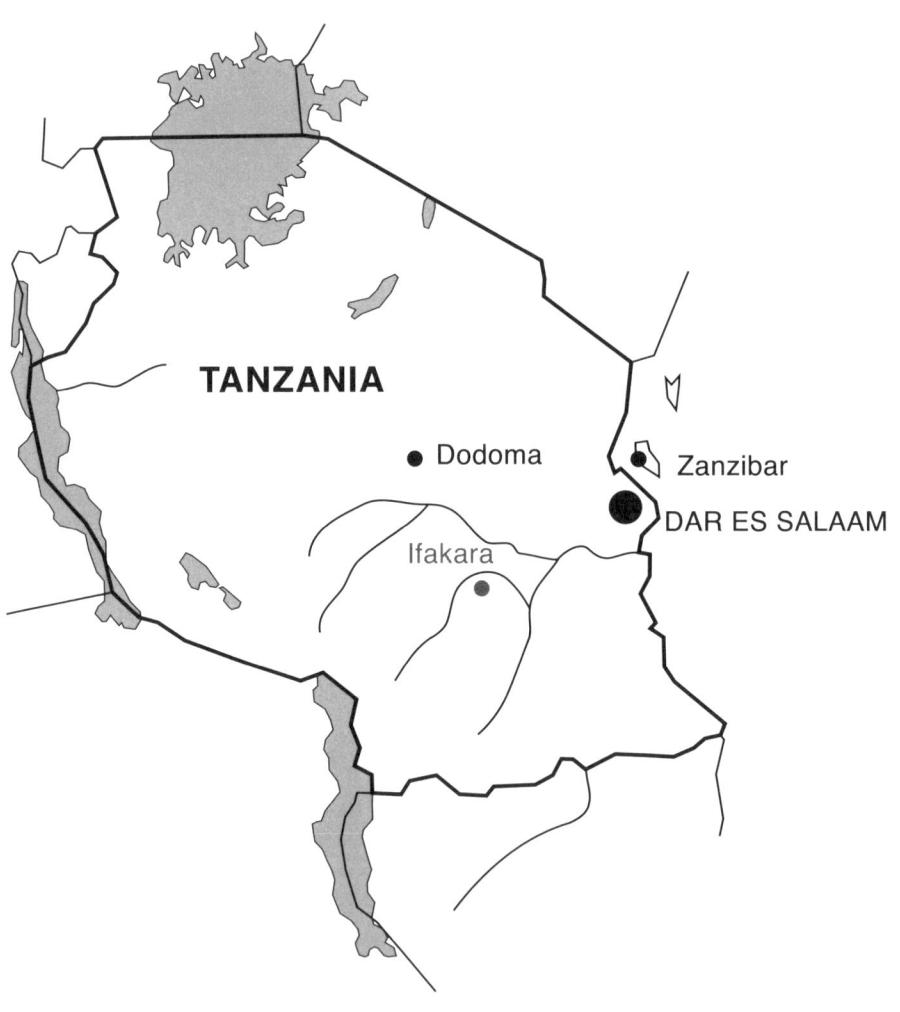

Chapter 1
Decolonization, Development and Geographies of Knowledge

This chapter serves as an introduction to familiarize the reader with time and places. It starts from the assumption that, at the end of the 1930s and from the beginning of World War II, the relationship between the French and British empires and their respective colonies was fundamentally re-shaped. Science and technology played a special role in the reconfiguration of empire, both as a tool for the development of the vast territories in Africa and as an instrument of power inherent in the production of knowledge. The historical context of what has been called the "imperialism of knowledge" (Frederick Cooper) and the "second colonial occupation" (Anthony Low and John Lonsdale) is important for a better understanding of Swiss scientific policy and the emergence of the Swiss Tropical Institute (STI), the main subject of the next chapter.[1] Despite enhanced state control over the colonial scientific enterprise in both Britain and France towards the end of the 1930s, the assumption that science provided a power base for a reinvigorated colonialism after World War II needs careful consideration. The African continent has never been a vast "laboratory" or a veritable testing ground for the scientist's zeal, as recently claimed by several authors. Rather, it is assumed here that scientific interventions within the colonial context of domination have to be read as a set of different – sometimes contradictory – constellations of protagonists who were themselves shaped by local constituencies.[2] The aim of this chapter is to retrace science's regained strength in the developmentalist project of the French and

---

1 Anthony Low, John Lonsdale, *Towards the New Order*, 1945–1963, in: Anthony Low and Alison Smith (eds.), History of East Africa, Vol. 3, 1976, pp. 12–16.
2 David Wade Chambers, Richard Gillespie, *Locality in the History of Science. Colonial Science, Technoscience, and Indigenous Knowledge*, in: Osiris, Vol. 15, 2001, pp. 221–240; David Turnbull, *Local Knowledge and Comparative Scientific Traditions*, in: Knowledge and Policy, Vol. 6, No. 3–4, 1993/94, pp. 29–54; David Livingstone, *Putting Science in Its Place. Geographies of Scientific Knowledge*, Chicago 2003. For empirical studies in the field of history of health, see: Nancy Rose Hunt, *A Colonial Lexicon* and Luise White, *Speaking with Vampires*.

British empires during the 1930s and 1940s.[3] It compares two techniques of scientific domination employed by the French and the British at two sites in their respective territories – Adiopodoumé (Côte d'Ivoire) and Mahenge (Ulanga) District (Tanganyika). While Adiopodoumé had been selected by the French Office de la Recherche Scientifique et Technique Outre-Mer (ORSTOM) as the most suitable place for creating a large-scale scientific complex, British science had established itself in Mahenge District in order to tackle a specific problem – the spread of trypanosomiasis.

Refashioning Science: Science for Development

At the Brazzaville Conference in 1944, France reaffirmed its claim over its vast empire. The domination of colonial subjects and the mastery of human bodies and nature was especially important for the former *grande nation*, humiliated by what Marc Bloch called the "étrange défaite" of 1940.[4] The reinvigoration of the doctrine of empire, shaken by the devastating effects of war, rested on the widely shared assumption that the colonial territories were poverty-stricken and ready to be uplifted. The government now assumed a more proactive role in the areas of health care and welfare, emphasizing the promise of science and technology. This was not entirely unjustified: World War II was not only unsurpassed in the development of new technologies for mass destruction, it was equally a catalyst for major research projects in the field of public health.[5] However, the linking of colonial development to the scientific enterprise was not due to World War II but can be traced back to the interwar period. In the 1920s, science ranked high in Colonies Minister Albert Sarraut's project of "valorization" of the colonies, but it would be more than a decade before efforts to better coordinate the vast array of French colonial science came to fruition. In 1937, the then Colonies Minister Marius Moutet was unambiguous about the benefits of such coordination:

---

3   While conventional wisdom links developmentalist thinking to the end of World War II, with Truman's Point Four Program speech as the foundational document, development projects can be traced back at least to the 1930s; see, for instance, Michael Havinden, David Meredith, *Colonialism and Development. Britain and its Tropical Colonies, 1859–1960*, London, New York 1993.

4   Marc Bloch, *L'étrange défaite. Témoignage écrit en 1940*, Paris 1946.

5   Leo B. Slater, *War and Disease. Biomedical Research on Malaria in the Twentieth Century*, New Brunswick, New Jersey, London 2009.

Scientific organization in the colonies is an urgent necessity. It is a prerequisite for economic valorization, but it is also a duty of our colonization, an example to be set, a light to illuminate the path we are pursuing.[6]

Moutet's vision of a coordinated approach was taken a step further when, in 1943, the Office de la Recherche Scientifique Coloniale (ORSC) was founded and placed under the direction of the Colonies Ministry. The Office had the threefold aim of "guiding, coordinating and monitoring scientific research in France's overseas territories".[7] For Raoul Combes – one of the major architects in the refashioning of French science and the Office's director between 1943 and 1956 – the enhanced government involvement in French colonial science was not least a question of scale:

The overseas territories are no longer … a museum, a laboratory or a vast reserve of scientific material. Such an attitude reveals a sort of "scientific colonialism" which is inconceivable given the huge task of the twentieth century to completely take possession of nature …[8]

During World War II, the Vichy regime embarked on a substantial, albeit discriminatory, welfare policy scheme that resulted in increasing state activities and rising numbers of social beneficiaries.[9] This emphasis on the "social" and "modernity" in domestic policies appears to have entered the realm of colonial policy, too, where the Office promoted the concept of applied research with a special focus on improving the poor agricultural output of the overseas territories.[10] This reorientation was reflected in the fact that the Office was renamed ORSOM (Office de la Recherche Scientifique Outre-Mer) in 1949 and ORSTOM (Office de la Recherche Scientifique et

---

6 Marius Moutet, Ministre des Colonies, quoted in: Archives Nationales Fontainebleau (ANF), Archives de l'ORSTOM, 19900236, Art. 2, Conseil supérieur de la recherche scientifique, Raoul Combes, Office de la Recherche Scientifique Outre-Mer. Exposé des activités pour les années 1948–1949–1950, p. 7.

7 Ibid., p. 3.

8 ANF, 19900236, Art. 1, Création et Organisation de ORSTOM, Exposé fait par M. Le Professeur Combes à la 1ère réunion du Conseil d'Administration de l'ORSC, pp. 1–5, here: p. 3; Raoul Combes held a chair of plant physiology at Sorbonne University.

9 Philippe-Jean Hesse, Jean-Pierre Le Crom (eds.), *La protection sociale sous le régime de Vichy*, Rennes 2001, p. 359.

10 Christophe Bonneuil, Patrick Petitjean, *Les chemins de la création de l'ORSTOM. Du Front Populaire à la libération en passant par Vichy, 1936–1945*, in: Petitjean (ed.), Les sciences coloniales. Figures et institutions, Paris 1996, série sous la direction de Roland Waast, pp. 113–161, here: p. 137.

Technique Outre-Mer) in 1953.[11] Apart from focusing on agricultural re-search, the Office pursued the dual aim of educating researchers and agri-cultural technicians, and establishing new research institutes throughout the overseas territories.[12] This latter aim was only feasible with the aid of the Fonds d'Investissement pour le Développement Economique et Social des territoires d'outre-mer (FIDES) – in 1946, France ended the "tradition of colonial self-sufficiency … making available metropolitan funds for de-velopment projects".[13] In the decade following World War II, the Office created thirteen new research institutes in the overseas territories, the first of which was the Institut d'Enseignement et de Recherches Tropicales (IDERT) in Adiopodoumé.[14]

Similar tendencies to attach growing importance to research for the de-velopment of the colonies, and signs of the ideologies of a new imperial-ism, can also be detected in the British case. Major catalysts for a reconsid-eration and internationalization of the "colonial question" were events in the West Indies, where the depressed socioeconomic situation culminated in widespread labor riots in 1937 and 1938.[15] The same year saw the pub-lication of Lord Hailey's massive African Survey, a large-scale project (1929–1939) evaluating the knowledge required for imperial administra-tion.[16] The Survey was published in three volumes – *An African Survey* by Lord Hailey himself, *Science in Africa* by Edgar Barton Worthington and *Capital Investment in Africa* by Sally Herbert Frankel.[17] The African Sur-vey had a strong influence on the future organization and institutional set-ting of colonial research. Lord Hailey was eager to put an end to science in Africa as almost entirely a private endeavor, and he argued that the gov-ernment should make substantial funds available for research on African

---

11   Marie-Lise Sabrié, *Histoire des principes de programmation scientifique à L'OR-STOM (1944–1994)*, in: Petitjean (ed.), Les sciences coloniales, pp. 223–233, here: p. 226.
12   Ibid.
13   Cooper, *Modernizing Bureaucrats*, p. 70.
14   The IDERT was originally known as the Institut Intercolonial de Recherche Scien-tifique (IIRS).
15   Michael Havinden and David Meredith mention Mussolini's claim over Ethiopia, Germany's demands for colonial restitution, and Japanese expansion in East Asia as further reasons for Britain's willingness to "protect" its colonies, see: Havinden, Meredith, *Colonialism and Development*, p. 195.
16   Tilley, *Africa as a Living Laboratory*, p. 3.
17   Ibid., pp. 73–74.

problems.[18] The Colonial Development and Welfare Act of 1940 (the counterpart to the French FIDES of 1946) permitted the expenditure of £5 million per year over a period of ten years for development and welfare projects in the colonies, as well as a sum of £500,000 per year for research activities with no time limit attached and with the minimum possible interference from government administrators.[19] Aside from the establishment of the Colonial Research Fund, the African Survey also gave rise to the setting-up of the Colonial Research Committee, which Lord Hailey agreed to chair in 1942. Alongside the existing Imperial College of Tropical Agriculture in Trinidad and the Agricultural Research Station at Amani in Tanganyika, a variety of new scientific institutions emerged, mostly in Africa.

Establishment of the IDERT at Adiopodoumé

In 1945, the botanist Georges Mangenot (later director of the IDERT), the zoologist Pierre-Paul Grassé and ORSOM's first director-general, André Nizery, traveled along the coast of the Ebrié Lagoon in southern Côte d'Ivoire to prepare the ground for the future site of the IDERT. Their exploratory tour included the inspection of a large plateau close to the Ebrié village of Adiopodoumé. Near the shores of the lagoon, the area was covered by a cocoa plantation, while a dense secondary forest marked the plateau's natural inner boundary. Several anthropologists described the Ebrié people as having originated from the northeast of the country and – compared to their immediate neighbors, the Atié, Alladian and Adioukrou – they were said to have been the last to arrive on the lagoon's shores.[20] One of the lagoon's principal traits as a cultural space was its adaptation to outside change.[21] The arrival of the French scientists in 1945 demanded a great deal of these skills.

---

18 Charles Jeffries, *A Review of Colonial Research, 1940–1960*, London 1964, p. 20; see also: Sabine Clarke, *A Technocratic Imperial State? The Colonial Office and Scientific Research, 1940–1960*, in: Twentieth Century British History, Vol. 18, No. 4, 2007, pp. 453–480.
19 Havinden, Meredith, *Colonialism and Development*, p. 218.
20 G. Niangoran-Bouah, *Les Ebrié et leur organisation politique traditionnelle*, in: Annales de l'Université d'Abidjan (Ethnosociologie), Vol. 1, No. 1, 1969, pp. 51–91, here: p. 60. The most detailed ethnographic description of the region is Marc Augé, *Théorie des pouvoirs et idéologie. Etude de cas en Côte d'Ivoire*, Paris 1975.
21 François Verdeaux, *Du pouvoir des génies au savoir scientifique. Les métamorphoses de la lagune Ebrié (Côte d'Ivoire)*, in: Cahiers d'Etudes Africaines, Vol. 26, No. 1–2, 1986, pp. 145–171, here: p. 155.

The location – distant enough from Abidjan to avoid distraction by the allures of a burgeoning African city, but close enough not to be entirely cut off from the centers of political decision-making – convinced ORSTOM to claim the territory as a site for its future scientific activities. The Ebrié could hardly ignore this wish. Jean Logon, who started working for ORSTOM in the late 1940s, recalls the negotiations between the French and the Ebrié about the conditions for ceding the villagers' land to French science.[22] The central figure in making a place for French science in Adiopodoumé was Félix Houphouët-Boigny (subsequently President of Côte d'Ivoire), whose opinion the Ebrié found it difficult to reject. Born to a family of chiefs in 1905, Houphouët held a degree from the School of Medicine in Dakar and became a successful cocoa farmer in Côte d'Ivoire. After the end of the Vichy regime, he founded the African Agricultural Union (SAA), which became the vehicle for his election to the French legislature in 1945.[23] At the beginning of 1946, Houphouët-Boigny, with a number of other key figures in African politics, was the driving force behind the abolition of forced labor in all French colonies (the Loi Houphouët-Boigny), which earned him widespread popularity and a reputation as the uncontested father of the nation. Raoul Combes invited Houphouët-Boigny to campaign with "all his authority" for the French cause, and in 1947 the agreement between the Office and the villagers stated that "the villages of Adiopodoumé and Abadjidoumé are willing to allocate 199 ha of land for the benefit of the Office de la Recherche Scientifique Coloniale".[24]

Initial construction work on what would become ORSTOM's largest scientific complex outside France had already been started a year before the official agreement between France and the Ebrié villagers was signed. Over time and on a total area of 228 ha, there emerged several large laboratories, accommodation for researchers and their families, a hostel for students, a club with a swimming pool and later a tennis court, schools and a dispensary, as well as a quarter for the essential African workforce, who soon started to call the site "petit plateau" in analogy to the "plateau" – the exclusively European residential area of Abidjan.

22   Interview with Jean Logon in Adiopodoumé, 6 August 2011.
23   Cooper, *Africa since 1940. The Past of the Present*, Cambridge 2002, p. 46.
24   ANF, Archives de l'ORSTOM, 19900236, Art. 52, Raoul Combes to Félix Houphouët-Boigny, 11 March 1947 and Georges Mangenot, Convention entre l'Office de la Recherche Scientifique Coloniale (Institut Intercolonial d'Adiopodoumé) et les villages d'Adiopodoumé et d'Abadjidoumé, 17 September 1947, p. 1.

With the IDERT, scientific practices in the colony were closely tied to metropolitan aspirations. Unlike other ORSTOM establishments, the IDERT had no funds of its own but was dependent on the ORSTOM budget.[25] Focusing on the training of young tropicalists, the IDERT was placed within an institutional framework that allowed for a controlled transfer of knowledge between Paris and Adiopodoumé. Research activities in 1946 started with agricultural entomology. Towards the end of the year, the botanist Jacques Miège, by then director of the Bouaké research station, joined the ORSC team as director of the laboratory of plant genetics.[26] Apart from entomology and botany, the scientific disciplines that blossomed in Adiopodoumé also included soil science and phytopathology. ORSTOM created a highly organized and highly efficient scientific bureaucracy in one of France's most valued colonies. Its existence was due to the close links between French and African politicians that would be one of the main features of the whole decolonization process in Côte d'Ivoire. As we will see later, a considerable number of African politicians owed their later careers to the training acquired at Adiopodoumé. With ORSTOM, France for the first time invested in the conduct of proper studies and the collection of statistical information about the countries they ruled. Several of the villagers regarded ORSTOM as a foreign imposition: the geographical isolation of the site and the racial separation between Africans and Europeans in day-to-day activities instilled a sense of "otherness". At the same time, with 100 French scientists and over 300 African collaborators, ORSTOM emerged as a powerful employee for a large number of technicians, laboratory assistants and gardeners, providing an image of modernity that could either be emulated, resisted or nostalgically remembered long after ORSTOM had disappeared.[27]

25 It was only in 1977 that ORSTOM (Adiopodoumé) and ORSTOM (Paris) were separated; see: Farma Marie Madeleine Chourouba, *Histoire de l'ORSTOM en Côte d'Ivoire, 1946–1994*, Mémoire de maîtrise, Université d'Abidjan, 1993/1994, p. 26.
26 Miège would later become director of the Botanical Gardens in Geneva. As a member of the Commission for the CSRS, he was the link between Swiss science and the French tradition epitomized by ORSTOM.
27 Chourouba, *Histoire de l'ORSTOM*, p. 19.

Science and Expertise in Mahenge (Ulanga) District, Tanganyika

The rural Mahenge (Ulanga) District in Tanganyika also witnessed the advent of science and development as manifestations of a more interventionist state in the interwar period.[28] After the defeat of German rule, Tanganyika became a British mandate of the League of Nations in 1922. The status of a trust territory was important insofar as the British were accountable in their duty to guarantee the "material and moral well-being and the social progress" of the territory's inhabitants.[29] British economic interests were, however, modest. As historian John Iliffe bluntly stated, "Tanganyika had been Germany's most valued colony. The British wanted to deny it to others."[30] With the end of World War I, a new protagonist entered the Mahenge scene: in this backwater of the British empire, the Swiss Capuchin mission, Baldegg Sisters and Italian Consolata Sisters took the place of the German Benedictines, whose project of evangelizing "heathen" Africans ended abruptly after the defeat of Germany. Inexperienced in colonial matters, the Capuchins established a stronghold in the district and complemented the spread of the gospel with Christian education and the delivery of health services.[31] In Mahenge, the missionaries encountered an ethnically diverse populace, resulting from a complex history of warfare, resettlement and boundary-crossings dating back to the nineteenth century. The main ethnic group living in the area consisted of people who, on the basis of a common language and customs, defined themselves as Wapogoro. Less numerous, but equally considering themselves as belonging to the district (whether or not these origins were acknowledged), were

28   As an administrative unit, Ulanga District came into existence on August 7, 1899. Since then, it has been renamed several times. From 1899 to 1917, it was known as Mahenge Military District. Between 1918 and 1936, it was officially called Mahenge District. From 1936 to 1974 (until its division into two separate districts, Kilombero and Ulanga), it was known as Ulanga District; see: Mkeli Mbosa, *Colonial Production and Underdevelopment in Ulanga District, 1894–1950*, Dar es Salaam 1988, p. 23; Lorne Larson, *A History of the Mahenge (Ulanga) District, 1860–1957*, PhD Study, University of Dar es Salaam, Dar es Salaam 1976.
29   Quoted in John Iliffe, *A Modern History of Tanganyika*, Cambridge 1979, p. 247; see also: Margaret Bates, *Tanganyika. The Development of a Trust Territory*, in: International Organization, Vol. 9, No. 1, 1955, pp. 32–51.
30   Iliffe, *A Modern History*, p. 261.
31   Marcel Dreier, *Healthcare, Welfare, and Development in Rural Africa. The Case of the Catholic Health Services in Ifakara/Tanzania in the 20th Century*, PhD University of Basel 2014 (forthcoming).

the Wandamba, Wangindo, Wabena, Wambunga and Wangoni.[32] In addition, a comparatively wealthy group of Indians was living in the mission's headquarters at Ifakara, whose power derived from their monopoly over the rice trading system based on African middlemen.[33] Despite the missionary society's active role in the provision of welfare services in the district, the colonial government also became more active in the interwar period. The colonial state's prime goal was to improve the district's agriculture. It more systematically endorsed regulations and tried to integrate the fertile Mahenge District into world market structures.[34]

The notion of "colonial government" in these transactions and processes is, however, misleading. The extent to which agricultural policies were applied in the countryside largely depended on the interests and capabilities of individuals who, as district commissioners and local experts, presided over the fate of their own area of influence. One of these individuals was District Commissioner Arthur Theodore Culwick, who – with his wife Geraldine Mary Sheppard, an Oxford-trained anthropologist – administered the district between 1930 and 1945.[35] Given her professional background and his broad interests in local culture, the Culwicks carried out anthropological field research on the health and diet of the Wabena – their "preferred tribe" in the area. At the end of the anthropological field work, Culwick was left with the belief (widely shared) that Africa's most pressing problem was a steady population decline due to widespread infertility. He was, however, convinced that these problems could be addressed, if not overcome, by a more systematic application of science and technology. Culwick's writings during the period reveal a shift from a liberal position of non-interference towards support for more interventionist solutions towards the end of the decade. Having, at the beginning of the 1930s, vetoed the introduction of cotton as a cash crop and defended local African indus-

---

32   Maia Green, *Priests, Witches and Power. Popular Christianity After Mission in Southern Tanzania*, Cambridge 2003, p. 16; Jamie Monson, *The Tribal Past and the Politics of Nationalism in Mahenge District, 1940–60*, in: Gregory H. Maddox and James Giblin (eds.), In Search of a Nation. Histories of Authority and Dissidence in Tanzania, Oxford, Dar es Salaam, Athens 2005, pp. 103–113.

33   Larson, *A History of the Mahenge (Ulanga) District*, p. 234.

34   Jamie Monson, *Rice and Cotton, Ritual and Resistance. Cash Cropping in Colonial Tanganyika, 1920–1940*, in: Allan Isaacman and Richard Roberts (eds.), Cotton, Colonialism and Social History in Sub-Saharan Africa, Portsmouth, London 1995, pp. 268–284; Larson, *A History of the Mahenge (Ulanga) District*, p. 298.

35   Veronica Berry (ed.), *The Culwick Papers, 1934–1944. Population, Food and Health in Colonial Tanganyika (now Tanzania)*, London 1994, pp. 14–15.

try against the creation of trade monopolies in Asian hands, he later supported more state-centered policies:

> The recent policy of the British Empire has been built up on the doctrine of "the sanctity of the individual", one which in my view represents the high-water mark of political thought. We believe the individual is more important than the state ... But while the idea of the sanctity of the individual is growing in importance, many are wondering whether he is best served by being left to his own devices. Are there not abundant signs all over the world that the free struggle of individuals for survival produces chaos, and that individuals themselves are clamoring for a co-ordination of their efforts?[36]

One of the sources of Culwick's plea for more government regulation and social engineering was the rural population itself, whose calls for better welfare services in the 1930s could not be ignored. The health sector was a case in point. The doctrine of indirect rule and the ideology of self-sufficiency of British colonies led to the creation of Native Administrations (NA), consisting of a native authority (chief/council), native courts and a native treasury; the latter was in charge of collecting taxes, some of which were transferred to the central government while the rest were used for welfare expenditures.[37] Given the fact that the Medical Department in Dar es Salaam mainly dealt with urban health care and the major hospitals – neglecting the need for adequate rural health care delivery – the NA system not only created double standards in health but also an effective means to address inadequacies in welfare provision. In 1936, Ifakara's Indian community complained about the deplorable quality of health care provided by the mission and asked for a government hospital in town. The discussions between the Indian community and the Tanganyikan government would continue over the next decade. They reached a climax in the context of a political-administrative reform which saw Kiberege cease to exist as the head of the relevant administrative unit in 1944. Apart from the mission-led dispensary in Ifakara (which charged user fees), there was an NA dispensary staffed with a dresser, whose quality of care was considered inadequate given the burden of disease.[38] Culwick declined the re-

---

36 Arthur T. Culwick, *New Beginning*, in: Tanganyika Notes and Records, Vol. 15, 1943, pp. 1–6, here: p. 2.
37 Iliffe, *A Modern History*, pp. 319–320.
38 Tanzania National Archive (TNA), 450, 653, Ifakara Station, 1936–1948, K. Truth, Boma Wanted, in: Tanganyika Standard, 23 January 1941.

quests on the grounds that Ifakara would not be a suitable place for investment: "If Ifakara grows, or if the Lumemo [the nearby river] defeats our efforts to prevent it changing course, the settlement will probably have to be moved. It would therefore be most unwise to sink money in buildings there at present."[39] Culwick's reluctance to invest in Ifakara was thus due more to the village's uncertain future than to a fundamental opposition to investments in the rural dispensary system. It was the outbreak of sleeping sickness that not only made it possible to combine the goals of biomedical research and rural development, but also offered Culwick an opportunity to put his ideas about health and general progress into practice.

Health Policy as Social and Economic Policy: The Case of Sleeping Sickness in Tanganyika

On December 12, 1942, Mbakala binti Kameta, a thirteen-year-old girl, died in a missionary dispensary in Ifakara. Having arrived in Ifakara only half a year earlier, she had been staying with a man called Anton Mtemaneja. Shortly before her premature death, she suffered from a high fever and was diagnosed with sleeping sickness by a Swiss physician, Dr. Alois Gabathuler, who was in charge of the government hospital in Mahenge and happened to be residing in Ifakara at the time.[40] Cases of human trypanosomiasis were not new to Tanganyika. In the aftermath of World War I, major outbreaks of the disease had been reported in Mwanza (1921–23), Liwale (1924) and Ufipa-Tabora, and the disease soon attracted colonial and metropolitan attention in the form of scientific action as well as public funding.[41] At the beginning of the twentieth century, there was widespread confidence that the disease was caused by the parasite *Trypanosoma brucei gambiense*, transmitted by the tsetse fly *Glossina palpalis*.[42] But the complex vector-parasite-man interactions and especially the role of game had yet to be fully

---

39   Ibid., A.T. Culwick, 27 January 1941, p. 1.

40   TNA, 61/104/G, Sleeping Sickness Mahenge, K. Dougal to the Sleeping Sickness Officer in Tabora, 7 January 1943.

41   Eleanor Fisher, Alberto Arce, *The Spectacle of Modernity. Blood, Microscopes, and Mirrors in Colonial Tanganyika*, in: Alberto Arce and Norman Long (eds.), Anthropology, Development and Modernities. Exploring Discourses, Counter-Tendencies and Violence, London, New York, 2000, pp. 74–99.

42   Michael Worboys, *The Comparative History of Sleeping Sickness in East and Central Africa, 1900–1914*, in: History of Science, Vol. 32, 1994, pp. 89–102, here: p. 90.

understood. In response to the disease, colonial governments adopted differ-ent strategies, which of course varied over time: isolation of patients, the kil-ling of game and environmental modifications – or a combination of these – were the favored approaches. One of the advocates of the environmental approach was Charles Swynnerton, a Rhodesian settler and naturalist, who became intrigued by the ecological aspects of the spread of sleeping sick-ness. After extensive studies on the tsetse fly in Mozambique, Swynnerton was appointed director of the Tsetse Research Department in Tanganyika and assigned to Shinyanga; here, he continued his research on the effects of controlled bush burning and fly extirpation and advised the government during the Mwanza outbreak in the 1920s.[43] Given the importance of game as a reservoir for parasite reproduction and the fact that *Glossina* could only traverse a short distance without bush cover, Swynnerton was convinced that the most effective way of tackling the disease was to create a natural barrier between people and game. This idea persisted into the 1930s and 1940s, when sleeping sickness provided the colonial government with legit-imate grounds for intervening more actively in Ulanga District as soon as the first fatalities were recorded in the mid-1930s. The official response to the emerging threat was to resettle the population in sites known as sleeping sickness concentrations and to clear vegetation around the new settlements so as to reduce the risk of new infections. But disease prevention was always just one argument for the resettlement schemes – other arguments, such as better administration or better access to medical care or educational facili-ties, also loomed large. Culwick, who was the driving force behind these schemes (involving over 20,000 people) in Ulanga, defended the project not so much on the grounds of disease prevention as in terms of the benefits these interventions would provide: "… freedom from the depredations of animals, easier access to medical and educational facilities, easier adminis-tration, more varied social intercourse and so on. Freedom from Sleeping Sickness cuts no ice at all, but the other benefits definitely do."[44]

In recent years, a growing body of scholarship has focused on sleep-ing sickness operations in order to deconstruct the "benign" aspects of co-lonial medicine.[45] For instance, writing about sleeping sickness policy in

43 Tilley, *Africa as a Living Laboratory*, p. 194.
44 TNA, 61/104/H, Sleeping Sickness Ulanga-District, A. T. Culwick, 2 July 1943.
45 This tradition of scholarship can be traced back to the 1980s; see especially: Roy MacLeod, Lewis Milton, *Disease, Medicine and Empire*, London 1988; Michael Wor-boys, *Science and British Colonial Imperialism, 1895–1940*, PhD Study, University of Sussex, Sussex 1979.

the Uele District of the Belgian Congo between 1903 and 1914, Maryinez Lyons argued that the colonial government's major concern with regard to the spread of the disease was declining economic performance, and that the government's response resulted in numerous interventions seeking to regulate the African body and the movement of people across the territory.[46] In a similar vein (and in line with the writings of John Ford), Helge Kjekshus argued that sleeping sickness policies in Tanganyika destroyed the long-established ecological balance between man and his natural environment and actually promoted the spread of the disease.[47] This line of argument, however, was not the achievement of critical historians writing in the 1970s and 1980s, but was foreshadowed by observers within Tanganyika's medical services. In 1959, James M. Liston wrote:

> It is now considered more practicable and constructive to allow and to encourage development within a sleeping sickness area. For example, the building of new roads to open it up and the welcoming of settlers rather than the establishment of sleeping sickness settlements or "concentrations" of the old type … [These older settlements] lead to over-use of the land and soil impoverishment within small heavily settled areas, with all the surrounding empty country abandoned to the tsetse fly.[48]

For Liston, and to a much greater extent for Culwick too, the sleeping sickness concentration might not have been effective in terms of disease prevention, but it satisfied their understanding of a "modern" African society, in which processes of economic production and social reproduction, the movement of people and the distribution of germs could be brought under control. Linking the idea of the concentration with the prerequisites of development exemplified what Giorgio Agamben analyzed as the very essence of modernity – the transformation of a state of emergency into normality.[49]

What interests us in the following is the interplay between the establishment of sleeping sickness concentrations in Ulanga District and the

46 Maryinez Lyons, *From "Death Camps" to Cordon Sanitaire. The Development of Sleeping Sickness Policy in the Uele District of the Belgian Congo, 1903–1914*, in: Journal of African History, Vol. 26, No. 1, 1985, pp. 69–91; Lyons, *The Colonial Disease. A Social History of Sleeping Sickness in Northern Zaire, 1800–1940*, Cambridge 1992.

47 Helge Kjekshus, *Ecological Control and Economic Development in East African History. The Case of Tanganyika 1850–1950*, London 1977; John Ford, *The Role of the Trypanosomiases in African Ecology. A Study of the Tsetse Fly Problem*, Oxford 1971.

48 Ministry of Health (MOH) Library, James M. Liston, Permanent Secretary (Director of Medical Services), Report on Health Services 1959, pp. 1–56, here: pp. 14–15.

49 Giorgio Agamben, *Homo Sacer. Die Souveränität der Macht und das nackte Leben*, Frankfurt am Main 2003, p. 30.

broader conceptions of rural development. The story emerging from the sources is, however, not one of an all-encompassing colonial state bureaucracy which, during World War II, continuously and comprehensively brought rural life under its own administrative logic. Rather, the colonial administration was divided up into modernization-minded social technocrats such as Culwick, who promoted a curative approach to health care, and people such as the Director of Medical Services, Alfred Turner Sneath, who considered preventive medicine to be more appropriate. Moreover, the colonial government had never been in a position to implement its far-reaching development utopias on the ground. Instead, it created geographically scattered "local situations of modernity", which satisfied the ideas of progress of those who supported the scheme most vigorously.[50]

Sleeping Sickness in Ulanga District

In 1936, the authorities of Ulanga District were alarmed by rumors of sleeping sickness taking its toll among the population of southern Liwale District. The latter had long been seen as fly-infested country, and the spread of the disease to neighboring Ulanga District along the major labor routes was considered just a matter of time.[51] Culwick's protective measures included the creation of settlements where the scattered population was to be concentrated, but it was only in 1939 that he was allowed to put his scheme into practice. In 1939, 3 cases of sleeping sickness were reported in Ulanga; a year later, there were 77 cases, with 17 in the first month of 1941 alone.[52] In 1940, large sections of the eastern and southern parts of the district were designated as a conservation area, incorporated into the Selous Game Reserve and closed to human habitation.[53] Indeed, all the Wapogoro and Wangindo people living in the area were resettled to the Luhombero Valley (1941) and Ruaha Valley (1942), respectively. Later, smaller concentrations were established at Kichangani-Lupiro (1943), Iragua (1943), Itete

50   Fisher, Arce, *The Spectacle of Modernity*, p. 94.
51   TNA, 461/16/2, Sleeping Sickness General, 1930–1940, anonymous, Sleeping Sickness, 22 May 1936.
52   TNA, No. 28446, Sleeping Sickness Concentrations in Ulanga, E. C. Baker, Provincial Commissioner Eastern Province and R.R. Scott, Schedule I, Ulanga-District – Mahenge Area, 9 March 1941, pp. 1–2, here: p. 2.
53   Larson, *A History of the Mahenge (Ulanga) District*, p. 302.

(1943) and Sofi-Majiji (1944).[54] Preceding the selection of the sites was a scientific study of local conditions in the new areas, their topographic characteristics and the fertility of their soils. Theoretically, the new settlements were to have been endowed with schools and dispensaries, each of the latter staffed with tribal dressers trained to "use the microscope to the extent of being able to recognize hookworm, roundworm, bilharzia, trypanosomes, filaria, relapsing fever, and malaria sometimes."[55]

From early on, such schemes also had their critics: in several memoranda and letters, the Canadian Paul Alfred Turner Sneath, who succeeded R. R. Scott as Director of Medical Services in 1944, eloquently expressed his displeasure over the uncontrolled proliferation of rural dispensaries that accompanied the sleeping sickness measures: "[The consequence of the spread of health infrastructure to the] African mind has been that his mystical susceptibilities have been enhanced with the idea that the European can provide by bottle, tablet, dressing and syringe a remedy to all his physical and mental disabilities without any effort on his part."[56] The mushrooming of health facilities in Ulanga District, as demanded by Ifakara's Indian community, and the uncontrolled distribution of drugs to rural sufferers ran counter to Sneath's conception of rural health care, which emphasized prevention and social medicine, thus anticipating later discussion on the focus of African public health care.[57] Interpreting Sneath's reactions more as a plea for a change of behavior on the part of the Africans than as a fundamental criticism of the resettlement schemes as such, the colonial government pursued its carrot-and-stick approach: compliance with the scheme was to be promoted through incentives such as tax exemptions. All those who tried to resist government measures, however, were forcibly removed. It was of vital importance to gain the support of the chiefs, and to convince them of the economic, medical and social advantages of the new sites. A concern often expressed by the government was that sufficient numbers of settlers should be attained so as to make the concentrations self-sustaining or even profitable as economic units. However, the achievement of this goal was constantly threatened by the responses of the local population to the resettlement schemes. In 1943, 15%

---

54   Ibid., p. 303.
55   TNA, 61/104/H, A. T. Culwick, 2 November 1942, p. 1.
56   TNA, 450, 653, P.A.T. Sneath to Provincial Commissioner Eastern Province, 1 September 1949, pp. 1–2, here: p. 1.
57   Bruchhausen, *Medizin zwischen den Welten*, p. 117.

of the Luhombero settlers deserted and crossed the border to Liwale, convincing the Provincial Commissioner that "if the ebb from the settlements continues, and there is no reason to suppose it will do otherwise, the settlement may become too small to keep out the fly and the urge to desert spread to other concentrations."[58]

Even though Culwick never ruled out the option of bringing deserters back by force, he was nevertheless convinced that the benefits of closer settlement would sooner or later make them return voluntarily. Similarly, the district's administrators never interpreted the desertions as a criticism of sleeping sickness interventions as such, instead attributing them to a "few turbulent spirits" who maintained close social contacts with communities in Liwale and Songea.[59]

The major resettlement schemes in Luhombero and Ruaha were not yet finished when Culwick accelerated the pace of social engineering and promoted the settlements as showcases of modern society for other regions too. The District's northern parts, especially, were to be subjected to sleeping sickness regulation, and Mgeta and Mbingu were identified as suitable places for closer settlement. Culwick's plea for more comprehensive political action went hand in hand with support for scientific investigation; science and policy were to be merged by all means, and Culwick was aware of the risks of a political-administrative apparatus which could be unreceptive to scientific knowledge:

> I am opposed to concentrating populations in this district unless it can be done properly. We have to deal with people living out of sympathy with their environment, and it is so easy to save them from sleeping-sickness only to kill them with numerous other diseases unless we plan carefully.[60]

However, the relationship between science and policy was never well balanced, and an administrative logic always seemed to prevail over scientific considerations. It was no accident that Culwick mentioned the importance of scientific planning in the pursuit of resettlement policies. The problem soon identified by politicians and agricultural experts alike was that, despite all claims to the contrary, the soils in the new settlements became exhausted, and people started to farm their crops outside the allotted areas.

---

58 TNA, No. 28446, Provincial Commissioner, 8 June 1943, p. 2.
59 Ibid.
60 TNA, 61/104/H, Sleeping Sickness Mahenge, 1941–1942, A. T. Culwick, 13 June 1942, p. 1.

There was a wide range of opinions as to how soil exhaustion could be brought under control. While Culwick seems to have preferred allowing the farmers to plant outside clearly demarcated areas, others – such as the Senior Agricultural Officer A. H. Savile – were more in favor of respecting the boundaries of the newly established settlements. According to him, there were still vast strips of fertile land within the settlements, and he was puzzled by the fact that Culwick seemed to be "prepared to accept the natives' excuses as having more weight than ... my training and expertise".[61] The gulf between science and policy became more accentuated in the newly planned settlements of Mgeta and Mbingu.

In 1942, the Provincial Commissioner for Eastern Province criticized the fact that the new home for thousands of people had never been subject to agricultural scrutiny, and he proposed that the work already undertaken should be suspended "until the end of the war unless an increase in the number of cases of sleeping sickness amounting to an epidemic, renders such a course imperative".[62] The voice of the Provincial Commissioner remained unheard: in summer 1945, a group of specialists including Paul Alfred Turner Sneath, H. Fairbairn (the Sleeping Sickness Officer in charge of the concentrations) and C. E. J. Biggs (Director of Agricultural Production and a member of the Tsetse Committee) met to discuss the ongoing activities at Mgeta and Mbingu. The reason for the meeting was that Biggs had vetoed the commencement of settlement activities in these areas before a sound agricultural survey had been conducted. At the meeting, however, he was informed that the movement of people had already been started, and that "it would be a matter of great political difficulty if settlement was held up for another year".[63] In the face of the government's determination to proceed rapidly, Biggs's veto vanished into thin air. Somewhat dismayed, he made clear:

> In these circumstances it seemed impossible to stick to the veto and settlement will now proceed, although I have made it perfectly plain that I can accept no responsibility if it is found that the area is unsuitable for agriculture or if the size of it is too small for the number of people it is proposed to settle in it. Neither have I accepted responsibility for any bad practices that may result through lack of planning beforehand.[64]

---

61   Ibid., A. H. Savile to A. T. Culwick, 17 December 1943, p. 3.
62   Ibid., E. C. Baker, 7 July 1942, p. 1.
63   TNA, No. 28446, C.E.J. Biggs, Director of Agricultural Production, 1 August 1945, p. 1.
64   Ibid.

It would appear that government officials such as Culwick or Biggs welcomed the resettlement schemes as important harbingers of modernity. From their perspective, resettlement meant the establishment of a new health infrastructure and would consequently lead to improved health care. More importantly, however, modernity was understood in economic terms. The resettlement of large parts of the population could only be justified if the whole process was meticulously planned, if the quality of the soil was assessed beforehand, and if the concentration would result in higher agricultural output. The fact that Culwick considered the resettlement schemes as nuclei for economic development becomes evident if one looks at the more comprehensive development plans he elaborated once the funds for fighting sleeping sickness started to dry up.

The Ulanga Rural Development Scheme, 1944–1951

The rural medical services in Ulanga District were mainly the result of a political-administrative logic that sought to contain the spread of sleeping sickness across the territory. Disregarding the many reports written by provincial commissioners on the mixed success of the sleeping sickness concentrations, Culwick heralded the measures as a turning point in the district's demographic development. While his scientific work on diet and health bore witness to decreasing fertility in Africa, the sleeping sickness concentrations were able to reverse this alarming trend:

> The policy of concentration is bringing an increasing number of people within easy reach of medical facilities, and is producing results which, although not unexpected, are proceeding with startling rapidity. Hospital attendances in the re-settled areas have outstripped the most sanguine hopes ... and the success of the treatment given, combined with a vigorous campaign to produce more and better food and to improve sanitation, is having a profound effect not only on the health, but also on the psychology of the community.[65]

Earlier rural health care efforts had produced a growing number of people "whose wants will be far more ambitious than the meager requirements of

---

65   TNA, No. 33041, Development and Reconstruction Ulanga District, A. T. Culwick, Memorandum on Education in Ulanga District, 28 August 1944, pp. 1–6, here: p. 1. For similar ideas, see: A. T. Culwick, *The Laborer and his Hire*, in: Tanganyika Notes and Records, Vol. 17, June 1944, pp. 26–33.

their fathers who were poverty stricken, diseased savages, picturesque in their semi-nudity, no doubt, but a disgrace to modern society".[66] The creation of a committee for postwar planning in Dar es Salaam in 1944 and the prospect of increased funds for development projects prompted Culwick to propose a more comprehensive Ulanga Rural Development Scheme (URDS). This, together with the Kilombero Valley Scheme and the Rehabilitation Scheme for the Uluguru Mountains, was approved by the Development Commission for the Eastern Province.[67] Culwick's efforts were motivated not only by his own observations of improved health in the district, but also by a report written by the Education Officer J. A. C. Blumer, who had visited Ulanga District in 1944 to inspect various government, mission and NA schools.[68] In the first paragraph of his report, Blumer admitted that the Ulanga District had been the "Cinderella" for many years, and that his analysis was not intended to overshadow the previous efforts of district officers "who have done all in their powers to deal with educational matters with the time and meager funds at their disposal".[69] What then followed was a harsh criticism of the government and NA schools, which lagged behind missionary-provided education both in physical appearance and in the quality of instruction. The new political situation created by seven newly established sleeping sickness concentrations – with almost 9000 taxpayers eager to obtain the promised benefits of closer settlement – called for increased efforts on the part of the colonial government.

Hence, education made up the core of Culwick's development project. However, with an additional focus on agricultural development and animal husbandry, it not only tried to be as comprehensive as possible but was also inspired by other major development projects, such as those planned in Sukumaland in Lake Province or the (notorious) Groundnut Scheme in what is now the Mtwara region.[70] Culwick's scheme had three major components: held together by a training center preferably located in Mahenge,

---

66 Culwick, Memorandum, p. 1.
67 TNA, No. 33041, A. McKenzie to the Deputy Chairman of Development Committee, 21 August 1947, p. 1. The Kilombero Valley Scheme, however, never received funds because the proposal was never worked out; see: Tanzanian National Library (NBA Section), F. H. Page-Jones, Annual Reports of the Provincial Commissioners on Native Administration for the year 1948, p. 33.
68 TNA, No. 33041, J. A. C. Blumer, Inspection Report-Ulanga District, 5 August 1944, pp. 1–5.
69 Ibid., p. 1.
70 Rohland Schuknecht, *British Colonial Development Policy after the Second World War. The Case of Sukumaland, Tanganyika*, Berlin 2010.

it aimed, first, to go beyond common efforts to increase yields through the mechanization of agrarian production by using industrial education to foster the transformation of natural goods into consumer goods:

> We need an army of skilled mechanics, carpenters, boat-builders, cycle repairers, masons, joiners, traders, etc and when I say "need", I mean that work is actually available for them now, and that the demand for them will grow rapidly provided the conditions are created to foster the economic expansion of this district, not only as an exporting community, but also as one in which internal trade plays a greater and greater part, which it undoubtedly could and should.[71]

Secondly – closely linked to the industrial education component – was animal husbandry, for which cattle would have to be moved from the plains to the Mahenge highlands. Thirdly, Culwick advocated the integration of the rural dispensary system into the overarching framework of the scheme. The several dispensaries that emerged within the enclosed spaces of the sleeping sickness concentrations throughout the 1940s were funded by the anti-sleeping sickness measures, but with the decreasing number of new infections, funds for rural health care fizzled out.[72]

The proposal to staff the training center with a European headmaster, a European farm manager, a European industrial instructor and a couple of African teachers and clerks faced outspoken criticism from various quarters. Unsurprisingly, Paul Alfred Turner Sneath, whose reservations concerning the material expansion of rural dispensaries have already been mentioned, could not fully support the scheme.[73] Others too were not enthusiastic about Culwick's proposal to maintain and expand rural medical services with the aid of colonial development funds. One of the critics was Conan-Davis, who was about to take over Culwick's post as District Commissioner in 1945. What Conan-Davis questioned, however, was not people's unrealistic expectations of health care (Sneath's concern), but the unrealistic assumptions about people's current health status on which Culwick's proposal was based. Conan-Davis could not find any references to support Culwick's claims of improved health in the district. According to the future District Commissioner, the NA dispensaries were "pathetic in their inadequacies"; the population of the Mahenge highlands, on whom

---

71   Culwick, Memorandum, p. 2.
72   NBA Section, F. H. Page-Jones, Annual Report for the year 1947, p. 38.
73   TNA, No. 33041, Sneath to the Deputy Chairman of the Development Committee, 26 August 1947, p. 1.

Culwick's hopes rested, were not able to produce grain surpluses but required food permits to survive, and there was not the slightest indication that "they have learned the first thing about proper feeding and wise cultivation".[74] To quote Conan-Davis in full:

> In his scheme, Mr. C. has let his imagination run riot and it is no more based on reality than is a fairy tale. There are errors, inaccuracies and false conclusions drawn from unproved hypotheses, and no wonder. The originator is neither qualified nor even trained, in veterinary science, dairy farming, medicine, engineering, forestry nor agriculture and has had very little administrative tuition in his more junior days. Frankly, it amazes me that the scheme has been so unconditionally accepted on the sole recommendation of an amateur.[75]

From today's perspective, Conan-Davis's reservations were fully justified. From the outset, the scheme suffered major setbacks, which led to a reduction of the approved funds from £97,000 to £47,000 over the ten-year period and a continuation of the scheme on a much smaller scale.[76] This reduction was due in particular to problems arising with the animal husbandry component of the project. As it turned out, the Mahenge highlands were not at all suitable for the settlement of cattle herds. In 1945, large numbers of cattle died as a result of East Coast Fever – "a disease which was understood not to be present in the Mahenge plateau".[77] On several occasions, the presence of tsetse fly was also reported, and after an in-depth survey made by the Veterinary Officer and the Pasture Research Officer, it was decided to postpone this component also because of a "lack of suitable grazing land for large scale development".[78] Culwick's plans for the education sector were also overtaken by reality: instead of a training center for an "army of mechanics and carpenters", the scheme provided for the establishment of a boarding school in Nawenge, comprising 60 non-Christian boarders. The original intention to challenge the Capuchin mission's monopoly in education was undermined by a decision to provide the Capuchins with funding to extend their school workshop for the training of a selected number of

---

74 Ibid., Conan-Davis, The Ulanga Rural Development Scheme, 12 December 1945, pp. 1–11, here: p. 2.
75 Ibid., p. 1.
76 NBA Section, F. H. Page-Jones, Annual Report for the year 1947, p. 42.
77 Ibid., Annual Report of the Provincial Commissioners for the year 1945, p. 32.
78 TNA, Microfilm (MF), 21, Ulanga District, Colonial Development Schemes, Ulanga Rural Development Scheme, p. 1.

non-Christian apprentices.[79] In 1951, the scheme collapsed altogether. The Nawenge boarding school was handed over to the Ulanga District's Native Authorities in 1952, as were the nine sleeping sickness dispensaries, each of which was equipped with a microscope and run by a dresser and an ayah (female helper). As the URDS report for 1951 dryly noted, "As far as can be foreseen at present, no development schemes will be operating in Ulanga District during 1952."[80]

The question of why the URDS failed is perhaps less difficult to answer than Conan-Davis's question of why it was promoted so vigorously in the first place, given the many critical voices raised. To start with the first question: one of the most striking characteristics the project shared with many others conducted at the time was a lack of cooperation with all those for whom it was originally designed. Development was something that was done *for* but not *with* Africans. Since development was supposed to "trickle down" from Europeans to Africans, such schemes were highly dependent on the presence of European staff, whose willingness to sacrifice a career in the colonial bureaucracy of Dar es Salaam for a life in far-away Ulanga was substantially overestimated. The importance and the impact of career patterns highlight the individuals at the core of such all-encompassing concepts as the colonial developmentalist state or the rural health system. In fact, health and development in 1930s and 1940s Ulanga were promoted by individuals to such an extent that it is hardly possible to speak of a "health system" at all. Culwick's replacement by the new District Commissioner, Conan-Davis. dealt a severe blow to the continuation of and support for the URDS.

Conan-Davis decried Culwick's ideas as a misjudgement of local needs and pointed to major flaws in the planning process. Why then was the project executed at all? As mentioned above, the URDS has to be seen in the wider context of late-colonial policies and the rise of the concept of rural development. Even though development never constituted a homogeneous discourse that could easily be translated into coherent rural policies, the concept nevertheless encompassed a number of specific ideas of what rural development was supposed to be – standardization of political and administrative processes, improvement of livelihoods through education and better health care, and rationalization of traditional agrarian systems through

---

79   Ibid., p. 2.
80   TNA, No. 33041, Ulanga Rural Development Scheme, Report for 1951, 14 December 1951, p. 1.

the application of science and technology. Emerging from the sleeping sickness concentration measures, the URDS is a good example of a policy that is path dependent, responsive to the claims of local populations, and involves the dual requirement of being scientific at its roots and progressive in its outcomes. Culwick, as its major proponent, was especially persuasive because he successfully deployed his local knowledge of the region as well as his strong belief in the power of science to remodel and transform African societies. It was this combination of local expertise (gained from living in the field for almost 15 years) and scientific vision that allowed the URDS to get off the ground.

Science and Decolonization

This chapter has argued that, from the late 1930s onwards, decolonization and science entered a mutually co-productive phase.[81] Policymakers in Paris and London considered scientific research in the colonies as an important factor in reshaping the increasingly strained relations between the colonies and the metropoles, and approved substantial funding. A growing scientific apparatus and the newly released metropolitan funds for colonial development and research did not, however, result in an all-encompassing "knowledge machinery" but created distinctive geographies of accelerated scientific action and social interaction in the colonies. Comparison of the two sites that emerged more or less by accident on the scientific landscape of the French and British empires reveals striking differences with regard to the motivation, function and social impact of the scientific efforts. The main motive for the creation of ORSTOM and its training center in Adipodoumé was to improve the coordination and monitoring of French science in the French colonies. ORSTOM-Adiopodoumé was just one of many newly created ORSTOM sites that were oriented towards Paris within the network of French postwar imperialism. Highly hierarchical in nature, the institute sought to research every hidden corner of natural and social life, compiling masses of scientific and statistical data about the colony. Although it unleashed a social dynamic in the nearby villages, ORSTOM never had the direct political impact that was experienced in Ulanga. There, disease prevention formed the basis of wider social and economic policies. The quest to contain the spread of the tsetse fly resulted

---

81 Lachenal, *Biomédecine et décolonisation au Cameroun*, p. 15.

in large-scale state interventions and the creation of several sleeping sickness concentrations, which were heralded as a model for rural development. For this reason, the position of Tanganyika within the larger project of empire says little about the character of colonial medicine or its impact on the local population. Sleeping sickness was considered a good opportunity to change rural African livelihoods and to accelerate the pace towards modernity. But the sudden exertion of state power within an area where governance lay in the hands of NA or foreign religious organizations was short-lived. The sense of emergency associated with sleeping sickness interventions could not be translated into sustainable development policies; this was due to local resistance, the lack of funds and, above all, differences within the colonial administration over the general objectives of the settlements. Whereas ORSTOM continued to operate in Côte d'Ivoire after a major reform in the 1960s, British colonialism in Tanganyika crumbled in the 1950s, opening the way to new international protagonists, of which Switzerland was not the least important.

Chapter 2
Switzerland in the World

The previous chapter proposed a reading of science and decolonization as co-productive social forces. Both colonial France and Britain played the scientific trump card – albeit with different local impacts – in a further round of the imperial game in the 1940s and beyond. As Raoul Combes insisted, the overseas territories were no longer to be seen as "a vast reserve of scientific material". Instead, in a powerful reinterpretation, they were neglected but potentially cultivable areas, with the seeds of progress waiting for science to make them flourish. Switzerland was not unaffected by this "imperialism of knowledge": World War II provided small niches for Switzerland to appear on the colonial stage. Here, too, science was the major vehicle used to step out of the enclosed laboratories of Switzerland and enter the African fields. Thus, in Switzerland as elsewhere, decolonization led to a variety of existing scientific disciplines being considered suitable for application in the colonies. However, the reconfiguration of science in Switzerland was not associated with colonial occupation – Switzerland had no colonial territory to subdue and no armies to protect from newly discovered pathogens. The institutionalization of tropical science in Switzerland was related instead to the specific domestic circumstances arising from World War II. Science and its many institutions were seen as a welcome stepping stone allowing young Swiss emigrants to leave the country for the colonies, and as an effective means of easing pressures on the postwar labor market. Paradoxical though it may sound, it was the strong focus on the nation that accounted for this transnational movement.

The first part of this chapter looks at the history of science policy in Switzerland. It concentrates on the historical processes that led to the establishment of the Swiss Tropical Institute in 1943 and the rise of novel forms of scholarly engagement with tropical environments. The second part focuses on the characteristics of "tropical knowledge" as a conglomerate of established branches of science. Lagging behind its French and British counterparts – after more than half a century of colonial scientific fieldwork – tropical science in Switzerland was not yet an established discipline but brought together fields such as medical parasitology, ethnography, agronomy and medicine. During the 1950s, scientific activities in these areas were brought to the colonial territories. The third part therefore examines the strategies employed by individual Swiss scientists to create a space for Swiss science in the tropics. It looks at how they joined the OR-STOM family working in Adiopodoumé, and how in 1951 they finally obtained what they longed for – a small research laboratory, known as the Centre Suisse de Recherches Scientifiques (CSRS), established on the OR-STOM site. The fact that colonial societies were not structurally divided into the social realms of "colonizer" and "colonized", but marked by various social hierarchies and hybrid identities, is now well established in the academic literature.[1] As the last part of the chapter aims to show, financial constraints meant that Swiss scientists could barely comply with the social obligations imposed by life among Europeans in the colony.

Science and the Postwar Economic Order

Until the interwar period, Switzerland largely lacked a national science policy. Science was organized locally and, with the exception of the Swiss Federal Institute of Technology (ETH Zurich), it was outside the reach of the federal government. Formalized connections between science, industry and the state – a major factor in the development of science policy elsewhere – were almost non-existent.[2] The medium through which the federal government first began to support science was the Swiss Society of Natural Science (Schweizerische Naturforschende Gesellschaft, SNG), the oldest federal scientific organization in Switzerland, which dated back to 1815.[3] However, during the economic recession of the interwar period and particularly during World War II, the Swiss government became more active in initiating a national science policy as part of wider economic measures.[4] The government's efforts to control scientific production within Switzerland were motivated by economic considerations. The war years

---

1   Homi Bhabha, *The Location of Culture*, London 1994; Ann Stoler, *Rethinking Colonial Categories. European Communities and the Boundaries of Rule*, in: Comparative Studies in Society and History, Vol. 31, No. 1, 1989, pp. 134–161.
2   Frédéric Joye-Cagnard, *La construction de la politique de la science en suisse. Enjeux Scientifiques, stratégiques et politiques (1944–1974)*, Neuchâtel 2010, p. 29.
3   Murray James Luck, *Science in Switzerland*, New York, London 1967, p. 97.
4   Antoine Fleury, Frédéric Joye, *Die Anfänge der Forschungspolitik in der Schweiz. Gründungsgeschichte des Schweizerischen Nationalfonds zur Förderung der wissenschaftlichen Forschung 1934–1952*, Baden 2002, p. 26.

left the country politically isolated and anxious about postwar depression. The fight against possible chronic unemployment, as experienced after World War I, became the foremost national priority. In 1940, Swiss President Marcel Pilet-Golaz announced in a radio broadcast that his government would do everything it could – "whatever the cost" – to prevent the Swiss labor market from nosediving.[5] Applied science controlled by the state and subordinated to economic requirements was considered a crucial instrument in reducing high unemployment rates. In the early 1940s, Arthur Rohn, President of the ETH Governing Board, and Johann Laurenz Cagianut, Federal Delegate for Employment Opportunities, met to discuss the idea of a Swiss National Science Foundation (SNSF). The project was biased towards the needs of the ETH, giving it disproportionate weight in the Foundation Board. Not surprisingly, the SNSF met with fierce resistance, especially from the cantons of Bern, Zurich and Basel, which saw it as violating the very principle of federalism. In addition, Basel was afraid that money would be channeled away from the pharmaceutical industry to the new foundation. Arthur Rohn's efforts therefore failed, and the project of an SNSF seeking to encompass all scientific disciplines in a nondiscriminatory manner was only realized in 1952, thanks to the efforts of Alexander von Muralt, a physiologist and President of the HFSJG Foundation (High Altitude Research Stations Jungfraujoch and Gornergrat). However, the failure of the Rohn-Cagianut project was not detrimental to the basic idea that the applied sciences could fuel the stuttering economic engine. Otto Zipfel, appointed Delegate for Employment Opportunities in spring 1941, launched a similar initiative. In a letter dated October 21, 1942 – based on the "Bundesratsbeschluss vom 29. Juli 1942 über die Regelung der Arbeitsbeschaffung in der Kriegskrisenzeit" (Federal Council Decree on wartime employment opportunities) – he urged all universities to submit research projects "that would generate job opportunities and benefits for the industrial, trade and agricultural sectors or that are suitable for stimulating exports and tourism".[6]

---

5   Quoted in: Erwin Bucher, *Zwischen Bundesrat und General. Schweizer Politik und Armee im Zweiten Weltkrieg*, Zurich 1993, p. 543.
6   Staatsarchiv Basel-Stadt (StABS), Universitätsarchiv I 71.1, (Schweizerisches Tropeninstitut), 1942–1944, Brief Otto Zipfel, 21 October 1942.

Creation of the Swiss Tropical Institute in 1943

Alfred Gigon, Professor of Internal Medicine at the University of Basel, felt that the creation of a Swiss Tropical Institute (STI) would be a suitable response to Zipfel's request. Though influential in the field of Swiss science policy and – with Alexander von Muralt – a major force behind the creation of the Swiss Academy of Medical Sciences in 1943, Gigon was more or less a stranger to the tropical world. Rooted in the social medicine tradition, he had published widely on relations between medicine and social policy, and nutrition among the working classes.[7] Why then did he promote the tropical cause in Switzerland? In a recent publication, Andreas Eckert reminds us that discourse on the tropics and tropicality emerged as a new feature during the process of decolonization. Rather than framing the tropical world as an earthly paradise or as the "white man's burden" (Rudyard Kipling), the term was increasingly imbued with the "concept of development, global tourism, commodity advertising and environmental politics".[8] However, Gigon did not yet conceptualize tropical spaces as targets for Western development initiatives. In his explanations of why Switzerland would need a tropical institute, earlier representations of the tropical world as overflowing with natural wealth loomed large.[9] According to Gigon, the possibilities deriving from such an institution were manifold and not at all restricted to medical research. In particular, the economic potential of a tropical school fired Gigon's imagination. A brief glimpse at the war-ridden European economies was sufficient to demonstrate that Switzerland could expect no salvation from trade relations with European countries. But while World War II left European economies in tatters, there were whole continents and subcontinents – Africa, Asia or Latin America – that would now self-confidently stake their claim in the postwar economic and political order, outstripping the old continent in political influence and economic

---

7 Alfred Gigon, *Etwas über Medizin und Sozialpolitik*, in: Sonderabdruck aus der Schweizerischen Medizinischen Wochenschrift, Vol. 75, No. 18, 1945, pp. 394–501; Gigon, *Die Arbeiterkost nach Untersuchungen über die Ernährung Basler Arbeiter bei freigewählter Kost*, in: Institut für Gewerbehygiene in Frankfurt (ed.), Schriften aus dem Gesamtgebiet der Gewerbehygiene, Heft 3, Berlin 1914.

8 Eckert, *"Tropics"*, in: Akira Iriye and Pierre-Yves Saunier (eds.), Palgrave Dictionary of Transnational History, Basingstoke, London 2009, pp. 1059–1061.

9 StABS, Universitätsarchiv I 71.1, Gigon, Exposé *"Schweizerisches Institut für tropische Wissenschaften und Wirtschaftsbeziehungen"*, 24 November 1942.

wealth.[10] As a country without a colonial past, Switzerland was well positioned in the race for new markets. Nonetheless, reconfigurations of global power relations called for readjustment of domestic economic structures, and the STI was a first step in this direction. As Gigon argued, "A tropical institute should mainly fulfill economic and scientific tasks, and the latter in the interests of the economy."[11]

Today's readers might be amazed about the power of Gigon's imagination in writing about rising Third World economies, especially on the African continent. It has to be acknowledged, however, that his plans reflected political necessities as well as economic realities at the time. The cautious optimism of his sentences encapsulates a specific historical situation: after the Battles of El Alamein and Stalingrad, the course of the war had taken a decisive turn in favor of the Allies. The more the military pendulum swung towards the Allied forces, the more Switzerland's "neutrality" and its wartime cooperation with Nazi Germany came to be internationally questioned. In particular, the Allies accused Switzerland of having sustained the German dictatorship through uninterrupted and intense trade relations. Given the chilly winds blowing from across the Atlantic, political realignment was one of Switzerland's main concerns. As early as 1942, a new division was created within the Department of Foreign Affairs, charged with working out strategies for integrating Switzerland into a postwar political system.[12] The country's foremost priorities were to smoothly take its place within a new political order and at the same time to remain competitive in entering new economic markets. Even before the outbreak of World War II, Third World markets were more important to Switzerland than to other small European open economies.[13] After the war, these economic relations were even more significant. While in 1938, 13.3% of all exports went to Third World markets, this proportion had risen to 22% by the mid-1950s.[14] The intensification of trade relations in the postwar period was mainly due to Switzerland's status as a neutral

---

10   Ibid., p. 3.
11   Ibid., Gigon to Zweifel, 10 February 1943.
12   Antoine Fleury, *La Suisse et la préparation à l'après-guerre*, in: Michel Dumoulin (ed.), Plans des temps de guerre pour l'Europe d'après-guerre, 1940–1947 – Wartime Plans for Postwar Europe 1940–1947, Bruxelles 1995, pp. 175–195, here: p. 176.
13   Etemad, *Structure géographique du commerce entre la Suisse et le Tiers Monde au XXe siècle*, in: Paul Bairoch and Martin Körner (eds.), Die Schweiz in der Weltwirtschaft – La Suisse dans l'économie mondiale, Zurich 1990, pp. 165–183, here: p. 173.
14   Ibid., p. 174.

country, completely devoid of imperialistic intentions.[15] It should be noted, however, that with the rapid recovery of Europe's postwar economies, European countries remained Switzerland's main trading partners. Moreover, among the newly emerging markets, there were sharp distinctions: Swiss exports flowed more abundantly to the markets of Asia and Latin America than to Africa.[16] However, the decision to create a tropical institute in Basel in 1943 cannot be attributed solely to economic reasoning. Equally important was the fact that the STI was a continuation of Basel's long-established colonial tradition.

Africa and Civic Culture

Gigon's choice of Basel as the future site of the STI was not wholly accidental. Switzerland in general and Basel in particular had a long history of encounters with Africa.[17] The discovery of "exotic" places and the collection of scientific specimens or ethnographic displays were deeply rooted in Basel's Protestant "patriciate".[18] Like many of Europe's imperial centers, Basel also witnessed the rise of a distinctive institutional network which organized the exchange and distribution of knowledge about the tropical world in the nineteenth century. The Basel Mission – founded in 1815 – became an important planning center, as it maintained missionary stations in West Africa, India, China and Indonesia.

---

15 David, Etemad, *L'expansion économique de la Suisse en Outre-mer (XIXe–XXe siècles). Un état de la question*, in: Schweizerische Zeitschrift für Geschichte, Vol. 46, No. 2, 1996, pp. 226–231, here: pp. 227–228.

16 Marc Perrenoud, *Guerres, indépendance, neutralité et opportunités. Quelques jalons historiques pour l'analyse des relations économiques de la Suisse avec l'Afrique (des années 1920 aux années 1960)*, in: Suisse-Afrique (18e-20e siècles). De la traite des Noirs à la fin du régime de l'Apartheid, Münster 2005, pp. 85–104, here: p. 94; see also: Etemad, *Le commerce extérieur de la Suisse avec le tiers monde aux XIXe et XXe siècles. Une perspective comparative internationale*, in: Les Annuelles. La Suisse sur la ligne bleue de l'Outre-mer, pp. 19–41, here: p. 32.

17 Minder, *La Suisse coloniale?*; Patrick Harries, Giorgio Miescher, *Immer etwas Neues aus Afrika. Einige Überlegungen zur Geschichte Afrikas in Basel*, in: Regio Basiliensis, Vol. 45, No. 2, 2004, pp. 87–97.

18 The term "patriciate" is borrowed from Philipp Sarasin, who defines patrician structures as being shaped by profession, income, property and familial bonds: see: Philipp Sarasin, *Stadt der Bürger. Bürgerliche Macht und städtische Gesellschaft. Basel 1846–1914*, Göttingen 1992 (2nd edition).

Sunday-morning jaunts to the tamed wilderness of the Zoological Gardens, or to the ordered displays of the ethnographic and natural history museums, were part of a deeply internalized cultural attitude. In addition, large numbers of scientific expeditions set off from Basel. Of paramount importance for the development of ethnography as a scientific discipline in Switzerland were the cousins Paul and Fritz Sarasin: in 1883–86, they explored Ceylon (Sri Lanka), meticulously describing the natural characteristics of the island and the behavior of the Veddas for a wider European public. Later, the Sarasins would venture into Celebes (Sulawesi), accompanied by an armed retinue to promote the expansion of Dutch colonial power.[19]

The chemical industry also had strong interests in the exploration of foreign territories. As Serge Reubi contends, there was a well-established tradition of industrialists financing scientific expeditions in exchange for testing of their products under tropical conditions.[20] Perhaps the most notable feature of African knowledge production in Basel was that, well into the second half of the twentieth century, these initiatives and institutions must be seen, not as single strands, but as connected by various interpersonal ties. As we will see later, the connections between different disciplines were exemplified, par excellence, by the zoologist Rudolf Geigy (1902–1995), who became the first director of the STI in 1943. Born into a wealthy industrial family, Geigy succeeded his father Johann Rudolf Geigy-Schlumberger (1862–1933) as a member of the Board of Directors of the pharmaceutical company J. R. Geigy AG in 1932. The Geigys belonged to a group of powerful families who shaped the city's cultural and political life. Even though this group's direct influence on Basel's politics declined during the interwar period, the social and cultural weight of these families remained intact at least until the 1960s.[21]

Given this rich tradition of close ties, the proposal to create a tropical institute was strongly endorsed by local academia. Even before Otto Zipfel had a chance to be inspired by the idea of an STI in Basel, Peter Von der Mühll, Vice Chancellor of the University of Basel and Professor of Greek

19   Zangger, *Koloniale Schweiz*; Schär, *Tropenliebe*.
20   Serge Reubi, *L'ethnologue, prestataire de service pour l'industrie dans la Suisse des années 1930–1960*, in: Hans-Jörg Gilomen, Margrit Müller and Laurent Tissot (eds.), Dienstleistungen. Expansion und Transformation des "dritten Sektors" (15.–20. Jahrhundert) – Les Services. Essor et transformation du "secteur tertiaire" (15e–20e siècles), Zurich 2007, pp. 319–327, here: p. 320; Reubi, *Gentlemen, prolétaires et primitifs*.
21   Sara Janner, *Rudolf Geigy (-Heese)-Hunziker (1902–1995)*, [unpublished typescript], 2010, pp. 1–7, here: p. 2.

Language and Literature, asked all faculty members to submit their responses.[22] The ethnographers, geographers, theologians and humanists all referred to the comprehensive insights about the tropical world that they would candidly share with the members of a future STI.[23] Ironically, outspoken resistance came from the Faculty of Economics. In their memorandum, the economists made it clear that they would prefer to support the project for an export promotion institute initiated by Basel's Chamber of Commerce, rather than endorsing an STI.[24] Fortunately for the proponents of the latter, however, an export promotion institute was already in the process of being created in St. Gallen, with the support of the Swiss government.

While all parties could more or less readily agree that the historical process of decolonization offered a good opportunity for Switzerland to reach out to the tropics, the organizational setup of the proposed institution proved to be more controversial. Zipfel and the political decision-makers in Bern envisaged the benefits of an STI mainly in economic terms. They wished to see the STI alleviating postwar labor market pressures by training a highly productive workforce for a sojourn in the tropics. Accordingly, they intended to finance the whole project through loans offered by the job creation program, which were granted for five years only. But Rudolf Geigy, personifying the strong network of business and scientific interests in Basel, had a long-term engagement in mind: the STI was not only to serve short-term economic interests but add a further element to Basel's scholarly tradition of relations with Africa. In 1943, thanks to Geigy's networking skills in Bern, the various parties finally agreed to establish the STI as an institution under public law, and to share the financial burden among the federal and cantonal government and private donors.[25] Geigy's ability to cater to the needs of different institutions in Basel was also apparent in the institute's daily academic activities. Geigy and his scientific colleagues at the STI had a broad understanding of the term "tropics", and their new object of investigation was to be examined by a variety of scientific disciplines.

22 StABS, Universitätsarchiv I 71.1, Brief Von der Mühll, 1 December 1942.
23 Ibid., Felix Speiser to Von der Mühll, 2 December 1942, as well as the head of the geography department and the deans of the faculties of theology and humanities, 4 December 1942, 4 December 1942, 5 December 1942.
24 Schweizerisches Wirtschaftsarchiv (SWA), Institute 196, Brief der nationalökonomischen Fachvertreter to Von der Mühll, 4 December 1942.
25 StABS, FD-REG 1d 37.2, (Schweizerisches Tropeninstitut), 1943–1959, Grossratsbeschluss betreffend Errichtung eines Schweizerischen Tropeninstituts in Basel.

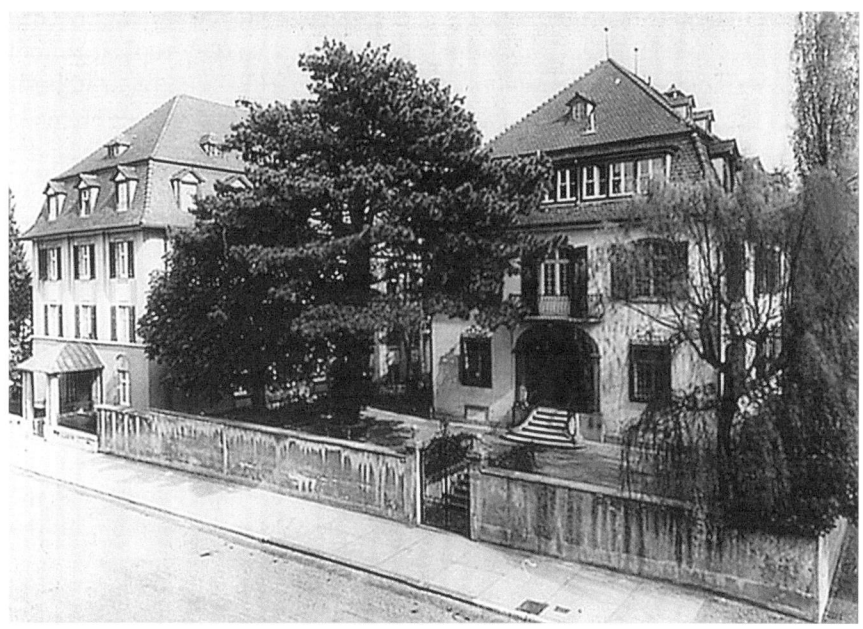

«Haus zur Föhre» and clinic Sonnenrain, 1940s, Archive STI

Encyclopedic Knowledge

Tropical science largely owed its progressive institutionalization to the dedication of Rudolf Geigy, who served as the STI's first director. In his tasks, he was assisted by a Board of Trustees composed of experts from politics, academia and private industry. Their function was to supervise the work of the institute, to approve the budget and to define its activities, "which had to be in accordance with economic interests, the provision of jobs and the promotion of exports".[26]

Everyday activities were administered by an Executive Committee, made up of Rudolf Geigy, Adolf Im Hof (a former member of the cantonal government and President of the Board of Trustees), Alfred Gigon and Rudolf Speich (Swiss Bank Corporation). Initially, the institute's various activities were widely scattered. The secretary, Walter Bodmer, had his headquarters at Stapfelberg 7, where he started to build up a large collection of

26 StABS, Universitätsarchiv I 71.1, Brief Von der Mühll to Zipfel, 15 December 1942.

major publications on tropical issues. Teaching activities were largely conducted at the main university building at Petersplatz, and a Tropical School
was housed in the cantonal school of commerce.[27] However, more important than the decentralization of activities was the fact that tropical science
was not yet a clearly demarcated "episteme". In other words, Switzerland's
lack of formalized colonial relations accounted for tropical science being
an amorphous body of knowledge. Accordingly, the STI tried to include as
many different disciplines as possible in their research and teaching activities, aiming at an encyclopedic knowledge of the tropical world. This aim
of focusing on the "entire tropical world" became especially evident in the
institute's teaching.[28] In the fall semester of 1943/44, the STI for the first
time offered a "general tropical course", designed for people with a general
interest in the tropics or, more specifically, for the missionaries, teachers,
traders and nurses who were preparing for a lengthy spell under the burning
tropical sun.[29] Given this heterogeneous audience, the topics covered in the
lectures ranged from anthropology, colonial history and geography to the
transmission of infectious tropical diseases.[30] However, participants were
invited not simply to consume prefabricated tropical knowledge but to re-
fine their practical skills in drawing and deciphering geographical maps,
first aid and various languages. In the fall semester of 1944/45, the organiz-
ers were overwhelmed by more than 100 applications, a third of which
came from students or members of the missionary societies. In the following years, the largest numbers of participants came from the industrial and
trading sectors, as well as the missionary societies.[31] Between 1945 and
1961, the initial rush abated, with annual numbers of enrollments on the
general tropical course finally averaging around 55.

Similar observations about all-encompassing tropical knowledge apply
to the STI's scientific journal, *Acta Tropica*. In his preface to the first volume, Geigy reminded readers that he had a very broad conception of tropi-

27 Marina Lienhard, *"Abenteurer sterben aus." Weisssein, Othering und Tropendiskurs
    in den Schriften und Korrespondenzen der Schweizerischen Tropenschule und ihrer
    ehemaligen Schüler (1943–1981)*, unpublished MA thesis, University of Zurich 2013.
28 StABS, FD-REG 1d 37.2, Broschüre *"Schweizerisches Tropeninstitut in Basel"*,
    Basel 1944, p. 17.
29 Later, the STI would add a medical course to the curriculum, specifically designed for
    physicians, veterinarians and biologists.
30 StABS, FD-REG 1d 37.2, Broschüre *"Schweizerisches Tropeninstitut in Basel"*,
    pp. 26–28.
31 SWA, Institute 196, Ratschlag 4246, pp. 10–11.

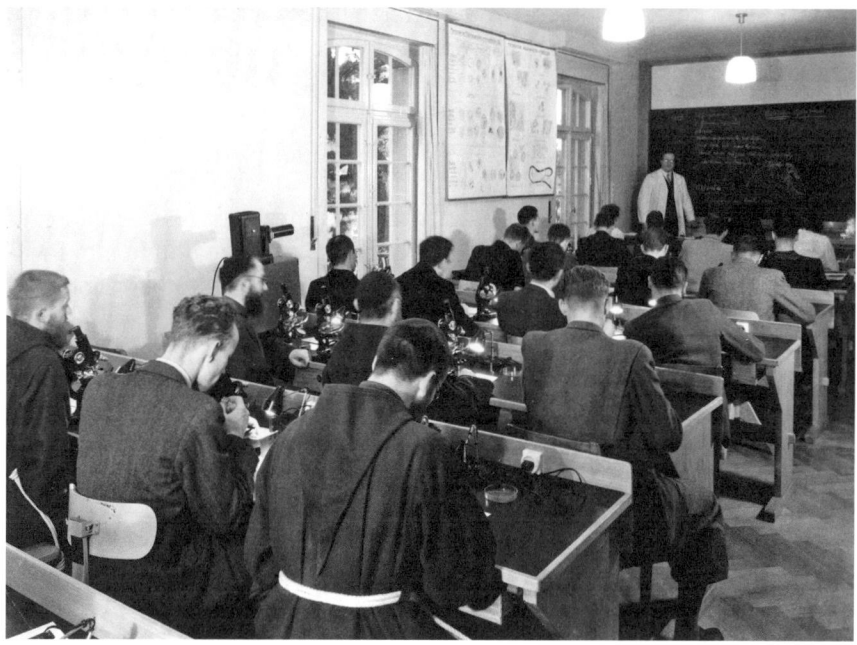

Rudolf Geigy teaching at the General Tropical Course, 1951, Atelier Eidenbenz

cal science.[32] The articles – many written by Geigy's students or scientific colleagues working in the colonies – reflected this approach. Contributions to the journal also dealt with the tropics from various angles and in various languages. Apart from the numerous articles on disease environments, popular topics included anthropology and art. For instance, Geigy himself ventured into the anthropological realm with a study of the initiation of girls in the Ulanga District of Tanganyika, co-authored with Georg Höltker in 1951.[33] Seven years later, art historian Werner Schmalenbach (whose doctoral thesis had examined the influence of primitive art on European art up to 1900) contributed an article on primitive art, while Thierry Freyvogel – one of Geigy's PhD students of whom we will hear much more later – contributed his reflections on a collection of plaited mats from the Ulanga Dis-

32 Rudolf Geigy, *Zum Geleit*, in: Acta Tropica, Zeitschrift für Tropenwissenschaften und Tropenmedizin, Vol. 1, No. 1, 1944, pp. 1–3, here: p. 1.

33 Rudolf Geigy, Georg Höltker, *Mädchen-Initiationen im Ulanga-Distrikt von Tanganyika*, in: Acta Tropica, Vol. 8, No. 4, 1951, pp. 289–344.

trict.[34] Amid this breadth of tropical knowledge, an inner core of what belongs to the academic field of tropical science started to crystallize.

Rudolf Geigy and a New Science for the Colonies

It could be argued that the desire for an all-encompassing representation of the tropics had its origins in the lack of a tropical science tradition in Switzerland. As we have seen, tropical science was a highly amorphous body of knowledge, open to a variety of intellectual influences. This was largely due to Rudolf Geigy, who almost single-handedly defined the contours of the new discipline. Over time, an inner core of sciences for the colonies emerged, mainly comprising ethnography, zoology (medical parasitology), agronomy and tropical medicine. What these disciplines had in common was their applied focus and their suitability for practice in the African field.

Zoology/Medical Parasitology

Of the four disciplines that dominated the tropical sciences in postwar Switzerland, zoology/medical parasitology had the greatest impact. Starting with Rudolf Geigy, most of the researchers populating the field of tropical science had a zoological background. Contrary to his father's wishes, Geigy opted for an academic career rather than a safe industrial career at J. R. Geigy AG. After graduating from the prestigious Humanistisches Gymnasium in Basel, he studied zoology, first under Friedrich Zschokke in Basel, and later under Emile Guyénot in Geneva, who familiarized him with physiological questions.[35] In 1931, he earned a doctorate in developmental biology, consolidating his international reputation as a skillful experimenter.[36] Back in Basel, Geigy accepted a post as a scientific assistant

---

34   Werner Schmalenbach, *Grundsätzliches zur primitiven Kunst*, in: Acta Tropica, Vol. 15, No. 4, 1958, pp. 289–323; Thierry Freyvogel, *Eine Sammlung geflochtener Matten aus dem Ulanga-Distrikt Tanganyikas*, in: Acta Tropica, Vol. 16, No. 4, 1959, pp. 289–301.

35   Janner, *Rudolf Geigy (-Heese)-Hunziker*, p. 1.

36   Geigy, *Action de l'ultra-violet sur le pole germinal dans l'oeuf de Drosophila melanogaster (Castration et mutabilité). Thèse présentée à la faculté des sciences de l'université de Genève pour l'obtention du grade de docteur des sciences naturelles*, Geneva 1931; see also: Janner, *Rudolf Geigy (-Heese)-Hunziker*, p. 2.

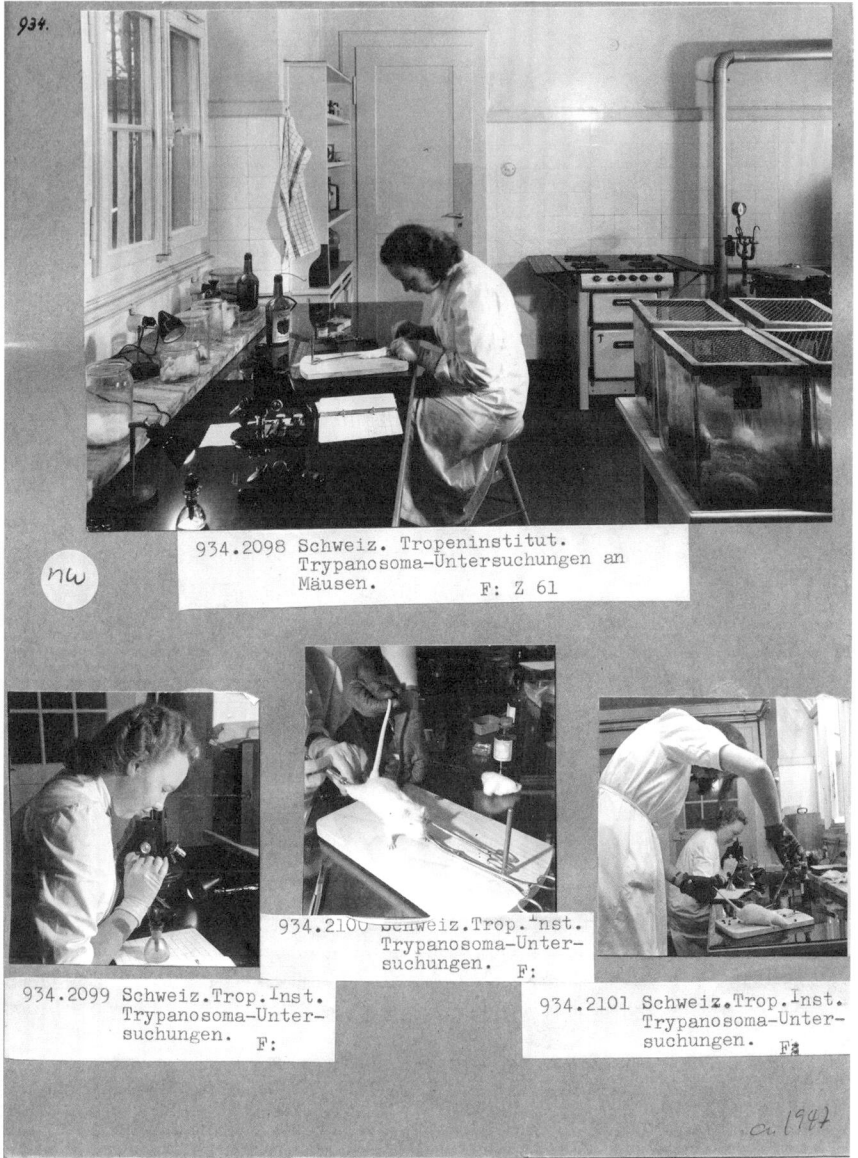

Sleeping sickness research at the STI, 1947, Archive STI

in the Department of Zoology, which from 1933 was led by Adolf Portmann. The two scientists' approaches to zoology were rather different.
Portmann, whose academic career was supported by Geigy's father, had a
flair for the philosophical: for him, nature manifested itself in a variety of
different forms (Gestalten), which provided certain insights into relationships and the development of species.[37] But natural phenomena could not
be entirely deciphered, however sophisticated one's methods might be.
There always remained an inexplicable residue, a hidden secret that nature
was unwilling to disclose.[38] Rudolf Geigy, in contrast, was more of an ex-
perimentalist. He worked in the tradition of Wilhelm Roux, who once pro-
claimed the scientific experiment as the key to scientific research. Only
with the aid of experimentation, Roux believed, could nature provide answers for the investigative mind.[39] During his time as an assistant, Geigy
occupied a small research laboratory in the Natural History Museum at
Stapfelberg, which owed its existence to the Basler Stiftung für experi-
mentelle Zoologie, a foundation initiated and financed by his father.[40] In
1935, Geigy took on a lectureship in experimental embryology and genetics. Three years later, he was awarded a full professorship. Research conditions improved considerably with the creation of the STI in 1943. Under
Geigy, zoological research was carried out at various sites: experiments
were conducted in the basement of the STI, morphology belonged to the
sphere of the Department of Zoology, systematized knowledge was the
province of the Natural History Museum, and applied zoology was the responsibility of the chemical industry.[41] True to his name, Geigy forged

37 Christian Simon, *Natur-Geschichte. Das Naturhistorische Museum Basel im 19. und
    20. Jahrhundert*, Basel 2009, p. 57.
38 Markus Ritter, *Die Biologie Adolf Portmanns im zeitgenössischen Kontext*, in: Basler
    Zeitung für Geschichte und Altertumskunde, Vol. 100, 2000, pp. 207–254; Joachim
    Illies, *Das Geheimnis des Lebendigen. Leben und Werk des Biologen Adolf Portmann*,
    Munich 1976.
39 Wilhelm Roux, *Die Entwicklungsmechanik der Organismen. Eine anatomische Wis-
    senschaft der Zukunft*, Vienna 1890, p. 9; see also: R. Weber, *The Beginnings of Devel-
    opmental Biology in Swiss Universities*, in: International Journal of Developmental Bi-
    ology, Vol. 46, 2002, pp. 15–22.
40 StABS, PA 1095, (A), Rudolf Geigy, Biographisches, -1995, anonym, Basler Stiftung
    für experimentelle Zoologie. Bericht aus dem Jahr 1942, p. 1.
41 Simon, *Naturwissenschaft in Basel im 19. und 20. Jahrhundert. Die Philoso-
    phisch-Naturwissenschaftliche Fakultät der Universität*, published online 2010, www.
    unigeschichte.unibas.ch/cms/upload/FaecherUndFakultaeten/Downloads/CSimon_
    NaturwissenschaftenBasel.pdf (accessed 16 February 2012).

close links with the biological laboratory of J. R. Geigy AG, which was established in 1937 to carry out research in the field of pest control.[42]

The above may have somewhat overemphasized Geigy's affection for scientific experiments. In his intellectual universe, the manipulation of nature went hand in hand with humble amazement at nature's diversity (and, one might add, concern for its protection). What he shared with Portmann was the inclination to urge his students out of the lecture halls and to acquaint them with the natural environment. The lesson to be learned was that the laboratory and the field were inextricably intertwined.[43] After 1943, pathogens and vectors of tropical diseases became Geigy's main objects of investigation.[44] He creatively combined the study of microorganisms with that of their pathogenic effects in humans, thus pioneering the field of medical zoology in Switzerland.[45] Whether Geigy conceived medicine as an applied branch of zoology is an open question.[46] What is more certain is that he sought to study tropical diseases within a wider ecological and social disease environment. Consequently, in combining an interest in the natural sciences with a fascination for ethnography, he was intellectually still deeply rooted in the nineteenth century, and probably closer to the research of the Sarasin cousins than to the field of developmental biology.[47]

Ethnography

After 1945, ethnography also contributed substantially to the field of tropical science. As has been briefly noted, collecting ethnographic material was common practice in Basel's civic culture. Private ethnographic collections had a highly symbolic value, indicating their owners' worldly wisdom. Anthropological efforts were largely born out of a conservationist spirit: modernity was no longer the privilege of the West but anchored in the harbors of Africa and Asia. Owing to increased contacts between "civ-

---

42 Janner, *Rudolf Geigy (-Heese)-Hunziker*, p. 2.
43 Geigy, *Erforschung der Natur im Feld und Laboratorium*, in: Verhandlungen der Schweizerischen Naturforschenden Gesellschaft (wissenschaftlicher Teil), 150. Jahresversammlung in Basel, 1970, pp. 9–20.
44 See his volume published together with Adelheid Herbig, *"Erreger und Überträger tropischer Krankheiten"*, Basel 1955.
45 Geigy's chair was renamed Medical Zoology in 1965.
46 Janner, *Rudolf Geigy (-Heese)-Hunziker*, p. 3.
47 Simon, *Natur-Geschichte*, p. 69.

ilized" and "uncivilized" cultures, the latter were increasingly endangered. The ethnographic collection of photographs still kept at the STI today is labeled "L'Afrique qui disparaît" (Disappearing Africa), and Fritz Sarasin's book on Melanesia was offered as a memorial to "one of the many populations of the Pacific Ocean steadily dwindling in the encounter with European culture".[48]

Geigy shared a strong fascination for ethnographic displays with many of his peers. In his early research as Director of the STI, the natural sciences and ethnography converged. Geigy minored in ethnography at university and closely followed the expeditions of the Sarasins, devouring their publications. In a letter to Fritz Sarasin, he wrote:

Dear friend

It was a special pleasure to receive the wonderful gift [i.e., the publication describing the results of the Sarasins' research expedition to Ceylon] you kindly gave me … You have long known how interested I am in your research and the stunning insights gained from your expeditions to foreign countries. You are also aware how much I am taken with ethnography, which prompted me to start touring the world myself. You cannot imagine the joy I felt while following your tracks in Colombo, hearing Swiss and German expatriates still talking about your stay there and recognizing the general interest in your work on this magnificent island and its inhabitants of older and recent times.[49]

Ethnographic knowledge circulated within Basel's high society; it was shared in the form of gifts and was very much part of people's mental luggage while visiting exotic places. Touring the world, it was natural that the zoologist Geigy should follow in the famous anthropologist's footsteps. In 1960, Geigy succeeded entomologist Eduard Handschin as a member of the Commission of the Museum für Völkerkunde (ethnographic museum).[50] This museum, like the Zoological Gardens, benefited from his generosity in financing the acquisition of ethnographic collections that would otherwise have been unattainable. His policy of patronage revealed an attempt to shift the ethnographic focus away from South-East Asia and Oceania towards Africa. From the 1950s onwards, his zoological students –

48   StABS, PA 212a, T2, Sarasinisches Familienarchiv, XLIV 92, Fritz Sarasin, Aus einem glücklichen Leben. Biographische Notizen von Fritz Sarasin, 1941.
49   StABS, PA 212a, T2, 28–28a, Rudolf Geigy, 1936, Rudolf Geigy to Fritz Sarasin, 27 September 1939, p. 1.
50   StABS, ED-REG 42a, 2–2-6 (10), Rudolf Geigy, 1960–1972, Ernst Staehelin to Rudolf Geigy, 4 February 1960, p. 1.

mainly working in Côte d'Ivoire and Tanzania – constantly purchased ethnographic objects and assured a steady flow of these items from Africa to the ethnographic museum in Basel.[51]

Agronomy and Technological Fixes

Featuring prominently in the wider array of tropical science institutions, discourses and practices was the Tropical School, also established in 1943. More than any other newly established institutions at that time, the school eased pressures on the labor market and put Geigy's zeal for applied science into practice. Organizationally independent of the STI – though closely monitored – it offered specialist courses for younger people with no previous professional qualifications who were interested in self-fulfillment and ready to set up their own business abroad.[52] As a general preparation for living abroad, the curriculum started with a two-year introduction to the tropical world. Students could subsequently enroll on a "sugar course", a "planter's course" or a "trading course".[53] Training at the Tropical School was geared towards ambitious aims. When they graduated, students were supposed to be able to manage a tropical plantation or sugar factory or to earn a decent living in the offices of a shipping company, a bank or private industry.[54] Teachers did not restrict themselves to imparting knowledge about the tropics but boosted students' networking skills to enable them to find employment. Of the almost 100 students who graduated between 1944 and 1951, 40 entered labor markets overseas as plantation assistants. Africa got the largest share, witnessing the arrival of 23 Swiss planters. Within Africa, the trust territory of Tanganyika attracted the largest number of graduates, followed by Morocco, Libya, Kenya, the Gold Coast, Algeria and

51 Archiv Museum der Kulturen Basel (AMKB), Museumskommission, Protokolle 1960–1964, R. Wildhaber, Kommission des Museums für Völkerkunde und Schweizerischen Museums für Volkskunde, Basel, Protokoll der Sitzung vom 17. November 1961, pp. 1–2, here: p. 1.

52 Interview with the President of the Verein ehemaliger Schüler tropischer Landwirtschaft (VESTI), Peter Betsche, 13 October 2006.

53 Over the years, the curriculum was modified several times: for instance, the training period was shortened, the sugar and planter's course combined, and the trading course discontinued.

54 SWA, Institute 196, Tropenschule des Schweizerischen Tropeninstituts in Basel, p. 32; StABS, Universitätsarchiv I 71.1, Frederik A. Rohn, Zur Gründung einer Schweizerischen Tropenschule, p. 1.

South Africa.[55] Though they were not necessarily employed by Swiss companies, their appointments were considered a success, at least strengthening Switzerland's trade relations with the European colonial powers.

Consciously or not, by joining plantation companies, Swiss emigrants became part of the economic system of colonial domination of which the plantation today remains the very metaphor. Taking the example of Tanganyika, Chapter 1 attempted to show that World War II gave rise to a novel form of "welfare imperialism" and fanciful ideas about modernizing African agricultural systems and increasing food production. These aims were shared by some of the Swiss planters, who became fervent advocates of changing "backward African minds" to allow modernity to set in.[56] However, the transformations unleashed by World War II were driven not only by modernizing tendencies but by the wider application of technological fixes, successfully marketed since the interwar period. The one that came to epitomize the technocentric approach to public health and the environment during World War II and thereafter was a cryptically named product released by J. R. Geigy AG – dichlorodiphenyltrichloroethane (DDT).

Virtually no other development more clearly symbolizes the transformations of World War II and its consequences for the postwar agricultural and health sectors than the advent of DDT.[57] DDT was cheap and could be applied extensively. During the interwar period, pesticide research in Switzerland had already expanded considerably, with the extension of pest control from small viticulture to larger cultivated areas, and applied entomology was of growing importance in science and industry. On the eve of World War II, this research entered a new dimension when Paul Müller, working at J. R. Geigy AG, identified the insecticidal properties of DDT while searching for a chemical compound to kill moths in clothing. As it turned out, DDT had a decisive advantage over conventional products in that it remained effective against insect pests for up to three months after initial application – the decisive *dis*advantage vis-à-vis nature, as later became evident.[58] Three years after the discovery of DDT, J. R. Geigy AG

---

55 StABS, FD-REG 1d 37.2, Geigy, Bericht zu Handen des Vorstehers des EDI, 1951, pp. 15–16.

56 StABS, ED-REG 1c 190–2-5 (1), Schweizerische Tropenschule, 1943–1964, Bericht über das Schuljahr 1957/58, 22 October 1958, p. 7.

57 Sunil S. Amrith, *Decolonizing International Health. India and Southeast Asia, 1930–1965*, New York 2006.

58 Margaret Humphreys, *Kicking a Dying Dog. DDT and the Demise of Malaria in the American South, 1942–1950*, in: Isis, Vol. 87, No. 1, 1996, pp. 1–17, here: p. 11.

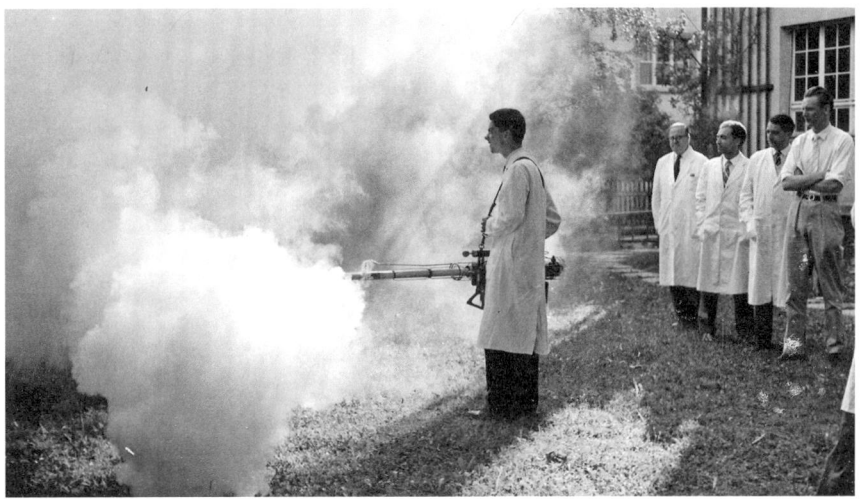

Deploying DDT in the STI garden, 1958, Archive STI

marketed the product under the trade names Gesarol and Neocid.[59] The "atomic bomb of the insect world" (as DDT has belligerently been called) became a decisive weapon in world warfare.[60] J. R. Geigy AG offered DDT both to the United States and to Nazi Germany. While mainly used as a crop protection agent in Germany, DDT was a crucial malaria-fighting tool in the Pacific Ocean theater for the United States.[61] Nor did the application of DDT subside in peacetime. After the war, it was widely embraced as a consumer product, continuing to leave its mark on insect pests in everyday domestic use.

When, in 1944, J. R. Geigy AG named Robert Wiesmann head of the Pest Control Division, the company's sales of this product line were at their peak. Wiesmann was one of the key figures in the discovery of the insecticidal properties of DDT and spurred the development of new chemical pest control agents.[62] At J. R. Geigy AG, Wiesmann supported the

59   Christian Simon, *DDT. Kulturgeschichte einer chemischen Verbindung*, Basel 1999, p. 173.
60   Humphreys, *Kicking a Dying Dog*, p. 12.
61   Lukas Straumann, *Nützliche Schädlinge. Angewandte Entomologie, chemische Industrie und Landwirtschaftspolitik in der Schweiz 1874–1952*, Zurich 2005, p. 206.
62   René Wyniger, *Dr. Dr. h.c. Robert Wiesmann*, in: Mitteilungen der Entomologischen Gesellschaft Basel, 22. Jahrgang 1972, pp. 69–70.

work of the young entomologist René Wyniger, who was about to move
from the Biological Laboratory to Wiesmann's research group in 1944.[63]
As a technical assistant, Wyniger laid the foundations for future research
by assembling large collections of insects. Both men collaborated closely
with Rudolf Geigy and the STI. As a vice-president of J. R. Geigy AG,
Wiesmann not only shaped the overall course of the company with Rudolf
Geigy, he also – with Wyniger – frequently taught applied entomology at
the STI and the Tropical School.[64] On several occasions, Wyniger in particular took his students out of the lecture theaters, trying to convince them
of the advantages of chemical pest control. In October 1959, the entomologist departed for East Africa to study large areas of cropland ravaged by
various pests. He was saddened to discover that, while many Western
plantation owners used chemical means to protect their crops, African
farmers were not yet sufficiently convinced to follow the Western model.[65]
In his view, instructing African farmers in applying chemicals and obtain-
ing higher yields was among the more important duties of Tropical School
graduates now working in Africa.[66] But DDT not only revolutionized the
world's agricultural sectors, it also became an important technological tool
in the rising field of postwar international health.

Tropical Medicine, DDT and Postwar International Health

Chapter 1 presented some of the dreams of a modern African society
dreamt by colonial officials such as Culwick. Seeking to control the spread
of trypanosomiasis, Culwick was an ardent advocate of the resettlement
schemes, from which more general socioeconomic development was to
derive. In this colonial logic, eradication of disease was never the only

---

63   Anon., *In Memoriam Dr. h.c. René Wyniger, 1921–2006*, in: Mitteilungen der Entomo-
     logischen Gesellschaft Basel, Vol. 56, No. 4, 2006, pp. 178–188, here: p. 179.
64   Schweizerisches Tropeninstitut in Basel, 1. Jahresbericht 1944, p. 7.
65   Wyniger, *Aus dem Tagebuch eines Entomologen*, in: Mitteilungsblatt der Tropenschule
     des Schweizerischen Tropeninstituts in Basel, No. 7, Basel 1959, p. 13.
66   Ibid., p. 16. It should be noted, however, that the widespread application of DDT also
     aroused criticism, in the context of Switzerland's notorious "cockchafer war" (Mai-
     käferkrieg), long before Rachel Carson's *Silent Spring* would arouse general indig-
     nation, rendering DDT a *materia non grata*. The first entomologist holding a chair in
     Zoology, Eduard Handschin, pointed out that the technology had detrimental effects
     on the environment: not so much the cockchafers, he claimed, but the new technology
     itself dangerously destabilized ecology's fragile balance.

goal. Instead, intervention in the fabric of society was a means to satisfy Western ideas of a modern society, more easily controllable by a bureaucratic apparatus. Despite the changes brought about by World War II, postwar international health showed many signs of continuity with the colonial past. Apart from the belief that interventions could easily be replicated in different settings, a military approach to such interventions and a woeful neglect of local knowledge, the postwar period was marked by a strong linkage between health and development. This linkage was nowhere more pronounced than in the case of malaria.[67] Stimulated by the success of efforts to eradicate smallpox and animated by a profound faith in Western technology, decision-makers based at international organizations in Geneva, Paris or New York believed that the eradication of malaria was feasible. This time, their prime targets were not Third World populations, but anopheles vectors. In 1947, the Rockefeller Health Foundation embarked on a large-scale malaria eradication campaign using DDT on the island of Sardinia.[68] While the ultimate aim of eradicating *Anopheles labranchiae* was not achieved, the intervention led to a reduction of malaria transmission and was therefore interpreted as a success story.[69] In 1955, the WHO – which had taken over responsibility for global antimalaria efforts from the Rockefeller Foundation – launched an ambitious malaria eradication campaign. Though the initiative achieved some successes, malaria morbidity and mortality returned almost to preintervention levels in many of the tropical territories where eradication was attempted.[70]

Even though J. R. Geigy AG had a large stake in DDT's global triumph, the STI's approach towards international health was not as technology-driven as one might expect. The STI had neither the logistical capacity nor the network that would have allowed for large-scale application of

---

67 Randall Packard, *Visions of Postwar Health and Development and Their Impact on Public Health Interventions in the Developing World*, in: Frederick Cooper and Randall M. Packard (eds.), International Development and the Social Sciences, pp. 93–115, here: p. 103.

68 Peter J. Brown, *Failure-As-Success. Multiple Meanings of Eradication in the Rockefeller Foundation Sardinia Project, 1946–1951*, in: Parassitologia, Vol. 40, No. 1–2, 1998, pp. 117–130; Brown, *Malaria, Miseria, and Underpopulation in Sardinia: the "Malaria Blocks Development" Cultural Model*, in: Medical Anthropology, Vol. 17, No. 3, 1997, pp. 239–254.

69 Ibid., p. 240.

70 Packard, *Malaria Dreams. Visions of Health and Development in the Third World*, in: Medical Anthropology, Vol. 17, 1997, pp. 279–296, here: p. 280; Packard, *The Making of a Tropical Disease. A Short History of Malaria*, Baltimore 2007, p. 159.

DDT in tropical countries. Instead, tropical medicine as it developed in Switzerland after the watershed of World War II had a clinical focus, driven by exaggerated anxieties about the possible re-emergence of tropical diseases in Switzerland.

While anthropological research sought to document cultures threatened by extinction abroad, tropical medicine strove to prevent tropical diseases from re-emerging at home. World War II was not just a catalyst for medical research and technology but nurtured people's feelings of living in an interconnected world.[71] In arguing for the establishment of the STI, Gigon had in mind Swiss people traveling to the tropics as well colonial officials and soldiers returning from hot climates. The problem with renewed mobility was that border-crossings were not the privilege of humans only: the introduction of pathogens could lead to outbreaks of tropical diseases in temperate climates if not carefully monitored. These anxieties – early signs of what Nicholas King would aptly call an "emerging disease worldview" – later proved not to be entirely unjustified.[72]

Italy was too close to Switzerland on the map not to share the burden of malaria with its neighbor. Italian parasitologist Bruno Galli-Valerio, Professor of Hygiene and Parasitology at the University of Lausanne, identified numerous regions throughout Switzerland which he assumed to have been breeding sites for *Anopheles maculipennis* and *Anopheles bifurcatus*.[73] During the nineteenth and the early twentieth century, malaria had been wiped out, which he attributed to an increase in animal husbandry and a shift in mosquitoes' preferences from humans to animals, as well as large-scale land improvement measures. Even during the late eighteenth century, major land improvement measures on the Linth Plain had been justified by pointing to the various health hazards arising from the numer-

71 Mark Lauterburg-Bonjour, *"Gedanken über das Studium der Tropenmedizin in der Schweiz"*, in: Schweizerische Ärztezeitung für Standesfragen, Vol. 28, No. 1, 1947, pp. 2–3.

72 Nicholas B. King, *Security, Disease, Commerce. Ideologies of Postcolonial Global Health*, in: Social Studies of Science, Vol. 32, No. 5–6, 2002, pp. 763–789; Laurie Garrett, *The Coming Plague. Newly Emerging Diseases in a World Out of Balance*, New York 1994.

73 He explicitly mentions the cantons of Geneva, Vaud, Valais and Neuchâtel, the region around Basel, the Rhine Valley, St. Gallen, the Linth Plain, Einsiedeln, the region around Thun, Interlaken, Brienz, around Alpnach and Flüelen, the Magadino Plain, and the Ticino and Maggia Valleys; see: Rudolf Geigy, *Malaria in der Schweiz*, in: Acta Tropica, Vol. 2, No. 1, 1945, pp. 1–16, here: p. 2.

ous swamps.[74] As historian Daniel Speich observed, the advocates of taming the Linth's waters claimed "civilization" to be on their side, while they portrayed the unruly swamps as symptoms of the moral decay of human society.[75] This binary rhetorical figure of "high moral standards = lack of disease" and vice versa is readily encountered during World War II, with one major difference: in this case, the moral decay/disease complex was threatening the Swiss population from beyond the nation's borders. Investigating the possibility of a re-emergence of malaria in Switzerland, STI employee Hans Gaschen (one of Galli-Valerio's students) declared:

> We have seen now the reasons for the retreat of malaria that formerly also existed in Switzerland and the surrounding countries. Could it reappear? Yes, and it is easy to prove. The authors agree unanimously that … the improvement of living conditions, in one word, general well-being, is the prime factor for malaria to disappear.[76]

Gaschen's reference to the improvement of living conditions as the determining factor for health and disease is important in the context of the overall history of malaria – largely dominated by vector control in the postwar years – as well as appealing to a contemporary audience: since the war reduced the general level of well-being, it created a space for the insidious return of malaria. This scenario was formulated against the backdrop of a specific historical incident. At the end of the war, a group of Italian and Yugoslav refugees entered Switzerland's neutral territory. They had deserted from their armies and had contracted malaria during their long odyssey.[77] As a precautionary measure, the Federal Commission for Internment and Hospitalization (EKIH) asked Rudolf Geigy and his staff to examine the infected refugees and to propose solutions for low-risk detention. In an improvised compound on the site of the Hilfsspital, the two malariologists André Perret-Gentil and Mark Lauterburg-Bonjour prescribed therapy

---

74 Daniel Speich, *Helvetische Meliorationen. Die Neuordnung der gesellschaftlichen Naturverhältnisse an der Linth (1783–1823)*, Zurich 2003, especially Part II, Chapter 2.
75 Ibid., p. 152.
76 Hans Gaschen, *Moustiques et paludisme dans le canton de Vaud à l'heure actuelle*, in: Bulletin de la Société Vaudoise des Sciences Naturelles, Vol. 62, No. 262, pp. 379–390, here: p. 389. The possibility of malaria re-emerging in Switzerland was already discussed in the years after World War I; see: Gustave Regamey, *Etudes relatives à la malaria. La distribution des Anophèles dans le Canton de Genève en relation avec les anciens foyers de malaria*, Thèse faculté des sciences, Lausanne 1927, pp. 5–6.
77 StABS, FD-REG 1d 37.2, Vorschlag des Geschäftsausschusses zur Weiterführung des Schweizerischen Tropeninstituts, 6 May 1946, p. 11.

consisting of cold baths as well as milk and quinine injections.[78] They were supported by the pharmaceutical companies Hoffmann-La Roche and Sandoz, who provided Vitaquin and Calgluquine tablets for efficacy tests.[79]

In the later postwar years, the STI promoted the professionalization of tropical medicine in Switzerland. By acquiring the Sonnenrain private clinic – rented out to the STI – the cantonal authorities created space for a tropical clinic capable of competing with other institutions in this field.[80] Soon after, the STI moved into the nearby Haus zur Föhre, which housed the institute's research laboratories, breeding spaces for insects, a lecture hall, a library and the administration.[81] However, it takes more than an institution to make a scientific discipline. It was felt that competitiveness in tropical medicine derives not just from high quality but equally from prestige – and in this respect, Swiss tropical physicians were somewhat deficient. Let us take the examples of the above-mentioned Lauterburg-Bonjour and Hermann Mooser. The physician Lauterburg-Bonjour was one of the early players in the field of tropical medicine. At Albert Schweitzer's famous hospital in Lambaréné (Gabon) in 1925, he gained first-hand experience of tropical health problems. Back in Switzerland, he shared his medical expertise with the nascent STI and within the Swiss Society of Tropical Medicine (founded in 1943), which he presided over from 1954 to 1966. Hermann Mooser's career was similar in some respects. Mooser studied medicine in Zurich and Lausanne. After graduating and working as an assistant at the University of Basel, he moved to Mexico in 1924, where he became head of the chemical-medical and the serological-bacteriological laboratory of the American Hospital.[82] His publications on Mexican typhus fever were widely discussed. He proposed the existence of a Mexican form of typhus (murine typhus, whose causal agent would later be called *Rickettisa mooseri*), which differed from European typhus in being transmitted by rat fleas rather than by body lice. Dismissing the possibility of humans serving as a reservoir for the disease, Mooser assumed that classi-

78   André Perret-Gentil, *L'observation des réfugiés malariens dans la section clinique et le laboratoire de l'Institut Tropical Suisse*, in: Acta Tropica, Vol. 2, No. 1, 1945, pp. 97–121, here: p. 104.
79   Ibid., p. 118.
80   SWA, Institute 196, Ratschlag 4246, p. 45.
81   Schweizerisches Tropeninstitut in Basel, 4. Jahresbericht 1947, p. 2.
82   Ernst Wiesmann, *Hermann Mooser 1891–1971*, in: Verhandlungen der Schweizerischen Naturforschenden Gesellschaft (wissenschaftlicher Teil), 152. Jahresversammlung in Luzern, 1972, pp. 322–324, here: p. 322.

cal (epidemic) typhus was also of murine origin.[83] In 1936, Mooser be-came Professor of Hygiene and Bacteriology at the University of Zurich. After the creation of the STI, he collaborated closely with Rudolf Geigy. In 1954, he would accompany him on an expedition to Tanganyika to in-vestigate the epidemiology of African relapsing fever.

Both of these physicians might have contributed substantially to the field of tropical medicine in Switzerland or elsewhere. What they lacked, however, was the reputation of the type of "tropical doctor" that had emerged in colonial France or Britain. Geigy believed that, if the STI wished to expand its efforts in the field of tropical medicine, then the trop-ical clinic would have to be led by a renowned personality who was deeply rooted within an administrative colonial African network. In Mé-decin-Général Adolphe Sicé, he might have found what he was looking for. Born in Martinique in 1885, Sicé graduated from the Ecole de santé navale in Bordeaux in 1910. During World War I, he served as a military physician in Morocco. The interwar period saw Sicé working in several different parts of Africa – including Haute-Sanga (Central African Repub-lic), Gabon and Madagascar – where he found rich material for the study of tropical diseases. In 1927, Sicé became director of the Institut Pasteur in Brazzaville, where he experimented with new methods of containing the spread of human trypanosomiasis – a tropical scourge which also aroused Geigy's interest. Sicé argued that the presence of the disease could only be confirmed by examination of cerebrospinal fluid obtained by lumbar punc-ture. In Brazzaville in the early twentieth century, this (painful) diagnostic procedure was so widespread that the verb "to lumbar-puncture" entered the vocabulary of the local population.[84] Sicé himself conducted over 10,000 of these procedures.[85]

Geigy managed to persuade Sicé to accept a chair as the first full pro-fessor of tropical medicine at the University of Basel. This appointment was welcomed by the medical faculty in Basel and did not go unnoticed by the Swiss expatriate community in French overseas territories: in particu-lar, commercial circles expected to see an improvement in Swiss-French

83   Hermann Mooser, *Die Beziehungen des murinen Fleckfiebers zum klassischen Fleck-fieber*, in: Acta Tropica (Supplementum 4), Basel 1945.
84   Hunt, *A Colonial Lexicon*, p. 93; for a detailed account of the various colonial prac-tices designed to contain sleeping sickness, see: Lyons, *The Colonial Disease*.
85   StABS, Universitätsarchiv X 3.5 158, Adolphe Sicé, 1946–1957, Alfred Gigon, Bericht über die Persönlichkeit und die wissenschaftliche Tätigkeit des Médecin Général Sicé, 3 January 1946, pp. 1–5, here: p. 1.

relations and more favorable sales figures. Jules Wanner, head of a fami-ly-owned Swiss import-export business in Douala (Cameroon), enthusias-tically wrote to Basel:

> Generally there was not just deep satisfaction about Sicé being welcomed at the STI. There is also an expectation of wider French recognition of Swiss emigrants living in Africa and therefore an improvement in business opportunities. General Sicé is much esteemed in government circles in Africa and, as I witnessed several times, the honors bestowed by Switzerland and especially Basel were very well re-ceived.[86]

However, even with a man of such dazzling colonial credentials as Sicé, tropical medicine in Switzerland waned before it really had a chance to take off. Sicé accepted the post of university professor but refused that of director of the tropical clinic, owing to obscure personal differences with Geigy. However, the tropical clinic's problems had less to do with whether or not it had an experienced practitioner as its head than with the structural problems of tropical medicine in the immediate postwar years. While the total number of patients treated rose from 184 to 246 between 1945 and 1947, it fell to 60 in 1950.[87] In 1957, the STI decided to abandon the Son-nenrain clinic and to integrate medical services (vaccination, consulta-tions, examinations) into the STI itself.[88]

   In summary, one could argue that, during and after World War II, trop-ical science in Switzerland was not yet an established scientific field but consisted of a heterogeneous body of scientific branches and scholarly tra-ditions. Tropical science was dominated by Rudolf Geigy, who juggled various subdisciplines and open the field up to economic influences. One major reason for this heterogeneity could be the absence of a Swiss colo-nial history. In contrast to European colonial powers, which spawned a growing body of colonial science, there was no such development in Swit-zerland. Though informed by the insights of the germ theory, there was neither an intellectual superstructure nor a set of agreed methodologies to control such a discipline. Tropical science in Switzerland was a field or a set of practices geared towards application. It centered on experimentation (medical parasitology), collections (ethnography), pest control (agronomy)

---

86 StABS, ED-REG 1a 1 1266, Sicé, Prof. Dr. Adolphe, – 1964, Jules Wanner to Adolf
    Im Hof, 18 February 1947, pp. 1–3, here: p. 1.
87 See the statistics in the annual reports, 1945–1950.
88 StABS, FD-REG 1d 37.2, Protokoll der Kuratoriumssitzung vom 20.03.1959, p. 3.

and clinical practice (tropical medicine). What tropical science in Switzerland shared with its French, British and Portuguese cousins was that it tended to leave the narrow confines of the nation, extending its sphere of action to the tropics.

Science on the Move

From early on, the STI operated within an imperial network. Geigy skillfully forged links with other tropical institutes working in the vast European empires or added secular elements to the gospel spread by the Basel Mission. However, the mission's various African outposts were unsuitable as a permanent base for the STI. Though part of the overall civilizing mission, scientific reason was not easily reconciled with evangelism. As one of the missionaries noted:

> The Basel Mission understands that in sending physicians and researchers to the tropics, the STI likes to use the mission's outposts. However, it cannot be disregarded that while the mission shares the institute's humanitarian aspirations, it has reservations about its economic zeal. Therefore, the missionary society has to distance itself from the institute's activities to some degree.[89]

Rather than being wholly dependent on the goodwill of the missionaries, Geigy and the STI were keen to establish contacts with scientific institutions working in Africa. In 1945, Geigy, his wife Nina, Hans Gaschen and the pathologist Frédéric Roulet boarded a US military aircraft, crossed the Mediterranean and headed for French Equatorial Africa. Their expedition was inspired by philanthropy as much as by colonial thinking – two phenomena best conceived as two sides of the same coin rather than as mutually exclusive.[90] The aim of the journey was to introduce the new institute to the colonial scientific authorities and, at the same time, to explore the possibility of having parasite-infected European colonialists hospitalized in Basel.[91] On a symbolic level, the expedition resembled previous scien-

---

89 StABS, Universitätsarchiv I 71.1, Protokoll des Initiativkomitees vom 12.11.1943, pp. 6–7.

90 Albert Wirz, *Die humanitäre Schweiz im Spannungsfeld zwischen Philanthropie und Kolonialismus. Gustave Moynier, Afrika und das IKRK*, in: Traverse, No. 2, 1998, pp. 95–110, here: p. 96.

91 Geigy, *L'expédition scientifique de l'Institut Tropical Suisse en Afrique Equatoriale*, in: La Revue Coloniale Belge, Vol. 6, 1946, pp. 10–12, here: p. 10.

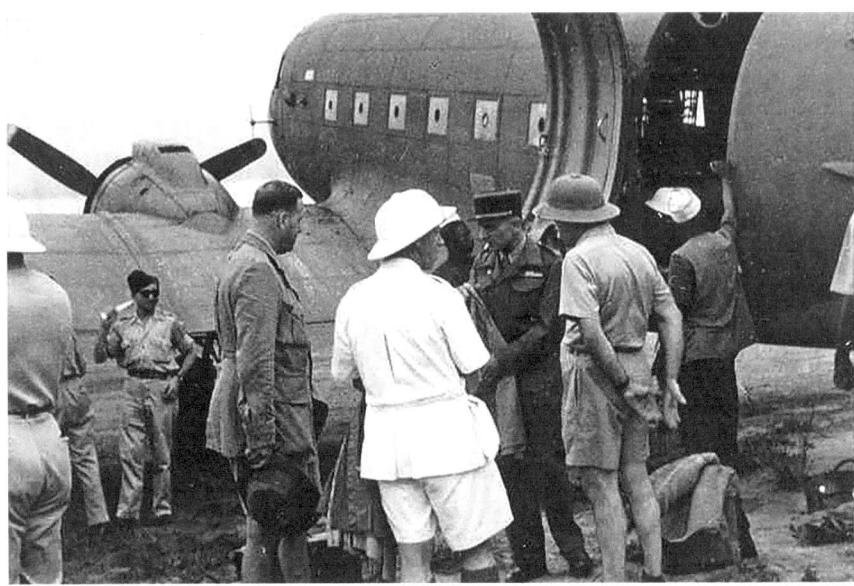

Boarding the plane for French Equatorial Africa, 1945, Archive STI

tific efforts to explore the African continent. In Dakar, the first stopover, the scientists lodged in the European quarter. In Accra, the capital of what is now Ghana, Geigy and his companions celebrated the Swiss national day with one of Africa's largest Swiss expatriate communities. Later, William Preiswerk-Tissot, the founder of the Union Trading Company (UTC) and a member of the STI's Board of Trustees, would familiarize them with the customs of the country and the activities of the UTC.[92]

The expedition reached its first scientific high point in Léopoldville – a burgeoning city, the economic center of the Belgian Congo, which turned out to be a veritable scientific El Dorado. Officially welcomed by Governor-General Pierre Ryckmans, Geigy and his entourage used a laboratory at the Institut Reine Astrid as a base for their daily search for scientific

92 StABS, PD-REG 1a, 1969–471 (Schweizerisches Tropeninstitut), 1945–1958, Geigy, Bericht über die wissenschaftliche Expedition des Schweizerischen Tropeninstituts nach Äquatorial-Afrika, p. 3; for the history of Switzerland's involvement in Ghana's health sector, see: Pascal Schmid, *Medicine, Faith, and Politics in Agogo. A History of Health Care Delivery in Rural Ghana, 1925–1980*, PhD University of Basel, 2013.

specimens. Frédéric Roulet visited the "natives' hospital" in order to "see interesting cases of tropical and other diseases and to conduct autopsies".[93] Geigy and Gaschen, for their part, toured the city's "native quarters" in order to "collect parasites and germs that transmit tropical diseases".[94]

Just a river cruise away from Léopoldville was Brazzaville, the capital of French Equatorial Africa. Here, the party's experiences were remarkably similar to those in Léopoldville – the hospitality of colonial governors, official receptions, the amassing of scientific material rather than extensive medical research. Among the items collected, a number of tsetse flies (*Glossina palpalis*) proved to be the most valuable. Surviving the passage to Basel, they surprisingly continued to reproduce in the basement of the STI, providing the scientific raw material for the institute's research on trypanosomiasis.[95] After a detour to Schweitzer's hospital in Lambaréné, Geigy and his colleagues returned to Basel, satisfied with what they had experienced. However, memories of the journey made the issue of their own field laboratory even more pressing than before.

Colonial Ties

In 1947, there was a clear wish to transcend the expeditionary nature of Swiss tropical research in Africa. Aware of French plans for a research station in Adiopodoumé, Rudolf Geigy, Jean-Georges Baer (Professor of Zoology at Neuchâtel University) and Claude Favarger (a botanist at the same university) went to Paris to conduct negotiations about the creation of a Swiss research laboratory within the large ORSC compound.[96] The Swiss scientists' resolve was strengthened by the close bonds existing between the two scientific communities. Jean-Georges Baer maintained a close friendship and a fruitful working relationship with Charles Joyeux, whose laboratory in Paris he had joined in 1927 for two years.[97] In 1952,

---

93 Geigy, *L'expédition scientifique*, p. 10.
94 Ibid.
95 Geigy, *Elevage de Glossina palpalis*, in: Acta Tropica, Vol. 5, No. 1, 1948, pp. 201–218.
96 Archives Nationales Fontainebleau, Paris (ANF), Archives de l'ORSTOM, 19900236, Art. 53, Raoul Combes, Note sur l'installation en Côte d'Ivoire d'un Centre Suisse de Recherche Tropicale. Lettre de M. le Professeur Grassé à M. le Président du Conseil, 6 November 1950, pp. 1–6, here: p. 3.
97 Jean-Georges Baer, *"Charles Joyeux" (1881–1966)*, in: Bulletin de la Société Neuchâteloise des Sciences Naturelles, Vol. 90, 1967, pp. 293–296, here: p. 294.

Baer dedicated his *Ecology of Animal Parasites* to his friend – later a professor at the University of Marseilles – acknowledging a steady flow of ideas which resulted in more than 200 joint publications.[98] Joyeux, in turn, co-authored with Adolphe Sicé his *Précis de médecine des pays chauds,* which was published in 1937 and soon became a classic in the genre of tropical medicine. More important, however, for the creation of a Swiss laboratory were the contacts between the botanists Claude Favarger and George Mangenot. After the war, Favarger studied at Sorbonne University under Mangenot and Alexandre Guilliermond, soaking up the "précieuse tradition française".[99] In 1949, he accepted Mangenot's invitation to join the French scientific community in Adiopodoumé, where he worked on the taxonomy of Melastomaceae in West Africa.[100] This invitation to the tropics was of great value for the Swiss botanist, who was seeking to defend taxonomy against other scientific disciplines such as chemistry and physiology. In his inaugural lecture at the University of Neuchâtel, he expressed his conviction that "the study of classification, i.e., attributing a place to each group in a fixed hierarchical framework, is of huge philosophical value and constitutes a useful effort of reasoning".[101]

Thus, in the aftermath of World War II, scientists from French-speaking Switzerland and their French counterparts established new contacts or revived earlier ones disrupted by the war. These interactions were facilitated by the scientists' common language. Perhaps even more advantageous was the fact that both professional groups belonged to the same "epistemic culture" of creating and justifying scientific knowledge.[102] They shared a common strategy to experience the natural world and to arrange nature's phenomena within a "hierarchical framework", to use Favarger's expression. But however important these scientific ties may have been,

98 Baer, *Ecology of Animal Parasites*, Urbana 1952.
99 Georges Dubois, *Naturalistes Neuchâteloises du XXe siècle (Cahiers de l'Institut Neuchâtelois)*, Neuchâtel 1976, p. 21.
100 Claude Favarger, *Recherches taxonomiques sur les Mélastomacées d'Afrique Occidentale*, in: Lyeuria, Vol. 10, 1952, pp. 53–56.
101 Favarger, *Systématique et morphologie dans la botanique moderne. Leçon inaugurale prononcée le 30 avril 1947 à son installation comme Professeur ordinaire à la chaire de botanique*, in: Bulletin de la Société Neuchâteloise des Sciences Naturelles, Vol. 70, 1947, pp. 21–32, here: p. 28.
102 Karin Knorr Cetina, *Epistemic Cultures. How the Sciences Make Knowledge*, Cambridge, London 1999, p. 1.

Switzerland also maintained direct links with Côte d'Ivoire through what historian Pierre Kipré aptly called the "petit monde des Blancs".[103]

Swiss Pioneers in Côte d'Ivoire

In a letter written in March 1952, Urs Rahm, the first director of the CSRS, confessed that he was puzzled by the large numbers of Swiss citizens living in Côte d'Ivoire.[104] This can be explained by the close-knit social network within which he and all subsequent Swiss researchers operated, for – compared to countries such as Egypt or the Gold Coast – Côte d'Ivoire never attracted large numbers of Swiss emigrants.[105] Even though Swiss emigration to Africa peaked in the aftermath of World War II, the compatriots Rahm encountered – who proved to be crucial in their support for the CSRS – belonged to the generation that left the country after World War I, escaping economic recession at home. Most of them found employment in French trading companies, such as the Société Commerciale de l'Ouest Africain (SCOA) or the Compagnie Française de l'Afrique Occidentale (CFAO), monopolizing the colony's foreign trade. Others were engaged in improving the colony's infrastructure.[106] Jules Vallon, for example, left his home in Payerne (Canton Vaud) and rose to the higher echelons of the SCOA. Victor Balet emigrated from Canton Valais in 1923, where he had been working in the timber industry for more than 13 years, and became one of the most important wood exporters in Côte d'Ivoire. Henri Vitoux, for his part, suffered the fate of the latecomer: arriving in 1934, he was engaged in public works until his business came to a standstill during World War II. After the war, he became a trustee and devoted much of his time to

103 Pierre Kipré, *Mémorial de la Côte d'Ivoire. La Côte d'Ivoire Coloniale*, Abidjan 1988, p. 230.
104 Fonds Urs Rahm (FUR), Correspondance Côte d'Ivoire 1951–1953, 13 March 1952, pp. 1–3, here: p. 1.
105 René Lenzin, *Schweizer im kolonialen und postkolonialen Afrika. Statistische Übersicht und zwei Fallbeispiele*, in: Studien und Quellen, Vol. 28, Die Auslandschweizer im 20. Jahrhundert – Les Suisses de l'étranger au XXème siècle, Bern, Stuttgart, Vienna 2002, pp. 299–326, here: pp. 302–303.
106 Catherine Coquery-Vidrovitch, *L'impact des intérêts coloniaux. SCOA et CFAO dans l'Ouest Africain, 1910–1965*, in: Journal of African History, Vol. 16, No. 4, pp. 595–621.

writing poems "admiringly evoking the heavy and hot atmosphere of the tropical countries where the tom-tom sounds".[107]

Of all the members of the Swiss community in Côte d'Ivoire, Gustave Meyer and Eugen Wimmer left the deepest historical imprints. In his auto-biography *Un demi-siècle en terre ivoirienne*, Meyer described the many obstacles facing those who accepted the burden of preparing the ground for the country's economic take-off. He tried to convince his readers that the life of a "pioneer" in the tropics was not necessarily crowned with eco-nomic success but marked by loss and privations. Looking back on his first period in the trading sector, he complains:

> Arriving in Côte d'Ivoire, my salary was 250 francs per month, which was not more than my sister earned as a household help for a physician in Berne. During my three years of loyal service, I touched the 425 franc threshold plus a small gra-tuity. By abstaining from everything, I was able to save the 10,000 francs that my brother had lent me but which I had lost in a financial affair before leaving Swit-zerland.[108]

Trying to raise his professional status, Meyer sought new employment: in 1927 he settled in Adzopé, where he cleared large areas of dense forest to set up a plantation business, which he had to start from scratch again when plant disease caused substantial crop failure. Looking back on his life in the colony, Meyer concluded: "I have not become a rich man. I had just enough to live a decent life because the work of a pioneer has never yielded much wealth. It is always those who come later who have the chance to get rich."[109]

While Meyer can be classified as belonging to what Harald Fischer-Tiné calls the "white subalternity", the same cannot be said of Eugen Wimmer.[110] After completing his engineering studies at the Swiss Federal Institute of Technology in Zurich in 1918, Wimmer moved to Paris, where he worked for René Dumoulin as an assistant engineer. In 1925, fascinated by the prospect of imbuing "backward" African colonies with the spirit of modernization, he moved to Abidjan, where he became director of the Cie. Africaine d'Entreprises (CAE). Six years later, he founded the Union

107 P. Laraisse, *La colonie Suisse en Côte d'Ivoire*, in: Echo. Zeitschrift der Schweizer im Ausland, Vol. 12, No. 33, 1953, pp. 28–29, here: p. 29.
108 Gustave Meyer, *Un demi-siècle en terre ivoirienne*, Paris 1975, p. 70.
109 Ibid., p. 305.
110 Harald Fischer-Tiné, *Low and Licentious Europeans. Race, Class and "White Subal-ternity" in Colonial India*, New Delhi 2009.

d'Entreprises Coloniales (UDEC). Wimmer was responsible for some of the major public work projects in the colony. The logic of the colonial economy – based on the extraction of products for metropolitan consumption – required reliable means of transportation between agricultural production sites and the ports.[111] On behalf of the French Colonies Ministry, UDEC constructed a railway line connecting Abidjan's emerging port to the granite quarries of Aké Béfiat, some 60 miles north of the bustling town.[112] The development of urban infrastructure became even more pressing with the decision to move the capital from Bingerville to Abidjan in 1934. Between 1930 and 1960, UDEC constructed several financial institutions, cinemas, hotels, factories, apartments, embassies and bridges – silent symbols of the colony's increasing economic and political importance for the Western powers.[113] Wimmer and – to a lesser degree all the members of the Swiss community –personified the various economic and political interests in the French territory. The boundaries between the political and economic spheres were porous, and successful businessmen were likely to be encountered on the political stage, too. In the year the UDEC was founded, Wimmer accepted a request to act as a representative in Côte d'Ivoire on behalf of the Swiss consulate in Dakar.[114] Switzerland did not maintain an embassy prior to Ivorian independence in 1960. All political issues concerning French West Africa (AOF) were dealt with by the consulate in Dakar. After World War II, Switzerland established a consular agency in Abidjan. In 1952, this was transformed into a vice-consulate, and Wimmer was awarded the title of honorary vice-consul.[115] In this ca-

111 Between 1924 and 1928, maritime traffic increased from 158,489 to 222,578 t, see: Zan Semi-Bi, *La politique coloniale des travaux publics en Côte d'Ivoire 1900–1940*, in: Annales de l'Université d'Abidjan, Vol. 1, No. 2, 1973–1974.

112 ETH Zürich (ed.), *Schweizer bauen und planen im Ausland – Les Suisses construisent à l'étranger. Ausstellung an der ETH-Hönggerberg Zürich – Exposition organisée par l'école polytechnique de Zurich*, Zurich 1978, p. 8.

113 Particularly famous was his first armored concrete bridge over the River Sassandra; see: Archiv Schweizerische Akademie der Naturwissenschaften, Depot Burgerbibliothek Bern (SCNAT), GA SANW 350, Zentralvorstand Lausanne, Korrespondenz 1953–1958, Notices biographiques sur G. Mangenot et E. Wimmer, pp. 1–2, here: p. 1.

114 Schweizerisches Bundesarchiv Bern (BAR), E 2200.5 (-), 1969/217, 4, Agence Consulaire de Suisse à Abidjan, Chef des Konsulardienstes (EDA) to Eugen Wimmer, 9 September 1931. In this role, he had (a) to report about job opportunities and general political and economic developments, (b) to organize the distribution of official documents from political institutions and (c) to help in the process of issuing Swiss passports.

115 BAR, E 2200.5 (-), 1969/217, 2, Correspondances officielles, 1952, EPD to Eugen Wimmer, 20 February 1952.

pacity, he was supposed to promote solidarity among the members of the Swiss community, as well as dealing with economic relations between his sphere of influence and Switzerland.[116] Not surprisingly for a person who maintained professional relations with business circles and ties with all levels of the French colonial administration, Wimmer was the driving force in providing the Swiss scientific community with a laboratory in the tropics. With this scientific initiative, Switzerland was likely to become a rival in the second scramble for Africa.

Colonial Rivalries

The Swiss zoologists who gathered at the STI in 1950 unanimously decided to accept the French invitation to establish a scientific laboratory in Adiopodoumé. Rudolf Geigy, who would support the center with money and a steady supply of young scientists, was however convinced that the CSRS could not be an STI-owned lab. Even though Wimmer's project was tailored to the needs of the STI, Geigy argued that his institute could not focus on one specific location in the tropics but must pursue scientific research in various regions.[117] The argument of the need for geographical flexibility is not overly convincing because three years after the creation of the CSRS, the STI established its own field laboratory in Ifakara.

The French response to the Swiss scientists' Paris mission of 1947 is a good indicator of science's symbolic status in sustaining the French empire after the war. Switzerland's move towards the colony did not meet with unmixed enthusiasm and was occasionally considered a threat to France's regained colonial vigor. One of the most authoritative figures to express concerns was Pierre-Paul Grassé, a giant in the world of French zoology. As mentioned in Chapter 1, Grassé was part of the French mission investigating the suitability of Adiopodoumé as a center for French scientific activities in 1945. His interest in the tropics was not entirely altruistic, however, since Adiopodoumé was under consideration as a new

---

116 Ibid.
117 BAR, E 2200.5 (-), 1979/93, 10, 0.2.23, Centre technique Suisse de Recherche Scientifique en Côte d'Ivoire, 1961–1965, Procès verbal de la séance du 7 mai 1950 convoquée à l'Institut Tropical à Bâle par les initiateurs du projet d'un Centre Suisse de Recherches en Côte d'Ivoire sous la présidence de Monsieur Jean G. Baer, Recteur de l'Université de Neuchâtel, 7 May 1950, p. 2.

site for his biology laboratory, which had been destroyed in the war. In a letter to the scientific committee of the ORSC, he wrote:

> the Swiss laboratory has undeclared aims that have nothing to do with science: medical trials for Swiss industry, trials with insecticides, impregnation of wood ... I can give you the proof. Without any colonial territory, Switzerland needs testing grounds for its industry. It believes it has found them in Adiopodoumé.[118]

Grassé raised one of the thorny issues that would continue to be the subject of permanent discussion between the two parties: what constitutes ideologically justifiable scientific practices in the colonies? While French scientific discourse heralded science's emancipatory role in the moral and material uplift of African people, Grassé suspected Switzerland of using the continent as a testing ground for the benefit of its domestic pharmaceutical industry. This subject will be discussed in more detail below. It suffices here to say that his arguments were formally taken up by former minister Marc Rucart, who, in a letter to François Mitterand (Minister of Overseas France in the Pleven government), wrote that Switzerland's arrival in Côte d'Ivoire would be "humiliating to French science".[119] In the internal dispute about the consequences of Swiss science in the tropics, the positive view of ORSTOM prevailed. Its director, Combes, rebutted Grassé's misconceptions as follows:

> the Swiss laboratory, with a staff of three, is not replacing any French organization. Far from constituting a threat to national prestige, the presence of the Swiss lab is rather a direct tribute to a French achievement.[120]

ORSTOM even went a step further in transforming Adiopodoumé into an international scientific center by officially requesting Wimmer to attract Norwegian and Danish research groups to Côte d'Ivoire.[121] In the end, it was the Dutch who established a research outpost under ORSTOM's direct administrative control. Thus, the reinforcement of French science and the strengthening of international scientific collaboration were not mutually exclusive. Rather, the invitation to noncolonial Switzerland and the Scan-

---

118 ANF, 19900236, Art. 53, Pierre Grassé au président du conseil scientifique ORSC, 14 October 1950, pp. 1–3, here: p. 2.
119 Ibid., Marc Rucart to François Mitterand, 13 November 1950, pp. 1–2, here: p. 1.
120 ANF, Combes, Note sur l'Installation, p. 4.
121 BAR, E 2200.5 (-), 1969/217, 2, Eugen Wimmer to the Swiss Consulate in Denmark, 16 October 1954; ibid., Eugen Wimmer to the Swiss legation in Norway, 17 October 1954.

dinavian countries indicates France's intention to interpret colonial science in the light of humanitarianism and as a unifying force. It left the door ajar for Switzerland's entry into the colonial realm.

Ordering Science

On August 1, 1951, a small group of Swiss and French scientists and colonial administrators gathered at the CSRS to inaugurate the new laboratory complex silhouetted against the muddy Ebrié Lagoon. Everyone was in celebratory mood given the impressive achievements and the prospect of future scientific collaboration. Gone were the dissonances that overshadowed the Swiss move to the tropics, as if the harmony of the natural surroundings was contagious. A series of speakers perpetuated the myth of a long tradition of scientific partnership between the two countries and praised the "Franco-Swiss family" that Adiopodoumé would come to stand for.[122] The image of harmonious familial bonds was taken up in Combes's speech:

> Many times the international character of scientific research has been underscored. The conditions of this collaboration between the world's intellectual elite, and the nature and the frequency of the relations established, allow one to speak of a huge global scientific family.[123]

The image of the Swiss-French family was deliberately chosen, perhaps not so much because of the personal friendships and scientific exchanges Côte d'Ivoire would offer, but because of the paternalistic nature of these relations. The Swiss laboratory – another building constructed by Eugen Wimmer – was too small to alarm even the most hard-pressed French colonialists. It offered laboratory space for three scientists and was modestly equipped, so that the scientists in residence had to ship their scientific material from Switzerland to the Ivorian coast according to their specific research agenda.[124] An agreement signed between the two parties in 1951

122 Archive Musée d'Histoire Naturelle de Genève (AMHN), 360.B.4.4, Mission scientifique en Côte d'Ivoire 1953–1957, Une émouvante manifestation d'amitié Franco-Suisse s'est déroulée le premier août à Adiopodoumé (à l'Institut de la Recherches Scientifique).

123 SCNAT, GA SANW 826, Kommissionen CSRS, Varia I 1951–1970, Premier août 1951, Discours de Monsieur le Professeur Combes, pp. 1–3, here: p. 1.

124 Urs Rahm, *La Côte d'Ivoire. Centre de Recherches Tropicales. Possibilités pour la participation suisse à l'exploration de la Côte d'Ivoire*, in: Acta Tropica, Vol. 11, 1954, pp. 222–295, here: p. 224.

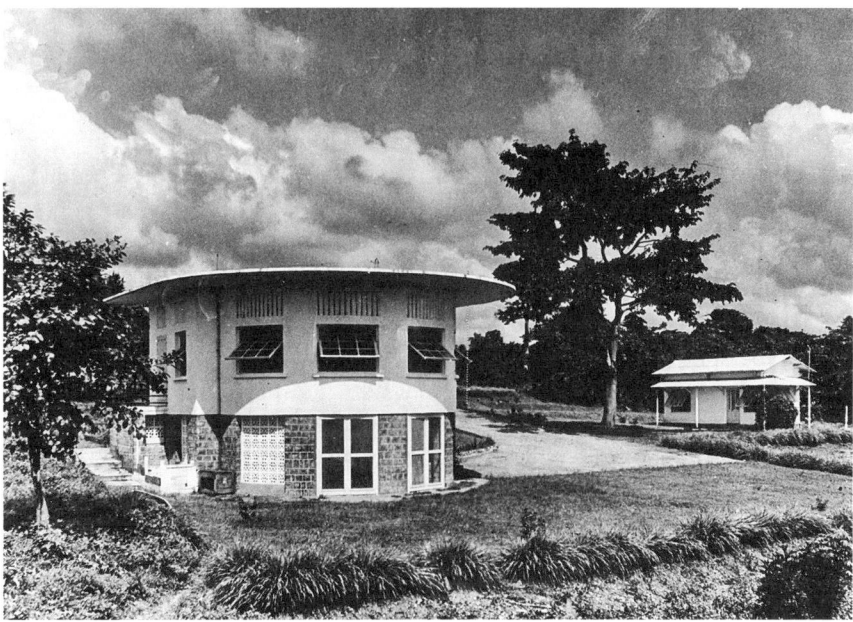

Centre Suisse de Recherches Scientifiques (CSRS), 1951, Archive STI

obliged ORSTOM to lease a strip of land to Switzerland for a period of 50 years and to provide running water and electricity to the laboratory.[125] On the other hand, the agreement codified the dependence of the CSRS on the powerful French research organization. The Commission for the CSRS had to ensure that research activities were restricted to the natural sciences, with the exception of geology and mineralogy, for France refused to tolerate any foreign activities in scientific fields that promised direct economic gains. Furthermore, ORSTOM maintained firm control over the Swiss scientific activities. The Swiss research agenda had to be approved by the Office, and all the researchers and Swiss visitors to Adiopodoumé had to be

125 SCNAT, GA SANW 829, Kommissionen CSRS, Akten Generalsekretariat 1984–1990, Convention entre l'Office de la Recherche Scientifique Outre-Mer, désigné ci-après par les initiales O.R.S.O.M., dont le siège est sis 20, rue Monsieur, Paris VIIe, représenté par son Directeur, Monsieur COMBES, d'une part et La Commission du Centre Suisse de Recherches Scientifiques en Côte d'Ivoire, représentée par son Président, Monsieur J. G. Baer, d'autre part, 20 July 1951.

announced in advance. This code of conduct was maintained even long after Côte d'Ivoire had gained political independence and was a source of constant resentment between the two countries because France suspected Switzerland of only partly meeting its demands.[126]

The unequal relationship that prevailed on a policy level overshadowed the politics of daily life. The tight financial constraints within which the CSRS operated hardly allowed the Swiss scientists to meet the social obligations that were more or less implicitly expected of white Europeans living on the "petit plateau". Quite naturally for demarcated spaces such as the ORSTOM compound, social contacts were restricted to the whites living on the spot. ORSTOM owned a small club with a swimming pool and a tennis court, where the scientists and their families would meet after an exhausting working day in the laboratories or the field. Swiss and French scientists celebrated the national days on July 14 and August 1, and Swiss directors were entertained by the French on several other occasions. But this hospitality could scarcely be reciprocated. As André Aeschlimann, director of the CSRS between 1959 and 1962, lamented:

> Our accommodation is about the size of a handkerchief. One single room ... I very much understand why the chief strongly recommended not having children. Where would one put them? ... But from the French perspective, this situation is lamentable. It is not very nice to hear during each visit: how small it is at your place. Couldn't you have built it with a little bit more room? Switzerland, the country of the banks which is so wealthy etc. ... I believe that if one accepts the establishment of research outposts abroad, which officially represent Swiss scientific research, one has to fully embrace the idea or leave it. We have done so to such a modest extent that we are not taken very seriously at ORSTOM.[127]

It is not surprising that science in the colonies did not have the same significance for Switzerland as it did for France. In striking contrast to France's intention to use scientific rationality to improve local economies, the CSRS was entirely designed to serve Swiss interests. It was considered a site where young Swiss biologists could broaden their minds in studying tropical nature, where new pharmaceutical products could be tested and from where scientific specimens and ethnographic objects could be sent home to enrich museums and scientific institutions. A possible role for the labora-

---

126 SCNAT, GA SANW 826, ORSTOM Korrespondenz 1951–1976, ORSTOM's Director General, Guy Camus to Jean-Georges Baer, 13 February 1969.

127 Fonds André Aeschlimann (FAA), Correspondance Côte d'Ivoire 1959–1962, André Aeschlimann to Thierry Freyvogel, 12 August 1959, pp. 1–2, here: pp. 1–2.

tory in serving a Third World country was explicitly rejected.[128] From a legal point of view, the CSRS was created as a foundation and accountable to the Swiss Department of Home Affairs. Administration and overall responsibility lay in the hands of the Commission for the CSRS, which was placed under the umbrella of the SNG. A local commission for the CSRS was also established in Abidjan, comprising Wimmer, Meyer, Vallon and other representatives of the Swiss community. They were asked to scrutinize the accounts and to facilitate the work of the scientific director in Adiopodoumé.[129] The organizational setup of the CSRS was a far cry from the scientific professionalism of the French neighbors. For young French scientists, Adiopodoumé occupied a firm place in the scientific curriculum. Having spent the first year of training at Bondy near Paris, young French tropicalists were invited to leave the confines of metropolitan lecture halls and to experience the tropics with all their senses. Their Swiss counterparts not only lacked tropical experience but, in most cases, those who went to Côte d'Ivoire did not know exactly what career paths they would pursue when they returned to Switzerland. The most striking difference, however, concerned financial resources. From the outset, the CSRS found itself in a precarious financial situation. The laboratory had to make do with contributions from various sources, with those from the pharmaceutical industry proving to be the most reliable.[130] This situation changed slightly in 1954, when the Swiss

128 Archive Swiss Tropical and Public Health Institut, Basel (ASTI), CSRS, Adresses, Commission, Principes, Ziele CSRS; see also: StABS, ED-REG 1c 190–4 (1), Schweizerische Forschungsstation Elfenbeinküste (Adiopodoumé) 1951–1968, Baer, Rapport adressé au Haut Conseil Fédéral à l'appui d'une requête en faveur d'une subvention destinée au Centre Suisse de Recherches Scientifiques en Côte d'Ivoire, pp. 1–6.

129 BAR, E 2200.5 (-), 1979/93, 10, 0.2.23, Henri Vitoux, procès-verbal de la séance du Comité local du Centre Suisse de Recherches Scientifiques en Côte d'Ivoire tenue au domicile de Monsieur Wimmer, le dimanche 12 Janvier 1952, pp. 1–3, here: pp. 2–3. The local commission was dissolved in 1956 and replaced by the vice-consulate; see: BAR, E 2400, 1000/717, 1, Abidjan, Jahresberichte 1953–1959, Eugen Wimmer, rapport de gestion du vice-consulat de Suisse à Abidjan 1956.

130 Between 1951 and 1954, CHF 104,000 was contributed by private institutions to support the construction of the Centre Suisse, while the Swiss cantons provided CHF 13,000; CHF 21,000 came from "other funds". Research activities were mainly supported by the Swiss National Science Foundation. See: SCNAT, GA SANW 458, CSRS, Gaston Clottu, Budget de la Confédération pour 1955. Augmentation de CHF 300'000.– à CHF 320'000.– de la subvention fédérale en faveur de la Société Helvétique des Sciences Naturelles, cette augmentation de Fr. 20'000.– étant destinée au Centre Suisse de Recherches Scientifiques en Côte d'Ivoire, 9 December 1954, pp. 1–4, here: p. 3.

parliament approved an initiative to increase subsidies to the SNG from CHF 300,000 to CHF 320,000, with the additional money allocated to the CSRS. The difficulties involved in raising money for Swiss research in the tropics and the perceived lack of interest among academia in Switzerland were to be persistent issues throughout the years to come.

Shifting towards Colonialism?

This chapter has dealt with two developments – the rise of tropical science within the broader framework of an emerging national science policy in Switzerland and the movement of Swiss science to the French colony of Côte d'Ivoire. The first development has to be seen in the context of the general tendency of European countries to pay increasing attention to the sciences during the interwar period. While science became meaningful within the wider empire for France and for Britain, it addressed domestic economic issues in Switzerland. Originally, there was nothing "colonial" about tropical sciences in Switzerland. Knowledge about the tropics derived from a variety of scientific disciplines and activities that had a long tradition in a noncolonial country such as Switzerland. However, in the decade following World War II, the growing internationalization of scientific activities, as well as contacts with a small but influential group of Swiss businessmen operating in Côte d'Ivoire, brought Switzerland into the colonial realm. In this respect, at least, Switzerland resembled other (colonial) countries. The CSRS was the first Swiss institution of its kind. Its organization was strongly dependent on ORSTOM, which exerted tight control over its scientific agenda and activities. Restricted by its powerful French neighbor, the CSRS was largely disregarded by Swiss academia. This was mainly due to Switzerland's changing scientific priorities in the context of Cold War politics. Nuclear physics, space research and molecular biology were more apt to forge international scientific ties in the Cold War context than activities which, according to Niklaus Stettler, can be classified as belonging to the "historical" tradition of biology, following a descriptive approach towards nature.[131] This shift in research priorities did not escape Jean-Georges Baer, who lamented:

---

131 Niklaus Stettler, *Natur erforschen. Perspektiven einer Kulturgeschichte der Biowissenschaft an Schweizer Universitäten 1945–1975*, Zurich 2002, p. 11, see also: Strasser, *The Coproduction of Neutral Science and Neutral State in Cold War Europe*.

Today there exists a tendency in Switzerland and elsewhere to favor research in the field of nuclear physics to the detriment of the biological sciences, whose results are generally not directly applicable. We however think that it would be wise to retain a certain equilibrium between the different scientific disciplines because no problem imposed by daily life will be solved by just one of them.[132]

Swiss scientific practices in Côte d'Ivoire did not correspond to the new trends at home and were perceived as anachronistic even by the French. It would appear that France had a more or less clear-cut idea of what science in the tropics after World War II should look like. The different forms of scientific practices are the subject of the next chapter.

132 BAR, E 3001 (B), 1978/30, 62, 07.149, Fondation pour un Centre Suisse de Recherches Scientifiques en Côte d'Ivoire, 1951–1954, Jean-Georges Baer to Ph. Etter (EDI), Monsieur le Conseiller fédéral, 28 April 1954, pp. 1–2, here: p. 2.

Chapter 3
Scientists in the Field

From the early 1950s onwards, with the creation of the scientific field station in Côte d'Ivoire and the Swiss Tropical Institute Field Laboratory (STIFL) in Tanganyika some years later, Switzerland constantly sent young scientists to the French and British overseas territories. Like their European colonial peers, they set out to explore the African continent, to conduct experiments and to collect scientific specimens.

This chapter follows several Swiss scientists to Côte d'Ivoire and Tanganyika and analyzes their ways of understanding the tropical world through their everyday fieldwork. It aims to show that the different local constituencies encountered in Côte d'Ivoire and Tanganyika led to two different colonial logics of scientific research. In Côte d'Ivoire, the French monopoly over the "mission to civilize" through science and technology impeded the pursuit of similar projects by the Centre Suisse de Recherches Scientifiques (CSRS).[1] Instead, Swiss scientists in Adiopodoumé started to discover the unspoiled nature and to amass scientific material, which was sent back home.

The story in Tanganyika is different. Here, in the absence of a network of colonial administrators or scientists, Swiss scientists had to rely on the knowledge provided by Swiss missionaries and the local population. It will be argued that these relations with Swiss development agencies and daily encounters with economic deprivation accounted for the more welfarist approaches adopted by Swiss scientists in Ulanga District. In other words, while in Côte d'Ivoire the ordering of nature according to fixed epistemologies was a major scientific goal, Africa's development and progress became the major concern for Swiss scientists working in Tanganyika. Of course, these two different social settings in which Swiss science took place are relevant to the overarching question of how the decolonization process impinged on Swiss scientific research in Africa. As we will see later, the Swiss scientists working at the two sites were influenced

---

1   Alice L. Conklin, *A Mission to Civilize. The Republican Idea of Empire in France and West Africa, 1895–1930*, Stanford 1997.

to different extents by political developments. The postcolonial pact concluded between France and the Ivorian elite and the striking continuities from the colonial to the postcolonial era did not impose changes for Swiss science in Adiopodoumé, and political developments went more or less unnoticed at the CSRS. By contrast, politics ruled the laboratory in Tanganyika. Not being able to sail in the wake of strong colonial interests, Swiss scientists in Ifakara closely observed how rural Ulanga District was slowly drawn into nationalist agitation. Through the lenses of Swiss researchers, the district became a "development laboratory" where the future political relationship between Europe and Africa could be studied.

The Discovery of Côte d'Ivoire

Arriving in Adiopodoumé in 1951, one of Urs Rahm's first priorities was to write an article with the telling title "La Côte d'Ivoire, Centre de Recherches Tropicales. Possibilités pour la participation Suisse à l'exploration de la Côte d'Ivoire"; this was to serve as an introduction to the new natural environment for future scientists working at the Ebrié Lagoon.[2] Rahm highlighted the immense richness of the natural surroundings, which provided endless possibilities for scientific exploration. With his description of the lagoon, the virgin forests and the nearby savannah, Rahm joined in a discourse of the tropics viewed as an earthly paradise or Garden of Eden, which had a long tradition in Western representations of the tropical world and which struck a chord with his European readership at home.[3] Pierre-Paul Grassé's fears about Adiopodoumé becoming a testing ground for the Swiss pharmaceutical industry were unfounded: the forces at play were romanticization rather than manipulation. Adiopodoumé was the fulfillment of a Swiss colonial desire or "colonial fantasy" (the term used by Susanne M. Zantop) and the confirmation of all the images that had been

2   Urs Rahm, *La Côte d'Ivoire. Centre de Recherches Tropicales. Possibilités pour la participation Suisse à l'exploration de la Côte d'Ivoire*, in: Acta Tropica, Vol. 11, 1954, pp. 222–295.
3   Philip D. Curtin, *The Image of Africa. British Ideas and Action, 1780–1850*, Madison 1964; Andreas Eckert, *"Tropics"*, in: Akira Iriye and Pierre-Yves Saunier (eds.), Palgrave Dictionary of Transnational History; Felix Driver, Luciana Martins (eds.), *Tropical Visions in an Age of Empire*, Chicago 2005.

associated with the African continent.[4] Working at the CSRS towards the end of the 1950s, André Aeschlimann, about whom we will hear more below, was perhaps more explicit about the significance of the site for Swiss science when he wrote:

> We live in a kind of paradise. Only the humidity is difficult to bear. It attacks everything, it drains one's strength. Everything is damp, everything goes moldy, everything rusts. But what a beautiful country! The nearby forest – so green that it seems almost black – is gorgeous. This huge virgin forest – the stuff of our dreams – with trees more than forty meters high and with its tangle of lianas, some of which are thicker than an arm … and its silence, this immense silence that increases the mystery.[5]

The widespread use of the paradise metaphor in relation to Côte d'Ivoire is interesting in itself and would merit further analysis. The point is raised here because this specific trope determined to a large extent scientific practices on the ground. Once they had arrived on the Ivorian shore, the scientists – most of whom embodied Geigy's tradition of experimental and medical zoology – did not necessarily continue their lab-based work but were attracted by the prospect of studying nature outside the laboratory and discovering unknown species. Urs Rahm himself is probably the most notable example. Working on his doctoral thesis in Switzerland, Rahm had studied the postembryonic development of alderflies (*Sialis lutaria L.* [Megaloptera]).[6] By means of ligation and extirpation experiments, he showed that metamorphosis of the larvae is dependent on a hormone secreted by a gland in the brain.[7] The new natural environment of Adiopodoumé, however, required a less interventionist scientific approach. At Rudolf Geigy's request, Rahm started to study the distribution of plankton in the Ebrié Lagoon. From an ecological point of view, this was a fascinating topic: with the opening of the Vridi Canal, which provided access to the salty ocean, the ecological conditions of the lagoon were likely to change.[8] But, despite the discovery of a new species of medusa, Rahm's

---

4 Susanne M. Zantop, *Kolonialphantasien im vorkolonialen Deutschland 1770–1870*, Berlin 1999, p. 11.
5 Fonds André Aeschlimann (FAA), André Aeschlimann, 18 April 1959.
6 Urs Rahm, *Die innersekretorische Steuerung der postembryonalen Entwicklung von* Sialis lutaria L. *(Megaloptera),* Inauguraldissertation Universität Basel, Basel 1952.
7 Ibid., p. 174.
8 Urs Rahm, *Zur Ökologie des Zooplanktons der Lagune Ebrié (Elfenbeinküste),* in: Acta Tropica (Separatum), Vol. 21, No. 1, Basel 1964.

trips on the lagoon were short-lived. His naturalist mind was not disposed to stick to one topic. Soon after his arrival in Adiopodoumé, he started to focus on the study of midsize mammals brought to the laboratory by local residents. The fauna of the African countryside was still considered uncharted territory, and Rahm – who was the only zoologist at the ORSTOM site at the beginning of the 1950s – became its ambitious cartographer.[9] His appetite for scientific discoveries resulted in numerous short publications on the main characteristics and behavior of the "unknown" animals.[10] In this tropical paradise, there was no time pressure for the study of nature, no research agenda to restrict one's own scientific interests and no expectations to be met. Rahm recalls:

> As soon as I arrived, I developed an interest in mammals and the like. We never had snakes but we had turtles and other animals. But I have to say that we did not have a research objective. That was impossible, because if you wanted to do research on one specific animal, then you would have been obliged to search for it and, if you were lucky, you would have found it a year later. I just lived from hand to mouth. I analyzed the animals as soon as they arrived at the Centre.[11]

Rahm's depiction of colonial life as "living from hand to mouth" reinforces the image of Adiopodoumé as a scientific paradise but conceals the practical aspects of fieldwork involved in the production of scientific knowledge. The research process also included expeditions to different parts of the country to collect specimens. These were not only important for the functioning of the CSRS, but "vital for the existence of the Swiss Tropical Institute in Basel".[12] Especially before *Glossina* could be bred un-

---

9   Fonds Urs Rahm (FUR), Urs Rahm, 14 February 1952.

10 See for instance: Urs Rahm, *Beobachtungen an* Atherurus africanus *(Gray) an der Elfenbeinküste*, in: Acta Tropica, Vol. 13, No. 1, 1956, pp. 86–94; *Beobachtungen an den Schuppentieren* Manis tricuspis *und* Manis longicaudata *an der Elfenbeinküste*, in: Revue Suisse de Zoologie, Vol. 62, No. 2/29, 1955, pp. 361–367; *Einige Schlangen des westafrikanischen Urwaldes*, in: Die Aquarien- und Terrarien-Zeitschrift (DATZ), Vol. 6, No. 11, 1953, pp. 292–294; *Einige Urwaldsäuger der Elfenbeinküste*, in: Leben und Umwelt, Vol. 9, 1952, pp. 1–5; *Einige Urwaldsäuger der Elfenbeinküste (II)*, in: Leben und Umwelt, Vol. 9, 1953, pp. 114–118; *Quelques notes sur le Botto de Bosman.* Extrait du Bulletin de L'Institut Français d'Afrique Noire (IFAN), Vol. 22, No. A/1, 1960, pp. 331–342.

11 Interview with Urs Rahm, 28 April 2009.

12 Staatsarchiv Basel-Stadt (StABS), ED-REG 1c 190–2-6 (1), Protokolle (Kuratorium, Geschäftsausschuss), 1944–1968, Eleonore Tschudin, Protokoll der Sitzung des Kuratoriums für das Schweizerische Tropeninstitut, 26 April 1954, pp. 1–6, here: p. 5.

der laboratory conditions, the STI's research on African trypanosomiasis depended very much on a steady flow of *Glossina palpalis* and *Glossina fusca* from Côte d'Ivoire to Basel.[13] Apart from scientific observations, collecting was the predominant "way of knowing".[14] As well as scientific objects, living animals were collected for zoological gardens, and ethnographic displays for Swiss museums, friends or private collections.[15] In the eyes of relatives in Switzerland, living in Africa automatically meant amassing scientific or exotic souvenirs. Given his own family's expectations, Rahm felt obliged to justify himself:

> It is wrong to say that I don't collect many objects. We do have some beautiful statuettes ... I will try to collect some minerals even though they are difficult to get. To create a herbarium is much too laborious and would consume all of my precious time ... I will however collect bugs and butterflies and that will keep me busy enough. There are some beautiful examples here but you have to work with chemicals, to soak the animals with DDT, and you have to constantly turn on the light in the box against the mold. Indeed, such a collection is not easy to create and everything takes a lot of time.[16]

Collecting was not just a tricky and time-consuming scientific practice. It was also inherently political and apt to stir up French colonial feelings. The delicacy of colonial relations was summed up by the activities of Villy Aellen, one of the many scientists working for a short period at the CSRS. Aellen, who studied zoology under Baer in Neuchâtel, was not a newcomer under the tropical sun: in 1946–47, he had joined the Swiss explorer Albert Monard on a scientific expedition to Cameroon, bringing back rich collections of scientific specimens to Switzerland.[17] In Côte d'Ivoire, Aellen developed a fascination for the study of small mammals. He found it deplor-

---

13 Archiv Schweizerische Akademie der Naturwissenschaften, Depot Burgerbibliothek Bern (SCNAT), GA SANW 826, Kommissionen CSRS, Tätigkeitsberichte Direktor 1952–1974, Urs Rahm, Rapport du Centre Suisse du 1er Janvier au 30 Juin 1952, 13 July 1952, pp. 1–4, here: p. 5; Rudolf Geigy, *Elevage de Glossina palpalis*, in: Acta Tropica, Vol. 5, No. 1, 1948, pp. 201–218.

14 John Pickstone, *Ways of Knowing. A New History of Science, Technology and Medicine*, Manchester 2000; Anke te Heesen, E. C. Spary, *Sammeln als Wissen*, in: Heesen and Spary (eds.), Sammeln als Wissen. Das Sammeln und seine wissenschaftsgeschichtliche Bedeutung, Göttingen 2001, pp. 7–21.

15 FAA, André Aeschlimann, 12 September 1961.

16 Fonds Urs Rahm (FUR), Urs Rahm, 28 April 1952.

17 Mémoires de l'Institut Français d'Afrique Noire (Centre du Caméroun), Série Science Naturelles, No. 1, *Résultats de la Mission Zoologique Suisse au Cameroun*, Dakar 1951.

able that most scientists before him had failed to recognize the specific characteristics of Ivorian fauna.[18] The money he received from the Swiss National Science Foundation (SNSF) for his seven-month stay at the CSRS was well spent: his final report to the Commission of the CSRS was outstanding evidence of the inadequacy of previous scientific observations in the colony. To the only known species of bat in Côte d'Ivoire Aellen added some fifty new ones. He was the first to report the presence of a red colobus monkey (*Colobus badius waldroni*) among the primates of Côte d'Ivoire, and he acquired many specimens of the royal antelope (*Neotragus pygmaeus*), "rarely to be seen in a museum".[19] Aellen, who enthusiastically shared his experiences with a wider readership in Geneva, was at the center of a small network of Swiss researchers working in Africa, as well as in Swiss natural history museums, through which the scientific trophies were traded.[20] It is interesting to note that while such practices were an inherent part of the epistemic culture of both France and Switzerland, they were perceived as outdated by the former. When Aellen reported his practices too openly in a letter to the SNSF, Baer felt impelled to intervene:

> It is thanks to the SNSF that you are in Adiopodoumé to pursue your scientific work. It is out of the question that you should provide Swiss museums with scientific specimens. I can even tell you that this is one of the reproaches we hear from Paris, where some people regard us suspiciously and look for any pretext to thwart us. You know very well that in the colonies, the smallest affair can grow to proportions that you could not have imagined before. We have to be very cautious, especially at the beginning. I can tell you in confidence that Paris has even ordered an inquiry into our activities, believing that our aims consist of nothing more than working for industry and providing our museums and zoological gardens with scientific material! We should not give any grounds for criticism, either in Côte d'Ivoire or in Switzerland at the SNSF.[21]

18   Archive Musée d'Histoire Naturelle de Genève (AMHN), 360.B.4.4, Mission scientifique en Côte d'Ivoire 1953–1957, Villy Aellen to Jean-Georges Baer, 7 June 1952, pp. 1–3, here: p. 2.
19   Ibid., Villy Aellen to Jean-Georges Baer, 13 November 1953, pp. 1–4; Villy Aellen, *Chiroptères Nouveaux d'Afrique*, in: Archives des Sciences, Vol. 12, No. 2, 1959, pp. 217–235; Villy Aellen, *Description d'un nouvel* Hipposideros *(chiroptera) de la Côte d'Ivoire*, in: Revue Suisse de Zoologie, Vol. 61, No. 24, 1954, pp. 474–483; Villy Aellen, *Animaux en Côte d'Ivoire*, in: Bulletin de la Société Neuchâteloise des Sciences Naturelles, Vol. 82, 1959, p. 329.
20   See his articles in the Swiss daily newspaper *l'Impartial*.
21   AMHN, 360.B.4.4, Jean-Georges Baer to Villy Aellen, 20 April 1953, pp. 1–2, here: p. 1.

As Baer's reaction suggests, there is no coherent notion of colonial science that would do justice to the wide variety of colonial scientific practices. What seems to have existed at that time was a set of rules, a standard set by the French for what constitutes accepted practice.[22] ORSTOM marked a new episode in the history of French scientific activities, and we may recall Raoul Combes's remark that the overseas territories were no longer to be seen as "a museum, a laboratory, or a vast reserve of scientific material", but the locus where France could prove the superiority of Western civilization through science. Moreover, there was a constant fear that the smallest incidents would be given the highest symbolic weight – to the detriment of the already fragile relationship between the "Orstomiens" in Paris and the members of the CSRS.

The success or failure of field science was not just a political balancing act but also largely dependent on African intermediaries. A central figure in the activities of the CSRS was Boukary Porgo, one of the many labor migrants coming to Côte d'Ivoire from Upper Volta. Porgo had been working for a French plantation company at Adiopodoumé when he was hired by the CSRS, where he then worked for over 30 years. Often called "the boy" by Swiss scientists, Boukary Porgo skillfully performed the functions of gardener, mechanic and laboratory assistant. His presence was indispensable, especially on scientific expeditions, where he acted as a cultural broker, introducing the Swiss scientists to rural village dignitaries. His support seems to have been largely taken for granted. André Aeschlimann's acknowledgement that "Thanks to you, I was able to observe all the mammals of Côte d'Ivoire (insectivores and rodents included)" is a rare expression of belated gratitude.[23] Swiss scientists relied heavily on Porgo's technical skills, knowledge of local geography and ability to speak various local dialects, but they were keen to maintain a rigid boundary between science and knowledge. This attitude was shared by ORSTOM, which also constantly redrew the boundaries between French science and African knowledge, on which the success of the scientific project ultimately depended. For instance, botanical explorations of Ivorian forests

22 Lukas Meier, *The Other's Colony. Switzerland and the Discovery of Côte d'Ivoire*, in: Patricia Purtschert, Harald Fischer-Tiné (eds.), Colonial Encounters of the Swiss Kind. Imperial Entanglements and Postcolonial Assemblages, Cambridge 2014 [forthcoming].

23 SCNAT, GA SANW 830, Centre Suisse, Varia, Korrespondenz, Geschichte der Station 1981–1987, André Aeschlimann to Boukary Porgo, 22 December 1986, pp. 1–2, here: p. 1.

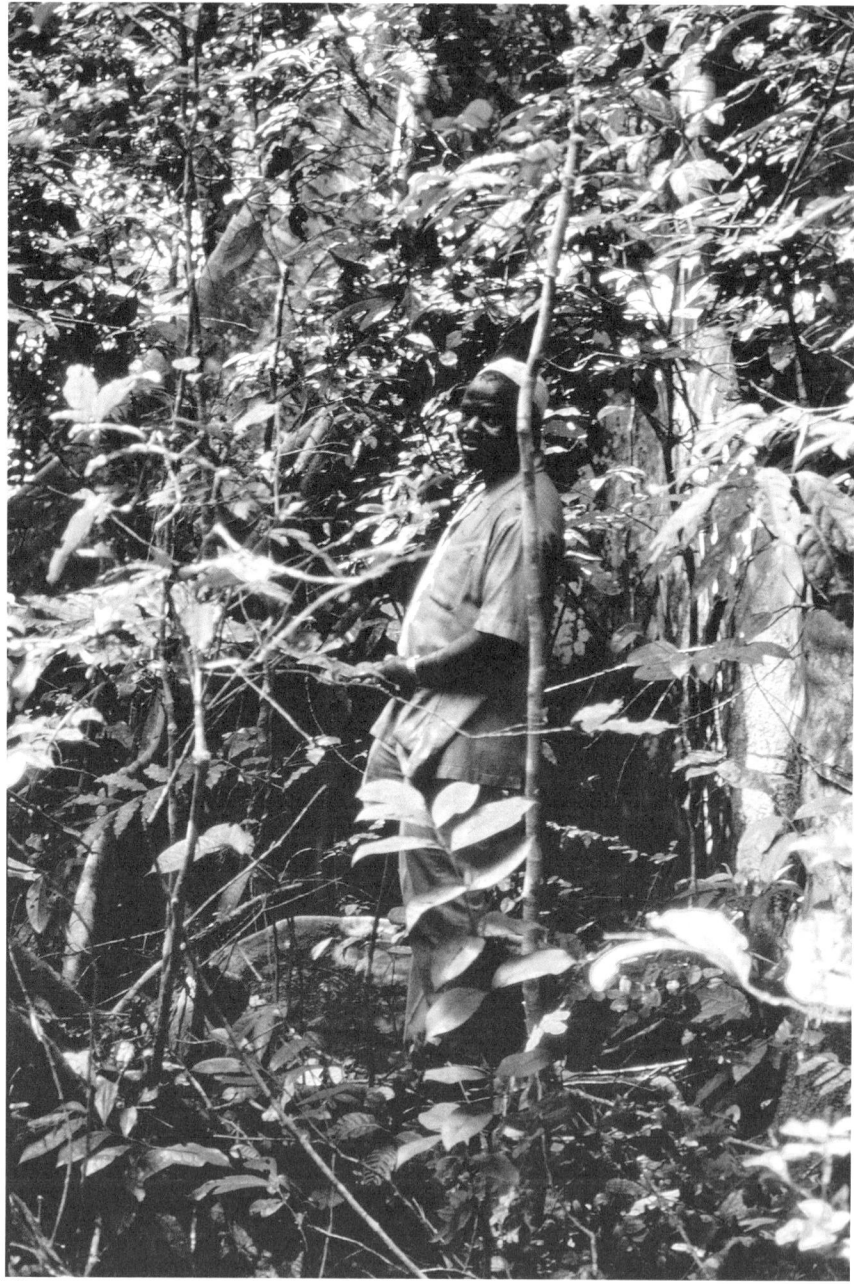

Boukary Porgo in the Tai Forest, picture: Jean-François Graf, 1978

owed much to the help of the young botanist Laurent Aké Assi – the son of Aké Anga, who had already assisted French botanist Auguste Chevalier in the classification of Ivorian forests.[24] However, as far as the training of young African scholars was concerned, ORSTOM took a different approach to that of the CSRS. The colonial ideology of remolding African individuals according to French "civilizing" standards – as well as a larger budget – allowed them to "cultivate the intrinsic qualities of certain black individuals and turn them into real observers and researchers".[25] It can be argued that, in the relationship between France and the African country, technical knowledge was the basic mechanism for social and economic mobility and one of the main features in the transition from colonial domination to a set of political and social rules that would constitute the laws of the postcolony. Political considerations were never foremost in the minds of the Swiss scientists: science was construed as a neutral and apolitical activity, and it is striking to what extent the colonial situation was taken for granted.

The Eclipse of Politics

On a personal and professional level, the boundaries between science and politics were porous. Hansjörg Huggel, who became director of the CSRS in 1955, was easily able to replace Eugen Wimmer as honorary consul while Wimmer recuperated in Europe. This does not mean, however, that science was understood as a political practice. For a better understanding of the power of knowledge production – and the eclipse of politics – in the colony, it is necessary to turn briefly to Lily and André Aeschlimann, whose directorship (1959–1961) coincided with the transition to Ivorian independence. André Aeschlimann was born in Geneva and raised in Delémont in Western Switzerland. After high school, he moved to Basel,

---

24 Laurent Aké Assi subsequently became one of the most renowned specialists in African botany. According to Auguste Chevalier, "[Aké Assi] can currently identify by their scientific and common names (in several languages) around 2000 Ivorian plant species and, better still, he can recognize them in dense forest, where the mixture of trees, shrubs and lianas is rather confusing. His knowledge and observational skills are truly prodigous." See: Auguste Chevalier, *Un jeune africain prodige. Aké Assi, préparateur à l'Institut biologique d'Adiopodoumé (Côte d'Ivoire)*, in: Revue internationale de botanique appliquée et d'agriculture tropicale, 1948, p. 279.

25 Ibid.

where he took courses in zoology at the university. Aeschlimann was fascinated by Geigy's concept of medical parasitology, which combined zoological studies of parasites with more practice-oriented research on health and disease. Aeschlimann's doctoral research was concerned with the embryonic development of *Ornithodoros moubata*, the vector of African tick-borne relapsing fever.[26] In Basel, he was immediately attracted by the tropical world, and especially Africa. He would occasionally browse through displays of African art in local secondhand shops, and he attended the ethnographic courses offered by Alfred Bühler on New Guinea and Papua New Guinea. He was also "very familiar with the museum's African art collection because Mr. Bühler allowed me to see it at a time when it was still locked up in the cupboard".[27] In 1958, with a grant from the Janggen-Pöhn Foundation, Aeschlimann went to Ifakara to carry out a systematic study of the distribution of ticks in the Ulanga District.[28] Having returned to Basel, however, he – together with his wife Lily – was sent by Geigy to the CSRS in Côte d'Ivoire to take over responsibility from Hansjörg Huggel. Apart from a basic interest in tropical nature, marriage was an essential requirement for the directorship of the CSRS. As Lily Aeschlimann recalled, "Côte d'Ivoire was not an easy place to live in". As well as the temperature – so unfamiliar for persons used to a European climate – there was the period of three years spent in near-isolation; marriage was therefore important for the "researcher's equilibrium".[29] From her childhood onwards, Lily Aeschlimann had shared her husband's fascination for the African continent:

> I always wanted to go to Africa … My father had a friend in Basel that he had studied French in Belgium with. This friend married a Belgian whose father had a business in the Congo. My father's friend also started a business in the Congo, in Léopoldville, and whenever he came to visit us in Basel, I begged him: "Uncle Charly, I want to go to the Congo with you!" But he always answered: "That's no place for little girls."[30]

---

26   André Aeschlimann, *Développement embryonnaire d'*Ornithodoros moubata *(Murray) et transmission transovarienne de* Borrelia duttoni, Inauguraldissertation Universität Basel, Basel 1958.

27   Interview with André Aeschlimann, 21 July 2010.

28   FAA, André Aeschlimann, Rapport du voyage de Monsieur A. Aeschlimann au Kenya et Tanganyika, à Messieurs les membres du comité de la Fondation Janggen-Pöhn, pp. 1–2.

29   Interview with Lily Aeschlimann, 21 July 2010.

30   Interview with André and Lily Aeschlimann, 21 July 2010.

Work at the CSRS was highly gendered. Lily Aeschlimann, who quit her job at the Sonnenrain clinic, helped out at the laboratory, typing letters to friends and other scientists, and dealing with administrative matters. Her presence was especially important from a social point of view. The highly political function of the CSRS was revealed by the various social activities and official meetings with the "Orstomiens", as well as with African politicians – including Félix Houphouët-Boigny and his wife: "In all modesty, I was the Centre Suisse's ambassadress."[31]

For André Aeschlimann in turn, Côte d'Ivoire offered the opportunity to follow Geigy in combining the study of basic parasitology with practical aspects of health and disease. "There are many species of Ixodides [ticks] in Côte d'Ivoire that are not yet classified," he wrote enthusiastically to the President of the SNG Research Commission, Jacques de Beaumont. In the same spirit as Swiss researchers before him, he started to compile an inventory of Ivorian ticks, which was to be "as complete as possible".[32] He discovered an unknown species which he soon named *Boophilus geigyi* in fondness for his patron at the STI. Aeschlimann was fascinated by the details of parasitism: what were the ticks' main hosts in the country, and why did some prefer a specific host while others were not at all selective? His work also had practical implications. The collection of ticks from villagers' domestic animals lowered the risk of disease transmission and thus had an immediate impact on the well-being of the African population. While Adiopodoumé may have been a confined space in terms of domestic life, this was offset by scientific expeditions and the global scope of scientific communications. During his years at the CSRS, Aeschlimann corresponded with other tick researchers, such as Harry Hoogstraal (in Cairo) or P. C. Morel (in France), about the latest discoveries in tick science. This orientation towards an international scientific community and the striking continuities in French-Ivorian relations during the 1950s and early 1960s may explain why scientific fieldwork in Adiopodoumé and relations with the rural population remained unaffected by the political upheavals. Like his peers, Aeschlimann commented only occasionally on these developments.

Switzerland's reluctance to comment on political events, and its tendency to take the social context for granted, says much about the trajectory of Ivorian decolonization, which became more heated after 1956, ending a

---

31   Ibid.
32   FAA, André Aeschlimann to Jacques De Beaumont, 27 May 1959, pp. 1–2, here: p. 1, also: Interview with André Aeschlimann, 24 January 2011.

period which has been described as "political sclerosis".[33] Many scholars writing about decolonization in French West Africa (AOF) would agree that, with the "loi-cadre" (Reform Act) of 1956 and France's new concept of territorialization, the "political endgame had begun".[34] Instead of being subject to the authority of the federal Government-General, each territory now had the power to administer its domestic affairs ("services territoriaux"), while France retained control over key policy areas such as foreign affairs and defense ("services d'Etat"). This distinction between "services d'Etat" and "services territoriaux" had far-reaching consequences for the individual African territories, as it put an end to the culture of demand and reduced the metropole's expenditure on African welfare to a minimum. Though this was mitigated by the ongoing provision of aid, it was now "foreign aid, a gift rather than an imperial obligation".[35] One of the factors underlying the Ivorian decolonization process in the 1950s was the personalization of official politics. France's foreign policy was shaped not only by éminences grises – such as Jacques Foccart who, as Secretary-General for African Affairs between 1958 and 1974, basically held African policy in his hands – but also by France's constant distinction between "real" and more doubtful African friends.[36] In this division of the African world, French anticommunism played a decisive role. Félix Houphouët-Boigny appears to have belonged to the former group and was most susceptible to French advances. In 1950, he met with René Pleven and François Mitterand and, in exchange for greater African influence over the colony's affairs and progressive reforms, he agreed to break openly with the French Communist Party and to renounce the "militant style of anti-colonial activism that had come to characterize the RDA [African Democratic Assembly]".[37]

33 Tony Chafer, *The End of Empire in West Africa*, p. 83; Yves Person, *French West Africa and Decolonization*, in: Prosser Gifford and William Roger Louis (eds.), The Transfer of Power in Africa. Decolonization 1940–1960, New Haven, London 1982, pp. 141–172, here: p. 143.
34 Frederick Cooper, *Africa since 1940*. p. 66.
35 Ibid., p. 82.
36 Alexander Keese, *First Lessons in Neo-Colonialism. The Personalisation of Relations between African Politicians and French Officials in Sub-Saharan Africa, 1956–66*, in: The Journal of Imperial and Commonwealth History, Vol. 35, No. 4, 2007, pp. 593–613, here: p. 599.
37 Timothy C. Weiskel, *Independence and the* Longue Durée. *The Ivory Coast "Miracle" Reconsidered*, in: William Roger Louis and Prosser Gifford (eds.), Decolonization and African Independence. The Transfers of Power, 1960–1980, New Haven, London 1988, pp. 347–380, here: p. 370.

During the empire-wide constitutional referendum of 1958, when the African population was asked to choose between the option of building a federation of African states and immediate political independence, Houphouët demonstrated his devotion to the ideal of a broader cooperative community with France. As Aristide Zolberg has shown, Houphouët's arguments in favor of a Franco-African community were based on economic considerations as well as problems of national unity. He was convinced that, without French economic support and investment, a decent standard of living would never be attained for the whole Ivorian population.[38] While many of the members of the Parti Démocratique de Côte d'Ivoire (PDCI) working in Africa rather than in France had reservations about postponing independence, Houphouët's power over the party was such that they would not have dared to raise their concerns publicly, or to draw attention to the coercion employed by the party leader during the referendum campaign.[39] The declaration of Ivorian independence on August 7, 1960, did not then mark such a historical break as in the case of Guinea, whose population voted in the 1958 referendum for immediate independence and against a constitution in which they saw their voices overruled by the will of the French.[40] In the case of Côte d'Ivoire, the postcolonial pact with France did not leave much room for maneuver for those who assumed political responsibility over the African country. The language of cooperation replaced the former discourse of assimilation, and, as Tony Chafer has argued, "This vision of a mutually beneficial relationship, in which independent Black African states would benefit from French support and cooperation in return for their support for France in the global arena, was to be the foundation stone for the maintenance of close Franco-African relations in the post-colonial era."[41]

With the smooth transition that would lead to a Franco-African family and the continuation of France's influence over the fate of Côte d'Ivoire, little changed on the ground and the Swiss saw no need to reflect on the implications of political independence. As has been shown before, the Swiss scientific activities of ordering the empire and filling gaps remaining in scientific knowledge of tropical parasitology were highly political, as

38 Aristide Zolberg, *One-party Government in the Ivory Coast*, Princeton, New Jersey 1969, p. 235.
39 Elizabeth Schmidt, *Anticolonial Nationalism in French West Africa. What Made Guinea Unique?*, in: African Studies Review, Vol. 52, No. 2, 2009, pp. 1–34, here: p. 20.
40 Ibid., p. 6.
41 Tony Chafer, *The End of Empire in West Africa*, p. 183.

they sustained the colonial order based on social hierarchies. Most important for Switzerland's shift towards development aid in the 1960s was the
fact that, after a decade of knowledge production in Côte d'Ivoire, Swiss
scientists emerged as new and highly esteemed development experts. Their
expertise in African problems had its roots in their efforts to order the natural world. Development was then perhaps not so much an intellectual
concept as it was directly derived from the practice of African fieldwork.
But before turning to the period of Swiss development aid and the role of
the STI in shaping official development policies in the 1960s and 1970s,
we should focus our attention once again on the practical aspects of science in Tanganyika.

The Permanent Expedition: Tanganyika 1954–1961

Leaving the CSRS under the tutelage of Jean-Georges Baer, Rudolf Geigy
found in Tanganyika a vast area most suitable for his research interests. In
1949, he had already been impressed by the many research opportunities
offered by the territory when, as a guest of the Capuchin mission in Ifakara, he worked on the mechanisms of transmission of trypanosomiasis,
malaria, relapsing fever and chiggers.[42] He had been introduced by Paul
Alfred Turner Sneath (Director of Medical Services) to Charles Swynnerton and John Ford working in Shinyanga, and to H. Fairbairn (a Sleeping
Sickness Officer, see Chapter 1) in Tinde.[43] Five years later, Tanganyika
was again host to a Swiss scientific expedition headed by Geigy. The
group also included Hermann Mooser and Thierry Freyvogel, one of
Geigy's students at the STI. While the latter studied the impact of high altitudes on the course of malaria infection, Geigy and Mooser resumed the
research on African relapsing fever which they had begun in 1949.[44]

    Investigations of African relapsing fever were especially attractive be-
cause knowledge of the mechanisms of transmission and the epidemiology
of the disease was still in its infancy. In fact, relapsing fever – caused by the

---

42 Tanzania National Archive (TNA), 450/87/20, Scientific (Tanganyika) Expedition by
    Profs. R. Geigy and H. Mooser and Dr. Freyvogel, 1954–1956, Rudolf Geigy to
    M. Meredith, 17 February 1954.
43 Ibid.
44 Ibid., Rudolf Geigy, Hermann Mooser, Programme of work for the scientific Tangan-
    yika Expedition in 1954 of Profs. Geigy (Swiss Tropical Institute, Basle) and Mooser
    (Institute of Hygiene, University of Zurich).

pathogen *Borrelia duttoni*, which is transmitted by the tick *Ornithodoros moubata* – had long been a neglected tropical disease. While human trypanosomiasis ranked high on the British research agenda and consumed the lion's share of British research funding, relapsing fever went almost unnoticed. At the beginning of World War II, Patrick Buxton, an entomologist at the London School of Hygiene and Tropical Medicine (LSHTM), felt that "the whole subject is one of the most serious gaps in medical entomology".[45] Fifteen years later, the situation remained unchanged:

> We have of course only too little detailed information on the incidence of the disease in Tanganyika in the past – my own feeling about this being that it is possibly better to adopt the point of view that relapsing fever has been widespread in the country for a very long time and to leave it at that, knowing that the records are pretty rough …[46]

The disease had been reported in Tanganyika since the interwar period and was usually associated with unhygienic conditions and increased mobility of the rural population.[47] However, at the beginning of the 1950s, Ronald Heisch and G. A. Walton, working at the Medical Research Laboratory in Nairobi, confirmed earlier observations that *Ornithodoros moubata* was to be found not only in human dwellings but also in the burrows of small wild mammals, such as porcupines, antbears and warthogs.[48] If this tick existed in the wild, then the most pressing research question was whether it carried *Borrelia duttoni*, and whether the wild mammals served as a reservoir for African relapsing fever.[49] As well as performing experiments with different strains of *Borrelia duttoni* in white mice, Geigy and his collaborators focused in particular on the "warthog hypothesis". Geigy's research objectives in Tanganyika not only revealed a shared interest be-

---

45 TNA, 450/66/Infectious Diseases, Spirillum Relapsing Fever 1948–1957, P. Buxton to R. R. Scott, 1 July 1940, p. 1.
46 Ibid., G. A. Walton, 16 November 1954.
47 Ibid., I. W. Mackchikan, 16 April 1956.
48 R. B. Heisch, W. E. Grainger, *On the Occurrence of Ornithodoros moubata Murray in Burrows*, in: Annals of Tropical Medicine and Parasitology, Vol. 44, 1950, pp. 153–155; R. B. Heisch, *Ornithodoros moubata (Murray) in a Porcupine Burrow near Kitui*, in: East African Medical Journal, Vol. 31, 1954, p. 483; G. A. Walton, *Ornithodoros moubata in Warthog and Porcupine Burrows in Tanganyika Territory*, in: Transactions of the Royal Society of Tropical Medicine and Hygiene, Vol. 47, 1953, pp. 410–411.
49 Rudolf Geigy, Hermann Mooser, *Untersuchungen zur Epidemiologie des afrikanischen Rückfallfiebers in Tanganyika*, in: Acta Tropica, Vol. 12, No. 4, 1955, pp. 327–345, here: p. 40.

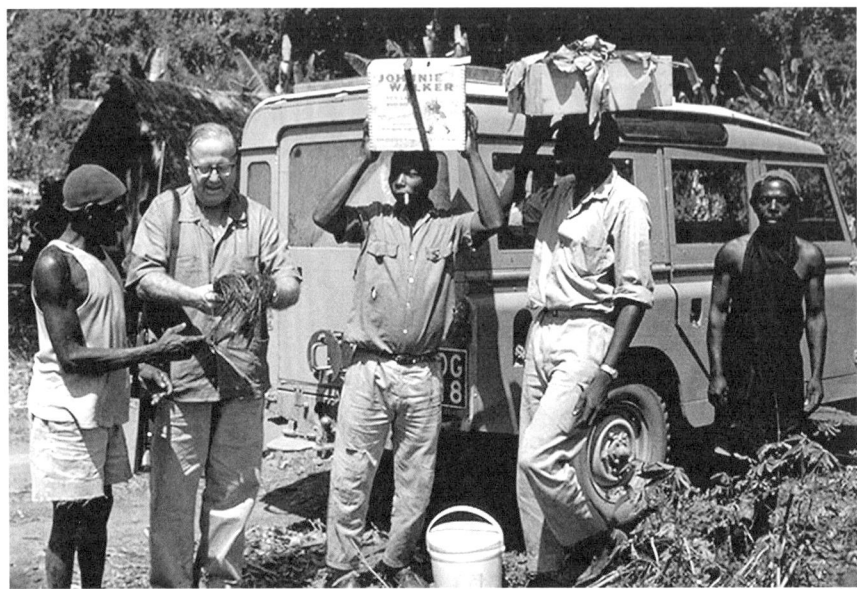

Rudolf Geigy, Pius Hermes and Ambros Mganda in the field, 1967, Archive STI

tween his group and British researchers working in East Africa, but also
the fact that tropical disease was understood within a larger epidemiological context: the STI was not just interested in the distribution of tropical
parasites or in narrowly conceived modes of disease transmission but in
the complex interplay between parasites' human and animal hosts, as well
as the impact of the natural environment.

Expeditions on this scale involved major logistical efforts and could
not have been carried out without the help of the Capuchin mission in Dar
es Salaam and Ifakara. From the mission's headquarters, Father Oswin
supported the STI by organizing import licenses for the scientific material
and dispelled British concerns that the Swiss would conduct "human experiments" with the African population.[50] The Capuchin mission was also
crucial in providing the expedition team with African personnel. Most of
the "boys" who were seconded to the team attended the mission school at
Ifakara and were selected from the classroom. Ambros Mganda, who was

---

50 Provincial Archive Dar es Salaam (PADSM), Father Oswin to Rudolf Geigy, 1 April
    1954, p. 1.

recruited in 1949 and would subsequently become one of the STI's closest collaborators, recalls the moment when Geigy entered the classroom and pointed at him because he was skinny and would easily be able to enter warthog holes.[51] Injecting white mice with brain liquid from warthogs could not confirm the hypothesis according to which these animals were reservoirs of relapsing fever in Ulanga District.[52] But for Geigy – nicknamed "Bwana Ngiri" (Mr. Warthog) by the local population – the expedition was still a success, as it put an end to the peripatetic nature of Swiss knowledge production in East Africa. In 1954, Karl Schöpf, the medical superintendent of St. Francis Hospital, came up with the idea of offering Geigy a space to establish his own scientific laboratory in a wing of the hospital under construction in Ifakara.[53] The idea was also well received by the head of the Swiss Capuchin mission, Edgar Maranta, who was aware that many of the missionary brothers and sisters in Ifakara had received their introduction to the tropics through the STI's General Tropical Course in Basel. However, the provision of laboratory space for STI scientists should not be interpreted as a mere returned favor. Maranta (later archbishop) was well aware that his missionary society would probably also benefit from these research activities. In a letter to Father Superior Hieronymus Schildknecht, he wrote:

> The missionary society has a strong interest in this field laboratory. Should it be successful in fighting malaria, relapsing fever or sleeping sickness, then we also will benefit. It seems to me that the mission could also contribute something towards scientific research.[54]

At the end of the expedition, Geigy asked his student Freyvogel whether he could imagine himself with a future in the tropics, building up what would become the STIFL. The young and talented Freyvogel – for whom the African territory offered an opportunity to "achieve many new things in scientific branches as various as biology, botany, zoology, ethnology and psychology" – did not refuse Geigy's offer. Before moving into Ma-

---

51 Interview with Ambros Mganda, 9 January 2009.
52 Rudolf Geigy, Hermann Mooser, *Untersuchungen zur Epidemiologie*, p. 341.
53 Fonds Thierry A. Freyvogel (FTAF), Thierry Freyvogel, Tagebuch, No. 1, Expédition de l'Institut Tropical Suisse de Bâle au Tanganyika, Ifakara Mai 1954 – Juli 1954, pp. 1–85, here: p. 4.
54 Diocesan Archives Kwiro (DAK), Parish Ifakara 1956–1969, Edgar Maranta to Father Hieronymus Schildknecht, 16 January 1958. (I am grateful to Marcel Dreier for this quotation.)

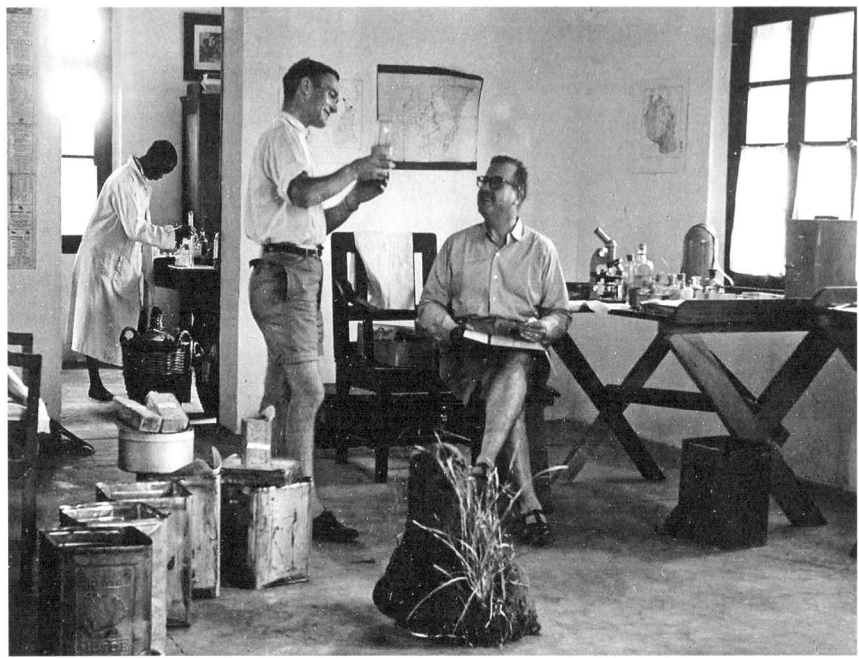

*STI's first temporary field-laboratory in the padres' house of the Swiss Capuchin
Mission, 1949, Archive STI*

ranta's house in Ifakara, however, Freyvogel spent some months in London with the malariologist Percy C.C. Garnham, whose discovery of the liver stage of the malaria parasite secured him a place in the annals of the history of malaria.[55]

As we will see later, the members of the Capuchin mission were not only actively involved in the research process, but sufficiently open to integrate a Protestant and exponent of a secular scientific community into their religious social life. As Freyvogel himself recalled, the regulations that structured daily life at the station were vital in providing stability in a somewhat chaotic African world. Days started at 6:00 a.m. with morning prayer in the nearby church; an hour later, all gathered for breakfast, which consisted of a bowl of milk and some maize and bananas. From there, ev-

---

55   H. E. Shortt, P. C. C. Garnham, *Pre-erythrocytic Stage in Mammalian Malaria*, in: Nature, Vol. 161, 1948, p. 126.

eryone rushed to their highly specialized daily work: one brother was responsible for the workshop, another for cattle-rearing, a third supervised the construction of the St. Francis Hospital, and so on. When the church bells sounded at noon, the brothers would gather at the church. After prayers, there was lunch, with lively discussions. Lunch was followed by a siesta and, after coffee at 3:00 p.m., everyone would return to their daily tasks. At 6:00 p.m., dinner was served, which was normally extended into an informal gathering on the baraza until 10:00 p.m., when the generators went off and the mission station was plunged into darkness.[56]

Malaria and the "Laboratory of Progress"

Scientific work did not enjoy the same predictability that the Catholics could attain through the structuring of their missionary lives, but was constantly destabilized by the unpredictability of the African field. Freyvogel traveled to Ifakara with two pressing research questions in mind: firstly, he wanted to investigate the impact of high altitudes on the course of malaria infection and secondly (more generally), he was eager to acquire a more in-depth understanding of mosquito behavior. This research program fitted well into the general research setting of the STI and was closely tied to a larger malaria research group working in Basel. In the 1950s, with the assistance of Alexander von Muralt – who was in charge of the Jungfraujoch research laboratories in the Bernese Alps – STI scientists were investigating the influence of high altitudes on the course of infection in chicken malaria (*Plasmodium gallinaceum*).[57] Avian models were key to malaria research from the 1930s up until 1948, when rodent malaria (*Plasmodium berghei*) superseded *P. gallinaceum* as one of the most productive models in malaria research.[58] *P. gallinaceum* was especially attractive because of

56 Interview with Thierry A. Freyvogel, 21 January 2010.
57 Adelheid Herbig-Sandreuter, *Untersuchungen über den Einfluss des Höhenklimas auf Hühnermalaria (*Plasmodium gallinaceum *Brumpt)*, in: Acta Tropica, Vol. 10, No. 1, 1953, pp. 1–27; Thierry Freyvogel, *Zur Frage der Wirkung des Höhenklimas auf den Verlauf akuter Malaria. Malaria in tiefer und mittlerer Höhenlage. Untersuchungen in endemischen Gebieten Tanganyikas*, PhD Study University of Basel, Basel 1955; Rudolf Geigy, Thierry Freyvogel, *On the Influence of High Altitudes on the Course of Infection of Chicken Malaria (*P. gallinaceum*)*, in: Acta Tropica, Vol. 11, No. 2, 1954, pp. 167–171.
58 Leo Slater, *War and Disease*, p. 41.

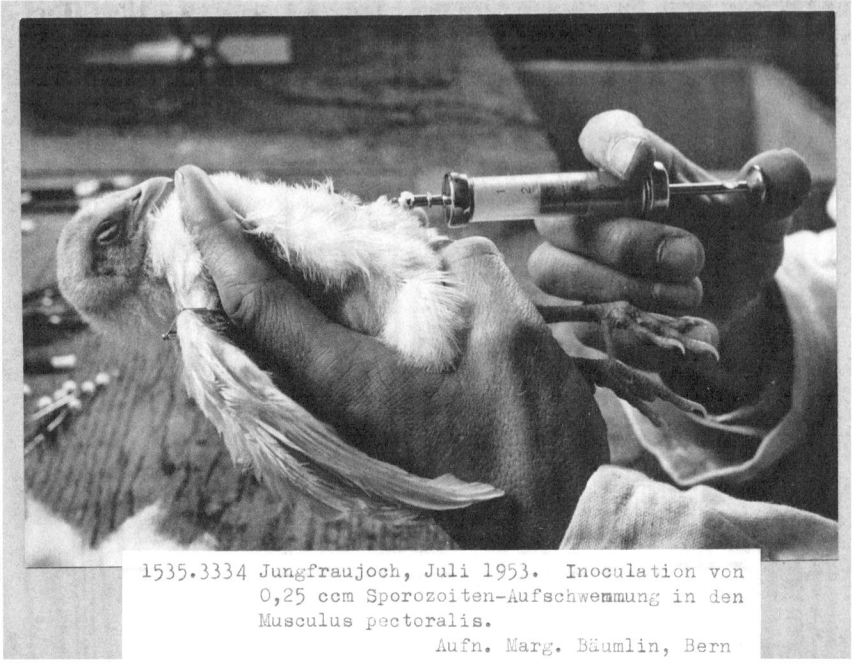

1535.3334 Jungfraujoch, Juli 1953.   Inoculation von
0,25 ccm Sporozoiten-Aufschwemmung in den
Musculus pectoralis.
Aufn. Marg. Bäumlin, Bern

Investigating the impact of high altitudes on the course of malaria at Jungfraujoch, 1953, Archive STI

the availability of its host, as well as its adaptability to a number of different hosts. Over time, avian malarias became the blueprint for mapping the disease in humans. Freyvogel's work in Ifakara involved two changes: firstly, he transferred the "experimental system" (Hansjörg Rheinberger) applied in the Bernese Alps and the STI to the rolling hills of Ulanga District and, secondly, he exchanged chickens for primates. However, the experimental work with primates, in particular, proved difficult. In order to make the animals more susceptible to malaria infection, Freyvogel had to excise the spleen and infect them with *Plasmodium cynomolgi* – a special strain he received from London. Freyvogel's experimental work was deeply anchored within the local community of Ifakara. The monkeys he used were captured by residents of Ifakara, who had been informed at mass about the Swiss scientists' needs.[59] At the operating table, Freyvogel

59   FTAF, Thierry Freyvogel, Lettres d'Ifakara, 19 July 1956, p. 2.

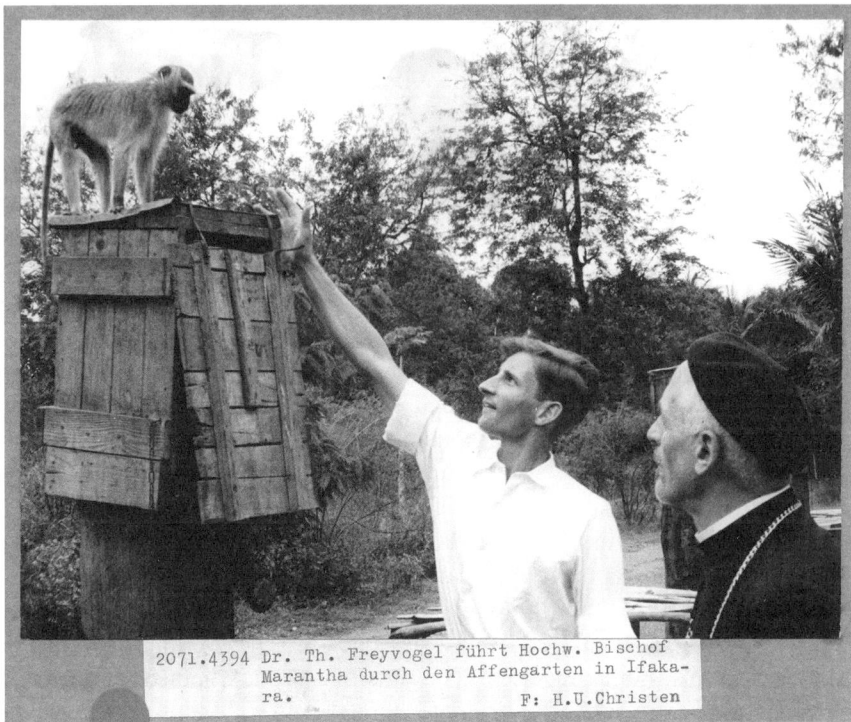

2071.4394 Dr. Th. Freyvogel führt Hochw. Bischof Marantha durch den Affengarten in Ifakara.   F: H.U.Christen

Thierry Freyvogel, Edgar Maranta and primate, Ifakara, 1950s, Archive STI

was assisted by African helpers: "some of whom were not clumsy at all. My assistant learned to anesthetize the monkey while I was performing the operations. Another one has now reached the stage that I can dare to stay away from the laboratory if I am sick or – what will hopefully be the case more often – away on business."[60] Despite all this valuable assistance, liver infection was never achieved in the primates. In addition, the logistical problems inherent in moving the animals to higher spots on the surrounding mountains and keeping them in captivity proved to be too challenging for the experimental work to be successful.

Studying mosquito behavior – the second item on Freyvogel's research agenda – was no less troublesome. Despite the numerous breeding sites of *Anopheles gambiae* that he encountered in Ulanga's wilderness, the mosquitoes could not be bred under laboratory conditions. Day after day, he

60   Ibid.

visited the houses of local residents to collect mosquitoes from the tattered
bed-nets. He brought them into his lab, as well as the larvae he found in
many wells between Ifakara and the Kilombero river, but they failed to reproduce:

> There was a time when I thought that it was probably because I fed them on animal
> blood instead of human blood, and so I went to the laboratory at night and let them
> draw my blood, but the wretched *Anopheles gambiae* refused to reproduce. Even
> today I don't know why this was so. It's just not easy to breed *Anopheles gambiae*
> under laboratory conditions.[61]

One of the reasons for the difficulties encountered was the simple fact that
Freyvogel's activities were performed while the laboratory was still under
construction. Supported by the Capuchins and African assistants, construction proceeded at a slow pace, as most of the building materials had to be
transported from Dar es Salaam to Ifakara, and progress was impeded by
the local climatic conditions. For Freyvogel, Ifakara was not just the building site for STI's future field research headquarters, but a "living laboratory" where Africans' ability to learn and to adopt Western rationality and
technology could be studied. He always declared the training of Africans
to be one of his main concerns.[62] His musings about whether the seeds of
Western rationality would germinate on African soil were prompted by
cultural preconceptions widespread on the European continent. On one occasion, for instance, Freyvogel came across an article by the Swiss psy-
choanalyst Fritz Morgenthaler – one of the founding fathers of ethnopsy-
choanalysis, who gained wide recognition through his book *Die Weissen
denken zuviel*.[63] In the article, published in the cultural magazine *Du*,
Morgenthaler argued that Africans cannot be trained, but only "drilled".
Freyvogel disagreed: his own experience working with African assistants
at the operating table and during the construction of the laboratory proved
the contrary:

> One of my assistants wears a pith helmet only when we are working under the
> burning sun for hours. So he has obviously understood the meaning of this hat,
> even though its use has not been recorded in the tradition of the local tribes. Many

---

61 Interview with Thierry A. Freyvogel, 21 January 2010.
62 (FTAF), Lettre d'Ifakara, 26 March 1956, p. 1.
63 Paul Parin, Fritz Morgenthaler, Goldy Parin-Matthèy, *Die Weissen denken zuviel. Psy-
    choanalytische Untersuchungen bei den Dogon in Westafrika*, Zurich 1963.

more examples of this ability to learn could be added, even where abstract thinking is involved. How else can the existence of Julius Nyerere, the leader of the Tanganyika African National Union, be explained? This is not to deny that Africans are deeply rooted in their traditional beliefs, but there is no doubt either that the impact of these beliefs is waning. I think that one of the reasons why Africans are denied access to abstract thinking lies in the fact that most of them live in a "me-you relationship" with the natural world, whereas we are used to emphasizing a "subject-object relationship". For Africans, things are imbued with life; they have their own will and temperament. For them, things cannot easily be manipulated as we are used to doing.[64]

It is not without a certain irony that Freyvogel adduced the wearing of one of the most potent symbols of colonial rule as evidence that Tanzanians would be able to adapt Western technologies and finally prove to be ripe for political self-determination. Freyvogel related his observations to wider political events on the global scene. He was especially interested in the question to what extent Europe could serve as a future model for African development. Freyvogel was convinced that Europe's influence could only be maintained through a moral and spiritual renewal at home. One telling indicator of the postindependence world order was the singular failure of the colonial government's efforts to date to develop and lift up the African population. While Freyvogel praised the missionaries' long-standing commitment and dedication to the material and moral improvement of the African rural community, he was shocked by British administrators' indifference to the development of "their" territory. In his diary, he noted ironically: "The administrators' lack of imagination and initiative is really admirable, and it is annoying to see how much money is wasted just in order to prevent budget cuts for the next year. The various missionary societies are doing much more for education and training [of Africans] than does the colonial government."[65] Freyvogel's comments on late colonial policies have to be interpreted against the backdrop of a rising nationalist movement in Ulanga District during the 1950s. Even though TANU only slowly gained a foothold in the district, many signs of the coming political turmoil were detectable, and some were recognized by Freyvogel. The 1950s not only saw the arrival of a new generation of administrators and the replacement of the ideology of indirect rule with the new concept of local government. The decade was also marked by local workers' claims for higher wages and a se-

---

64   FTAF, Lettre d'Ifakara, 5 August 1957, p. 1.
65   FTAF, Freyvogel, Tagebuch 1, pp. 70–71.

ries of protests which, according to Freyvogel, escalated into "strike-mania".[66] Even though most of what was achieved fell short of the protesters' expectations, the political movement had an impact on the organization of missionary work in Ifakara. In 1957, the mission raised workers' wages, while at the same time reducing the working week from five to four days and discharging nonessential staff.[67] Political consciousness impaired mission life in various ways. On several occasions, mission buildings were deliberately set on fire; Father Meinhard Inauen was harassed after having extolled the virtues of work at mass; and at a TANU meeting in 1960, attendees criticized the fact that African women were treated by dressers.[68] In a striking reversal of the Indian community's demands for better health services in the mid-1930s, it was now the African community that was no longer ready to accept the mission's unchallenged presence in the district, or the economic disparities existing between Africans and the Indian community. In the face of these political developments in the district, the Capuchin mission adopted various strategies, some more progressive than others from today's vantage point. One of these was the promotion of Capuchin-trained Elias Mchonde, who in 1956 was named Auxiliary Bishop of Dar es Salaam, and whose appointment was accompanied by Maranta's admonition: "If we want to have an African Church, then we must also have African clerics and African bishops. Otherwise, the Church remains a foreign body, and that we do not want."[69]

The dawning of political nationalism towards the end of the 1950s had a strong international dimension. As Ulrich Lohrmann observed, the period between 1954 and 1957 was the high tide of discussions between Julius Nyerere's TANU and UN officials.[70] In these interactions, Nyerere strengthened his position as the unchallenged leader of TANU. Moreover, he emerged as one of the most trusted African politicians in the West and sparked off discussions at the UN about when and under what conditions the trust territory should become independent, within a time frame of

66   Ibid., Freyvogel, Lettre d'Ifakara, 18 December 1957, p. 1.
67   Ibid., Freyvogel, Lettre d'Ifakara, 19 February 1957, p. 1.
68   Fonds Fritz Haerdi (FFH), Fritz Haerdi, Tagebuch 3 (9 February 1959), Tagebuch 2 (29 January 1959) and Tagebuch 5 (7 July 1960).
69   Cited in: Lorne Larson, *A History of Mahenge (Ulanga) District*, p. 331.
70   Ulrich Lohrmann, *Voices from Tanganyika. Great Britain, the United Nations and the Decolonization of a Trust Territory, 1946–1961*, Berlin 2007, p. 545; Cranford Pratt, *The Critical Phase in Tanzania 1945–1968. Nyerere and the Emergence of a Socialist Strategy*, Cambridge 1976.

about 20–25 years.[71] Freyvogel shared the admiration of a large number of Swiss politicians and scientists for Nyerere's education and modesty. Nevertheless, he regarded the planned schedule for Tanganyikan independence as unrealistic and as one of the UN decisions taken without sufficient knowledge of local realities:

> Anyway I would be blind if I did not admit that the country is undergoing a huge and accelerating development. I am also curious to see whether or not the country will be independent in twenty-five years as planned, and how the Africans will rule themselves. I think this is one of the UN's objectives that has been decided upon on the basis of a thin body of knowledge. Given the fact that, intellectually, even the Europeans and Americans have hardly been able to cope with scientific and technological progress, becoming more and more slaves of their own innovations, how could one expect the Africans to be able to adapt to our culture within sixty-five years, so as to be competitive as independent states? On the other hand, I am very interested to see what the Africans are going to do with our culture, with which they are now constantly confronted. As far as one can retrace the history of Black Africa, the Africans have always brought home elements from other continents, but have assimilated all the intruders and transformed these imported cultures into something new and typically Black – *qui vivra verra*.[72]

According to Freyvogel, the measure of whether or not the country was ripe for independence was the Tanganyikans' ability to adapt to Western culture and to master Western technology. However, the relationship between the West and the "rest" has always been more complex and multifaceted than would fit into the model of one-way diffusion of Western science to Third World countries implicit in the writings of George Basalla and others.[73] The transfer of Western scientific models to the tropics has not always been successful, as the difficulties encountered in Freyvogel's fieldwork demonstrate. Swiss scientists also borrowed extensively from local knowledge, as illustrated in particular by the case of Fritz Haerdi.

---

71   Ulrich Lohrmann, *Voices from Tanganyika*, p. 547; Susan C. Crouch, *Western Responses to Tanzanian Socialism, 1967–83*, Aldershot 1987; Ali A. Mazrui, *Tanzaphilia*, in: Transition, Vol. 31, 1967, pp. 20–26.
72   FTAF, Freyvogel, Lettre d'Ifakara, 8 July 1956, pp. 1–2.
73   George Basalla, *The Spread of Western Science. A Three-Stage Model Describes the Introduction of Modern Science into any Non-European Nation*, in: Science, Vol. 156, No. 3775, 1967, pp. 611–622; Ilana Löwy, *Yellow Fever in Rio de Janeiro and the Pasteur Institute Mission (1901–1905). The Transfer of Science to the Periphery*, in: Medical History, Vol. 34, 1990, pp. 144–163.

The Pitfalls of Local Knowledge

Africans were not just executors of scientific instructions or passive objects of study. As has been shown, Freyvogel's work was deeply embedded within local village life. Villagers provided him with vital study material, and laboratory assistants were crucial during operations and in the construction of the lab space. But medical research did not allow for extensive exchanges between different knowledge systems. Freyvogel attempted to show how Western malaria models work in the tropics, and the laboratory – however destabilized by the tropical environment – derives from a Western idea of the locus of scientific production. The fact that science in the tropics was constantly jeopardized and prone to failure was a lesson also learned by pharmacist Fritz Haerdi, who arrived in Ifakara in 1958.

Haerdi's investigations of the botanical aspects of traditional healing had their origins in a list of medicinal plants compiled by the Baldegg Sister Arnolda Kury, the pioneer of Swiss medical services in Ifakara. When Sister Arnolda (as she was known) started her work as a midwife in Ifakara in the 1920s, the health infrastructure was still very rudimentary: "Fearlessly, day or night, she would pedal, walk or wade to the houses of the women giving birth, and she slowly acquired the unshakeable trust of the Christians, Muslims and heathens."[74] Credited with saintly attributes, she attended the births of almost two generations in Ulanga District, had a good word for everyone and a special affection for all those suffering from leprosy or tuberculosis.[75] On her visits to the homes of women in labor or the sick, she was accompanied by Hermes Mlaganile, who had already served as a dresser under the German colonial administration.[76] Given the limited availability and impact of Western medicine, Sister Arnolda informed herself about the properties of medicinal plants and integrated local "vernacular knowledge" into her own treatment methods.[77] Over the years, her compendium listed over 100 medicinal plants, including their local names and applications.[78] While local "traditional knowledge" trav-

---

74   FTAF, Freyvogel, Lettre d'Ifakara, 4 September 1962.
75   Ibid.
76   Interview with Fritz Haerdi, 12 November 2010.
77   The notion of "vernacular science" is from Helen Tilley and suggests "the translation and, more important, appropriation of select dimensions of vernacular knowledge into scientific worldviews". See: Tilley, *Global Histories, Vernacular Science*, p. 117.
78   Fritz Haerdi, *Die Eingeborenen-Heilpflanzen des Ulanga-Distriktes Tanganjikas (Ostafrika)*, in: Acta Tropica (Supplementum 8), Basel 1964, p. 9.

eled between different epistemologies, the compendium itself fell into the hands of Rudolf Geigy, who asked Fritz Haerdi to undertake an exact classification of medicinal plants in Ulanga District. Haerdi's studies in Tanganyika were financed by J. R. Geigy AG, which had an interest in the chemical properties of natural products:

> You must see, until that moment no one had yet made an inventory of what belonged to the field of traditional medicine. I just arrived at the right moment, when you still could worm the information bit by bit out of the population. Later, with the rise of nationalism, it was much more difficult. But when they [the Africans] started accusing the West of stealing their things – which is not true of course – I was no longer in Ifakara.[79]

The appropriation of information involved a complex process of negotiation between the Western scientist and his African assistants. Hermes Mlaganile was as indispensable for Haerdi's botanical studies as he had been to Sister Arnolda. He was the "door opener", as he knew everyone and everyone knew that he had worked with Sister Arnolda. He introduced Haerdi to the traditional healers working in the region, and to a group of people well versed in botany. They were equally vital in assisting Haerdi on his expeditions through the country. As Haerdi recalls, he would never have left the mission station without someone who could repair his car in case of a breakdown or who was sufficiently familiar with the natural environment to avoid encounters with wild animals. On the one hand, intermediaries such as Hermes Mlaganile occupied a powerful position within Ulanga's society, given their ability to travel and to mediate between different epistemologies. On the other hand, their close relationships with the Europeans laid them open to all sorts of accusations. On November 3, 1959, one of Haerdi's collaborators was attacked by a group of armed villagers from Ilungwa. He was accused of having made an agreement with vampires and was believed to have come to the village to kidnap people. Similar vampire stories had already been noted by Freyvogel, who reported people's belief that Europeans drew their blood in order to fuel airplanes back in Europe. Historian Luise White invites us to interpret such rumors not primarily as African "superstition", but as an indication of: "the world of power and uncertainty in which Africans have lived in this century. Their very falseness is what gives them meaning; they are a way

---

79   Interview with Fritz Haerdi, 12 November 2010.

of talking that encourages a reassessment of everyday experience to address the workings of power and knowledge and how regimes use them."[80]

The privileged social position of African assistants – deriving from new sources of income through collaboration with Europeans – had to be traded off against a new role within their own societies, where the history of the colonial encounter was being played out. However, the position of the Swiss scientists in this complex scientific transaction was not necessarily one of strength. Haerdi's language skills at the beginning of his stay were only rudimentary, and he could never be sure what kind of information his assistants were conveying or concealing, deliberately or not. He referred to these issues on several occasions. On November 16, 1959, for instance, he noted: "Joseph once again made difficulties: he claimed not to know a specific tree, even though he had presented it to me several times before as 'dawa' [drug]. Sometimes I am really not sure whether he is trying to mess around with me or not."[81] Haerdi used various strategies to cope with the uncertainties of the cultural encounter: "Very often I double-checked the information and showed the specimens to different persons, and so I got to know what it really was."[82] However, this double-checking did not prevent him from mixing up different plant specimens, as he was informed by specialists in Nairobi or at Kew Gardens (London), where he sent his collections for exact classification.[83] While his African assistants had to cope with their ambivalent intermediary roles, Haerdi transformed his relative position of weakness into one of strength by mediating between different scientific fields. His expeditions through rural Ulanga District were never merely botanical but also involved the provision of medical treatment for the local population. On September 10, 1958, Haerdi diagnosed the community of a small village in the district as mostly suffering from "worms and costiveness".[84] Swelling of the glands was also widespread among his patients, and he was especially concerned with the treatment of small children.[85] Once, on his way to Kisawasawa (a small hamlet north of Ifakara), he stopped at the house of a relative of

---

80   Luise White, *Speaking with Vampires*, p. 43.
81   FFH, Fritz Haerdi, Afrika-Tagebuch, IV, 6 August 1959–20 March 1960, entry for 16 November 1959.
82   Interview with Fritz Haerdi, 12 November 2010.
83   Ibid.
84   FFH, Fritz Haerdi, Afrika-Tagebuch II, 1 September 1958–5 February 1959, entry for 10 September 1958.
85   Ibid.

one of his assistants, who was suffering from severe pneumonia. The family members asked for medication because the patient did not seem to be in a condition to be moved to a hospital. Haerdi rushed back to Ifakara to get drugs, but, as he noted in his diary: "It is very questionable whether I can help. I will give them some instructions for a cure. Otherwise there is nothing I can do."[86] The strategies employed by Africans and Swiss scientists to deal with the uncertainties and misunderstandings of the colonial encounter were thus strikingly similar: Haerdi's medical efforts reflect Rudyard Kipling's notion of the "white man's burden" – seeking to treat patients with virtually no means of doing so but just because he believed that it was expected of him. This self-ascribed role still reverberates today. As Haerdi confirmed: "Listen, as a European, I was automatically the trustworthy source of information, which obliged me to do the triage … and I always carried enough drugs around with me and knew what they were good for. And then you gave some aspirin, knowing that it would not necessarily improve the condition, but the patient was satisfied."[87]

For those who wish to analyze the practices of science in categories of "weak" and "strong", it is safe to say that botanical and medical research in the 1950s was contested knowledge. The Swiss Capuchin mission, far from being the powerful protagonist in health care delivery, was just one among many providers of health care in the district. Science's strength, however, lay in its ability to draw on various sources of trust and legitimacy. As Fritz Haerdi demonstrated, scientists apparently found it easy to shift from botany to medicine, from the study of plants to the treatment of people. Science and medicine in the 1950s was not effective in terms of its impact on people or its ability to restore health, but in promoting the circulation of people and objects around the world, which compensated for science's weaknesses on the ground:

> As a European – and this is the case everywhere in Africa – you have to have a certain stock of things that you can deliver. It is assumed that a white person has so many skills, even though this is not true, but what can you do?[88]

---

86 FFH, Fritz Haerdi, Afrika-Tagebuch IV, 6 August 1959–20 March 1960, entries for 1/2/3 September 1959.
87 Interview with Fritz Haerdi, 12 November 2010.
88 Ibid.

Inventorizing and Improving Africa: Swiss Science in the Field

This chapter has argued that the different social and political realities encountered by Swiss scientists in Côte d'Ivoire and Tanganyika gave rise to two particular paradigms of field research – discovery and improvement. The first concept applies to the CSRS in Côte d'Ivoire. Unable or unwilling to join in the French project of valorization of their colony, Swiss scientists in Adiopodoumé believed they had entered an earthly paradise. They lived "from hand to mouth", as Urs Rahm recalled, filling scientific gaps by naming and describing new species, creating scientific collections and providing Swiss scientific institutions with exotic specimens. In so doing, they prepared the ground for the scientific careers they would pursue on returning to Switzerland. The paradise metaphor also applied to the social realm: the political context of decolonization and nationalist agitation in Côte d'Ivoire was considered a French affair and hardly commented on.

Local networks and the process of decolonization in Tanganyika had a different impact on Swiss knowledge production in Ifakara, where the prospect of embarking on a "civilizing mission" seemed more realistic. One of the main characteristics of science in the field was its weakness, as well as its local rootedness. Despite the cautious attempts to establish the laboratory as the preferred site of medical research, the field as a space of "cultural translations" took precedence over laboratory work.[89] The uncertainties of field research matched the openness of the political process of decolonization in Tanganyika. In striking contrast to the "Franco-African familiarity" which characterized France's postcolonial relations with Africa, Britain's neglect of Tanganyika left Swiss scientists musing about its uncertain future.[90] For researchers such as Thierry Freyvogel, science became the lens through which African progress could be studied. As we will see in the next chapter, on the eve of independence, Tanganyika became one of the favored targets of the international aid industry, in which Switzerland played a prominent role.

89 Henrika Kuklick, Robert Kohler, *Introduction*, in: Kuklick and Kohler (eds.), Science in the Field, Osiris, Vol. 11, 1996, pp. 1–14, here: p. 4.
90 Guillaume Lachenal, *Franco-African Familiarities. A History of the Pasteur Institute of Cameroon, 1945–2000*, in: Mark Harrison, Margaret Jones and Helen Sweet (eds.), From Western Medicine to Global Medicine. The Hospital Beyond the West, New Delhi 2009, pp. 441–444.

Chapter 4
The Charitable Impulse: Development and Nutritional Research in Switzerland and Africa

This chapter turns away from the scientific practices that were central to the Swiss presence in late-colonial Côte d'Ivoire and Tanganyika to focus on the rise of the development apparatus in Switzerland, the emergence of a new dispositive with its own set of rules and practices, and the role played by the Swiss Tropical Institute (STI) and global charities in the new development paradigm. One of the main features of the new era was a strong diversification of the players who strategically placed themselves in – or were driven into – the web of development practices. Though their reasons for doing so varied, they all shared the belief that African societies must and could be transformed through the application of Western techno-science. There is a tendency, now all too familiar, to emphasize the faith in the transformative power of DDT or "miracle seeds" not only to revolutionize Third World agriculture, but also to set "backward" farmers on the path to modernity. It is, however, important to emphasize this because the lessons learned in the 1960s and the unfulfilled wishes of technoscience need to be borne in mind in order to understand what happened in the 1990s, when talk of "transforming societies" or "eradicating disease" was replaced by "improving health systems with the scarce resources available" or "cost-sharing" – the latter almost a faith in itself.

In what follows, it is argued that Switzerland occupied a privileged space in the global politics of the 1960s, unified by the belief in technological progress but divided by ideological differences. Switzerland's un-blemished (colonial) past and its humanitarian reputation made it a favorite partner for new African governments seeking to overcome development discrepancies and embark on substantial trade relations. However, as indicated in the previous chapter, Switzerland's opportunities to enter the post-colonial African stage were constrained by the contingencies of colonial histories and postcolonial actor constellations. While Swiss scientists' concerns about development and modernization in Tanganyika were followed by large-scale Swiss development projects in Tanzania, the ongoing French presence in Côte d'Ivoire inhibited such activities in the West African country. It should also be recognized that, in the context of global development efforts, the term "Switzerland" needs to be defined more precisely. Even after the creation of the official Swiss development agencies in the early 1960s, it was private-sector players such as the STI, the pharmaceutical industry, or the food giant Nestlé who were among the first to engage in development practices in the African health and agricultural sectors.

"A New Ethic of Giving"

In the 1950s. the landscape of Switzerland's charitable work – traditionally the domain of private organizations – was reconfigured. Charity took on a broader meaning, and development was considered a crucial instrument of Swiss foreign policy and an effective ideological weapon in global Cold War politics.[1] In the 1950s, financial and technical aid was limited to multilateral financial support for the UN Development Program (UNDP), as well as Swiss expert missions to India and Nepal.[2] The rise of the Swiss development apparatus, and the politicization and internationalization of development, was closely related to the process of decolonization sweeping through what was then known as the Third World. The Bandung Conference of 1955 – where 29 Asian and African nations unanimously opposed colonial rule and articulated their wishes for a new world order – marked a turning point in Switzerland's perceptions of global power relations. As a country with a "small open economy", Switzerland was traditionally deeply enmeshed in world trade and subject to the vagaries and inconsistencies of world markets.[3] With the process of decolonization, Switzerland gradually reinter-

---

1   Christoph Graf, *Die Schweiz und die Dritte Welt. Die Anerkennungspraxis und Beziehungsaufnahme der Schweiz gegenüber dekolonisierten aussereuropäischen Staaten sowie die Anfänge der schweizerischen Entwicklungshilfe nach 1945*, in: Studien und Quellen, No. 12, Bern 1986, pp. 37–112, here: p. 89; Ulrich Kägi, *Die Schweizerische Entwicklungshilfe*, in: Entwicklungsländer (BRD), Vol. 5, 1960, pp. 150–152, here: p. 150; Regula Renschler, *Die Entwicklung der Entwicklungshilfe zur Entwicklungspolitik*, in: Richard Gerster (ed.), Die Entdeckung der Schweiz. 25 Jahre Helvetas. Jubiläumsschrift, Basel 1980, pp. 113–123, here: p. 113; Monica Kalt, *Tiermondismus in der Schweiz der 1960er und 1970er Jahre.*

2   René Holenstein, *Wer langsam geht kommt weit*, p. 49; Rolf Wilhelm, *Gemeinsam unterwegs. Eine Zeitreise durch 60 Jahre Entwicklungszusammenarbeit Schweiz-Nepal*, Bern 2012.

3   Peter J. Katzenstein, *Corporatism and Change. Austria, Switzerland and the Politics of Industry*, New York 1984, p. 24.

preted its restrictive policy of neutrality, which – as one of the major ideological pillars of Swiss identity during World War II – lingered on in the 1950s. Development aid was not just a response to the feelings of solidarity awakened among large parts of the Swiss population, but a means of overcoming Switzerland's postwar isolation on the global political stage.

However, the concept of development did not command a consensus, as regards its content or the practical political implications for Switzerland's relations with the Third World. It was made up of affirmations of solidarity and Switzerland's humanitarian tradition, the belief that the achievements of the Swiss welfare state after 1945 should be applied globally, and also less altruistic political and economic considerations.[4] Perhaps the most widely held assumption was that African, Asian and Latin American populations were living in "poverty" – commonly defined as a lack of material wealth. The solution to this state of deprivation was the transfer of technology to these countries, as well as the re-establishment of sound trade relations, from which economic growth would follow. The assumption of congruency between development aid and trade relations was reflected in the institutional setup of development aid in Switzerland. Before 1960, responsibility for technical aid was shared among the Federal Office for Industry, Trade and Labor (BIGA), the Department of Economic Affairs (EVD) and the International Organizations Division (part of the Department of Foreign Affairs), which often led to disputes about the allocation of rights and duties.[5] This situation changed in 1960, with the creation of the Service for Technical Cooperation (DftZ), which a year later was placed under the direction of the Department of Foreign Affairs and the Federal Council's delegate for technical cooperation. The main architect of this new conception of development aid was Federal Councillor Max Petitpierre, for whom technical cooperation was a highly political endeavor and who tried to shift the emphasis from multilateral aid towards more bilateral and project-based development work.[6] Petitpierre's vision was carried a step further in 1961, with the Swiss parliament's approval of a global credit for development aid amounting to CHF 60 million over a three-year period, and in 1963, with

---

4   René Holenstein, *Was kümmert uns die Dritte Welt*, pp. 91–98.
5   Branka Fluri, *Umbruch in Organisation und Konzeption. Die technische Zusammenarbeit beim Bund, 1958–1970*, in: Peter Hug and Beatrix Mesmer (eds.), Von der Entwicklungshilfe zur Entwicklungspolitik, Studien und Quellen, Vol. 19, Bern 1993, pp. 382–39, here: p. 382.
6   Ibid., p. 383; Daniel Trachsler, *Bundesrat Max Petitpierre. Schweizerische Aussenpolitik im Kalten Krieg*, 1945–1961, Zurich 2011.

the appointment of August R. Lindt to replace Hans Keller as the Federal Council's delegate for technical cooperation.[7]

A former Swiss ambassador to Washington and UN High Commissioner for Refugees, Lindt had to maneuver carefully between the concept of neutrality (in the sense of equal treatment of Third World petitioners) and the financial constraints that necessitated a choice of future beneficiaries of Swiss development aid. Initially, the criteria for determining who was most in need and should therefore benefit from Swiss attention were not yet clearly defined.[8] Rolf Wilhelm, one of the pioneers of Swiss development aid, who joined the DftZ in 1962, recalled:

> evenings … sitting at the round table and in front of the map of Africa, contemplating and considering where the best chances and the biggest obstacles would lie. What were the arguments for or against the various African coastal countries where Swiss missionary societies were also active? What was the position of the former colonial powers? What were the arguments for or against Guinea, and what about the Sahel country Mali? There was a lot to discuss though and I often returned home very late.[9]

In the discussions held in front of the empty map of Africa, economic and political considerations did not necessarily prevail over other criteria. Taking the example of Rwanda, historian Lukas Zürcher has identified the degree of identification with the target population as a vital factor in the targeting of development aid. Rwanda became a showcase for Swiss development not least because the more Swiss development planners studied the character of this African country, the more it seemed to reflect Switzerland's own identity – a small, mountainous country with modest politicians and a comparatively large agricultural sector.[10] History also played

---

7   Rolf Wilhelm et al. (eds.), *August R. Lindt, Patriot und Weltbürger*, Bern, Stuttgart, Wien 2002.

8   DftZ employee Roy Preiswerk listed several positive criteria for possible Swiss support, including the special role Switzerland could play as a neutral state, limited territorial expanse, geographical proximity to Switzerland, the existence of a Swiss community in the country concerned and existing activities of Swiss private organizations. See: Roy Preiswerk, *La coopération technique. Dimension nouvelle de la politique étrangère Suisse,* in: Annuaire Suisse de Science Politique, Vol. 6, 1966, pp. 75–97, here: p. 90.

9   Rolf Wilhelm, *Aus der Anfangszeit der schweizerischen Entwicklungshilfe*, in: Wilhelm et al. (eds.), August R. Lindt, Patriot und Weltbürger, pp. 127–138, here: p. 129.

10 Lukas Zürcher, *"So fanden wir auf der Karte diesen kleinen Staat."* Globale Positionierung und lokale Entwicklungsfantasien der Schweiz in Rwanda in den 1960er Jahren, in: Büschel and Speich (eds.), Entwicklungswelten, pp. 275–309.

its part. Third World countries with which Switzerland had traditionally maintained ties automatically came into the focus of the DftZ. The selection of Tanganyika as one of the focal points for Swiss development aid was justified by the many Swiss missionary societies working in the country, as well as the comparatively large Swiss community (around 650 people).[11] The question of who should benefit from development aid overlapped with the more practical one of how such policies could be implemented. In addition to the selection of target societies, there was a concentration on core topics of Swiss expertise, such as agriculture, dairy farming, tourism and the hotel industry, banking and insurance, mechanical engineering, and public administration.[12]

Two points should be noted about the concept of Swiss development aid in the first years of the existence of the DftZ. Firstly, the health sector did not feature prominently as a domain of technical expertise. The improvement of people's well-being was considered charitable work and not readily compatible with the new credo of transfer of technical knowledge. Secondly, and equally importantly, the DftZ lacked the requisite expertise in most of the core areas mentioned above. This was acknowledged by the DftZ itself, which did not wish to challenge the many private organizations traditionally active in the field of international solidarity, and saw its function as that of subsidizing existing efforts undertaken by private players, such as the STI. August Lindt, a friend of Rudolf Geigy, was unambiguous about this point. At a meeting with representatives of private organizations in 1963, he declared:

> Because in Switzerland we lack the required personnel, it is of vital importance to collaborate closely with all the existing organizations and institutions, such as the Swiss Tropical Institute or the Graduate Institute of International Studies, as well as all the private organizations present at today's meeting.[13]

11 Schweizerisches Bundesarchiv Bern (BAR), E 2200.83 (A), 1983/26, 3, B. 8.6, Dienst für technische Zusammenarbeit, Agricultural Development (Lumemo), 1962–1963, August R. Lindt, Schweizerische technische Zusammenarbeit mit Tanganyika, 4 March 1963, pp. 1–2, here: p. 2.

12 Diplomatische Dokumente der Schweiz [Dodis], Notiz an Herrn Bundesrat Wahlen über Richtlinien für unsere technische Zusammenarbeit mit den Entwicklungsländern, Bern 12 February 1962, pp. 1–4, here: p. 4.

13 BAR, E 2200.83 (A), 1983/26, B 8, 771.1, Technische Zusammenarbeit 1961–1965, August R. Lindt, "Die bilaterale Entwicklungshilfe der Schweiz aus der Sicht des Eidgenössischen Politischen Departements." Referat von Dr. A. R. Lindt, Delegierter des Bundesrates für Technische Zusammenarbeit (Resumé), 28 May 1963, pp. 1–7, here: pp. 3–4.

Towards the end of the 1950s, the STI was at the forefront of Swiss development aid and about to become a close partner of the DftZ in planning and executing development projects, especially in Tanganyika. Rudolf Geigy and his collaborators at the institute were deeply drawn into the Third World euphoria that prevailed in Switzerland in the 1960s. Geigy was convinced that African decolonization would usher in a "new era in the history of mankind", and that the "unchallenged Western hegemony" in Africa would probably come to an end.[14] He saw his new concept of solidarity as divorced from economic and religious reasoning, which until then had loomed large in the arguments for development aid. In a lecture held in 1963, he stated:

> We have to see our aim in the creation of a new ethic of giving, driven neither by political or economic considerations nor by Christian values … The new giving I am talking about derives exclusively from a sense of international responsibility and the motive of bringing people closer together, as has been practiced successfully by the absolutely independent Red Cross through its long history. [15]

Like many others, Geigy strongly believed that the privileged West had a moral obligation to assist the undeveloped and the needy on the intricate paths towards modernity. In his publications, however, Geigy stressed that it was important not to exploit the hierarchies and unequal power balance inherent in this relationship: Switzerland's assistance should take place within an "atmosphere of trust" and be devoid of "pitiable dependence" and "submissive gratitude".[16] It is not suggested here that Geigy's emphasis on a new ethic of giving, devoid of political and economic interests, was mere rhetoric, or a more or less deliberate strategy to distance himself from the J. R. Geigy AG with which he was usually associated. It will be argued, however, that the development alliances he skillfully forged were held together by more than humanitarian motives. In 1960, Geigy initiated the establishment of the Basel Foundation for Aid to Developing Countries – involving the six pharmaceutical companies Ciba, Durand & Huguenin,

14 Rudolf Geigy, *Der Sprung in die Selbständigkeit. Entwicklungshilfe und Menschheitsproblem.* Rektoratsrede gehalten an der Jahresfeier der Universität Basel am 23. November 1962, Basel 1962, pp. 1–22, here: p. 4.
15 Entwicklungshilfe in Tanganjika. Ein Vortrag von Prof. Rudolf Geigy, in: Neue Zürcher Zeitung (NZZ), 5 December 1963.
16 Rudolf Geigy, *Lehrzentrum Ifakara in Südtansania. Völkerverbindende Entwicklungshilfe*, in: Basler Nachrichten, 31 January 1976.

J. R. Geigy AG, Hoffmann-La Roche, Lonza and Sandoz – whose deed of foundation expressed the wish to help underdeveloped countries, especially in the vital areas of medicine, hygiene and agriculture.[17]

The Basel Foundation for Aid to Developing Countries and the Rural Aid Center in Ifakara

In striking contrast to Rudolf Geigy, Arthur Wilhelm – Vice-President of Ciba and President of the Swiss Society of Chemical Industries (SGCI) – made no secret of the economic and political interests underlying the companies' possible engagement in Tanganyika. Wilhelm was well aware of the changing atmosphere in Switzerland and the political and social pressures facing private industry. Indeed, several Swiss companies had already highlighted their participation in the development sector. As early as 1949, Gebrüder Volkart in Winterthur embarked on a technical aid project under the direction of the newly established Volkart Foundation. The Swiss Foundation for Technical Development Aid was established in 1959, and both Ciba and Sandoz were already collective members of the Swiss Association for Technical Assistance (SHAG).[18] Ciba's vice-president shared the widespread view that it was in the newly independent African countries that the groundwork should be laid for future economic competitiveness, and the threat of an emerging communist ideology countered. In the company's newspaper, Wilhelm wrote:

> I don't want to call Switzerland's youth to the twentieth-century crusade in the underdeveloped countries. But I think that more young people – scientists, technicians and business people – should go to the front line of the struggle to develop Africa, if we are to retain our prestige in the world. Only in this way can we sharpen the weapons that we will so desperately need in the future battle for the markets of the free world.[19]

17 Firmenarchiv der Novartis AG, Bestand CIBA, RE 15.04.1, Basler Stiftung zur Förderung von Entwicklungsländern, März 1960-Februar 1963, Akten Prof. Dr. M. Staehelin, Stiftungsurkunde, p. 2.

18 Albert Matzinger, *Die Anfänge der schweizerischen Entwicklungshilfe 1948–1961*, Bern, Stuttgart 1991, p. 170.

19 Arthur Wilhelm, *Von den kulturellen Aufgaben Europas in Afrika*, in: Ciba-Blätter, Vol. 170, 1960, pp. 2–11, here: p. 8.

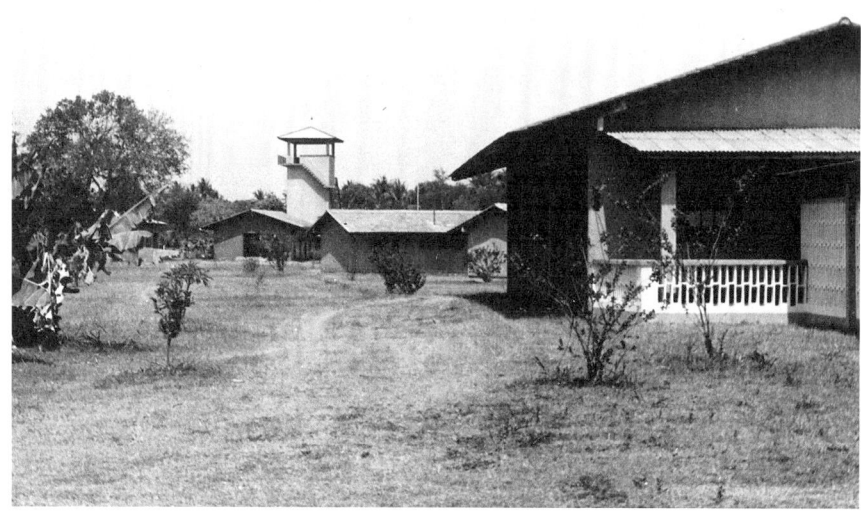

The Rural Aid Center (RAC) in Ifakara, 1960s, Archive STI

Since the battle evoked by Wilhelm was not just about economic transactions, but one that would ultimately be decided in the cultural sphere, European scientists, technicians and business people were the ideal phalanx to guarantee Africa's adaptation to Western values. According to Wilhelm, physicians were among the few foreigners in Africa "who enjoy the natives' respect" because they help them to "get rid of demons, charmers and sorcerers".[20] There was no doubt that the Western effort was wholehearted, but the outcome was uncertain. Were Africans capable of adapting to Western culture at all? Was the establishment of capitalist economic structures a wise strategy, or was it not more likely that nascent capitalist structures in Africa were especially liable to communist take-

20 Staatsarchiv Basel-Stadt (StABS), ED-REG 1c 190–2-8 (1), Ifakara Schulungszentrum 1959–1968, Ansprache Arthur Wilhelm anlässlich der 80. Generalversammlung der Schweizerischen Gesellschaft für Chemische Industrie, 27 October 1960, pp. 1–15, here: p. 7.

over?[21] Answers to these pressing questions were best to be found on the ground. In 1960, Geigy, Wilhelm, his wife Ria and Albert Meier (a young Ciba engineer) traveled to Tanganyika to discuss the chemical industry's development aspirations with Edgar Maranta, with high-ranking British officials and with the future Tanzanian president, Julius Nyerere.[22] The main reason for the journey was Geigy's proposal to the Basel Foundation to invest in the education of young Tanganyikans, especially in the fields of medicine and agriculture. One of the classical approaches to development widely adopted in the 1960s was to invite students to Switzerland, where – over a short period – they would acquire certain technical skills which could then be applied when they returned to their home countries. However, the members of the STI saw major weaknesses in this form of development aid – not least the risk that, having tasted the fruits of Swiss affluence, the young African scholars would remain in Europe or seek careers elsewhere, without feeling obliged to commit themselves to the economic and social advancement of their own countries.[23] More effective, in Geigy's eyes, was the concept of training on the spot, which he wanted to promote by creating a Rural Aid Center (RAC) in Ifakara, whose graduates would form the new middle class that the emerging nation urgently required.[24]

21 Firmenarchiv der Novartis AG, Bestand J. R. Geigy AG, VW 8, Protokoll Nr. 4/61 der Sitzung des Wirtschaftspolitischen Komitees, 16 August 1961, p. 1.

22 Rolf Wilhelm (in collaboration with Marcel Tanner and Thierry Freyvogel), *Das Projekt des* "Rural Aid Center" *in Ifakara, Tanzania*, [Typescript], 6 April 2004, pp. 1–9, here: p. 1.

23 Thierry Freyvogel, *Entwicklungshilfe in Tanganyika*. Separatdruck aus dem Schweizerischen Jahrbuch "Die Ernte", 1963, pp. 55–66, here: p. 64.

24 Rudolf Geigy, *Training on the Spot. Swiss Development Aid in Tanzania 1960–1976*, in: Acta Tropica, Vol. 33, No. 4, 1976, pp. 290–306; Rudolf Geigy, *Neue Aufgaben des Tropeninstituts,* in: Mitteilungsblatt der Tropenschule des Schweizerischen Tropeninstituts in Basel, No. 9, 1960, pp. 6–9; BAR, E 2003–03 (-), 1976/44, (Schweizerisches Tropeninstitut Basel), 1960–1963, Rudolf Geigy, Unmittelbare Entwicklungshilfe am Ort in Afrika. Vortrag gehalten am 17. Januar 1963 vor der Deutschen Afrika Gesellschaft und der Deutschen Parlamentarischen Gesellschaft in Bonn; Novartis Firmenarchiv, J. R. Geigy AG, SP 5, Spenden für Wohlfahrts- und Fürsorgeinstitutionen: Entwicklungshilfe/Entwicklungsländer 1960–1965, Arthur Wilhelm, Hilfe zugunsten von Entwicklungsländern (Exposé), Februar 1960, p. 10; BAR, E 2200.83 (A), 1983/26, 4, C 9.1, Rural Aid Center Ifakara, 1960–1965, Bericht über die Reise der Herren Dr. Arthur Wilhelm, CIBA, und Prof. Rudolf Geigy, Schweizerisches Tropeninstitut, zum Studium der in Ostafrika bestehenden Möglichkeiten für Schweizerische Entwicklungshilfe – zu Handen des Basler Initiativ-Komitees, 19 September 1960.

Building the Tanzanian Nation

As regards Switzerland's wish to train paramedical personnel in Ifakara, three points should be noted: firstly, Tanganyika remained dependent on foreign donors, and especially on Britain, in major areas of public life; secondly, there was a mismatch between Switzerland's focus on the middle class as the moral pillar of the nation and Nyerere's attempt to integrate the rural populace into the overall nation-building project; and thirdly, the Tanganyikan health sector in the early 1960s was characterized by acute deficiencies in manpower, training and finances. With regard to foreign relations and public services, Tanganyika's political independence in 1961 did not necessarily mean a decisive break with the past: until 1963 – when various Western policy decisions led to what historian Cranford Pratt has called "the loss of innocence" in Julius Nyerere's political thinking – Tanganyika's foreign relations were still very much focused on its former colonial master.[25] Tanganyika's continued dependence was apparent, given the ongoing British financial contributions to its former mandate territory, as well as the structure of public services, where several key positions remained in the hands of British experts. One of the prime examples of a dependence strategy in action is the World Bank report of 1961, whose economic recommendations were entirely based on the reflections of Western experts, and whose conclusions were more or less directly translated into the First Development Plan (1961–64).[26] While the implementation of an orthodox Western development model – with its fondness for exploiting the untapped potential of African agriculture – can be interpreted as a colonial legacy, the rural development discourse was unprecedented. As Michael Jennings has shown, the new African elite's emphasis on raising socioeconomic standards, as well as the "moral betterment" of the rural population in particular, marked a decisive shift from colonialism to the postcolony.[27] In contrast to Geigy's emphasis on strengthening the middle class through education, Nyerere's political project mainly focused on the underprivileged

---

25 Cranford Pratt, *The Critical Phase in Tanzania*.
26 International Bank for Reconstruction and Development (ed.), *The Economic Development of Tanganyika*, Baltimore 1961.
27 Michael Jennings, *"A Very Real War." Popular Participation in Development in Tanzania During the 1950s and 1960s*, in: The International Journal of African Historical Studies, Vol. 40, No. 1, 2007, pp. 71–95, here: p. 87; Michael Jennings, *We Must Run While Others Walk. Popular Participation and Development Crisis in Tanzania, 1961–9*, in: Journal of Modern African Studies, Vol. 41, No. 2, 2003, pp. 163–187.

rural population. Development in postindependence Tanganyika mainly meant rural development, which – in contrast to the European experience – was integral to discourses of citizenship and nationhood.

Health featured prominently in the nation-building discourse: the "new" Tanganyikan citizen was healthy and able to contribute physically to the creation of the nation. In presenting the new Medical Development Plan of 1963, the Minister for Health, Derek Bryceson, stated:

> There is too apart from humanitarian reasons, another very good reason for want-
> ing a healthy population. This is because we need every bit of energy we have to
> put to the task of building the nation. Building a nation is not a job to entrust to
> chronically sick people.[28]

The relationship between nation-building and health was not just that the nation, as an "imagined community",[29] was made up of healthy citizens, but equally that the moral requirements of citizenship called for individual efforts to build up a healthy nation. The postindependence development planners acknowledged the vital importance of expanding rural health care through newly built dispensaries and especially health centers; perhaps even more important, however, was that these facilities were to be "built as nation-building projects with a resultant financial saving in capital expenditure", as noted in the Medical Development Plan.[30] As well as serving the goal of national unification, however, the nation-building discourse was a means to legitimize an austerity program in health care spending, since the lion's share of rural health expenditure was to be covered by the local authorities. Not surprisingly, despite the declared aim of improving the health status of rural dwellers, health care expenditure in the immediate

28 Tanzania National Archive (TNA), 450/HE/1172, Medical Development Plan, 1963, Speech by the Hon. D. N. M. Bryceson, M. P., Minister for Health, p. 2.
29 Benedict Anderson, *Imagined Communities. Reflections on the Origin and Spread of Nationalism*, London, New York 1991.
30 TNA, 450/HE/1172, Medical Development Plan, Second Draft of the Medical Development Plan. A Report of the Medical Development Committee, pp. 1–10, here: p. 5. The importance of providing a sufficient number of rural health centers offering both curative and preventive services had already been acknowledged in 1956 and was reiterated in the widely cited report by sociologist Richard Titmuss; see: Richard M. Titmuss, *The Health Services of Tanganyika. A Report to the Government*, London 1964, pp. 57–58; M.P. Mandara, *Health Services in Tanzania. A Historical Overview*, in: G. M. P. Mwaluko et al. (eds.), Health and Disease in Tanzania, London, New York 1991, pp. 1–7, here: p. 5; Wilbert Chagula, Eleuther Tarimo, *Meeting Basic Health Needs in Tanzania*, in: Kenneth W. Newell (ed.), Health By the People, Geneva 1975, pp. 145–168, here: p. 149.

postindependence period fell short of expectations. Compared to sectors such as agriculture and industry, the funds directed to health in the Three Year Plan (1961–1964) and the first Five Year Plan (1964–1969) turned out to be meager.[31] Government spending on health was mainly absorbed by larger hospitals and curative services, thus cementing the often-deplored colonial legacy of rural-urban inequalities in the provision of health care in Tanzania.[32] Only with the second Five Year Plan (1969–1974) came the shift from wishful thinking to a real per-capita increase in health care spending and the channeling of funds to the establishment of medical facilities in the country's vast rural areas.

One of the areas clearly indicating the problems of the Tanzanian health sector in the early 1960s was the training and availability of health care personnel. With about twelve registered doctors in government service in 1961, the Tanzanian health service after colonialism essentially had to be started from scratch.[33] On the eve of independence, there were several different levels of health personnel, each trained according to their specific functions within the health system. On the lowest echelon was the rural medical aide, in charge of a rural dispensary and replacing what had been known as the tribal dresser. The next level was occupied by the medical assistant, responsible for the curative and preventive services offered by health centers. The training of medical assistants constantly gave rise to heated political debate. In the years following independence, politicians were more inclined to increase the number of African doctors than of medical assistants – who threatened the professional ethos of the former. Medical assistant courses were discontinued in 1962 but restarted six years later. Makerere University in Uganda was the only institution offering full medical degrees to Tanganyikans, Kenyans and Ugandans. In 1961, the Tanganyikan government planned to supplement Makerere by establishing a Medical School in Dar es Salaam, while at the same time closing down the Medical Assistants School at Muhimbili Hospital. The Medical School

31 John Iliffe, *East African Doctors. A History of the Modern Profession*, Cambridge 1998, p. 130; W. Kilama, A. M. Nhonoli, W. J. Makene, *Health care Delivery in Tanzania*, in: Gabriel Ruhumbika (ed.), Towards Ujamaa. 20 years of TANU leadership. A Contribution of the University of Dar es Salaam to the 20th Anniversary of TANU, Kampala 1974, pp. 191–217, here: p. 198.

32 Oscar Gish, *Planning the Health Sector. The Tanzanian Experience*, London 1975, p. 24; Meredeth Turshen, *The Political Ecology of Disease in Tanzania*, New Brunswick, N. J. 1984, p. 194.

33 John Iliffe, *East African Doctors*, p. 119.

was opened in 1963 and awarded medical diplomas – rather than medical degrees – to assistant medical officers. In 1968, the School was incorporated into the University of East Africa and became the Faculty of Medicine, University College, Dar es Salaam University of East Africa.[34]

The STI's Rural Aid Center had been heralded as a showcase of development, not only because it shifted the focus to the less developed peripheral rural regions, but particularly because it employed a specific governance structure, including existing health and research institutions in Ifakara.[35] Between July and October 1961, members of the STI trained 40 rural medical aides, who had been selected by the Ministry of Health. Until 1964, the training also included several courses enabling medical assistants to upgrade to assistant medical officers, as well as courses for health assistants, who were trained at the request of the Tanzanian government and, it would appear, against the wishes of the Basel Foundation.[36] STI members were proud to show urban dwellers arriving from Dar the African hinterland and to introduce them to the medical problems encountered in the Tanganyikan countryside; they were also proud to offer courses where the students worked in the clinic, in the lab and on expeditions to the Tanzanian bush.[37] Even though the curriculum was geared towards biology, clinical medicine, pathology, rural health and hygiene, and epidemiology were also key subjects. Special attention was given to practical courses in laboratory techniques and the chemical control of ectoparasites. But efforts to modernize the agricultural sector also commanded a consensus among the industrial sector, the Swiss Development Agency and Tanzanian nation-builders.

Development's Utopias: the Lumemo Project

From the outset, strengthening the health sector through an "army against misery, disease and death" was never considered the sole or most effi-

---

34 Kilama, Nhonoli, Makene, *Health care Delivery in Tanzania*, p. 206.

35 Jürg Bürgi, Al Imfeld, *Mehr geben, weniger nehmen. Geschichte der Schweizer Entwicklungspolitik und der Novartis Stiftung für Nachhaltige Entwicklung*, Zurich 2004.

36 Archive Swiss Tropical and Public Health Institute, Basel (ASTI), Courses 1966–1971, Die Basler Stiftung zur Förderung von Entwicklungsländern, pp. 1–2, here: p. 1.

37 Thierry Freyvogel, *The Work at the Rural Aid Center (RAC) Ifakara, Tanganyika*, in: Acta Tropica, Vol. 21, No. 1, 1964, pp. 91–95, here: p. 94.

cient way of promoting Tanzania's socioeconomic progress.[38] In the early 1960s, health expenditure lagged far behind investments in agriculture and industry, which were also considered the genuine development areas by the DftZ in Bern. The Swiss proposals, discussed with Archibald (Archie) Forbes – Permanent Secretary of the Ministry of Agriculture & Cooperative Development and a veteran of the Tanganyika groundnut scheme – during the visit of Geigy and Wilhelm in 1960, reveal the primacy of agriculture and the desire of the Basel Foundation to open up new markets for its chemical products. The prospects for this endeavor seemed especially favorable given that Imperial Chemical Industries (ICI) was losing ground in the East African pharmaceutical market.[39]

The cooperative movement that arose in Tanganyika in the mid-1950s became the cornerstone of the revitalization of rural areas, and it was these cooperatives, as social and economic units, that were regarded by the Basel Foundation as beneficial to the import and exploitation of Western science and technology.[40] Forbes requested that training for rural medical aides should be accompanied by special courses for members of the Ministry of Agriculture. In particular, he strongly supported courses in laboratory techniques and training in the application of insecticides for field assistants. He also proposed the creation of a mobile unit that was to tour the northern part of the country, training coffee farmers in various spraying techniques.[41] The expansion of the work of the RAC from medicine into agriculture was also enthusiastically supported by the DftZ. In 1961, the agency was puzzled by the fact that medical missions to the Third World did not appeal to young Swiss doctors, and a first attempt to send out health professionals to Tanganyika had to be abandoned owing to the

---

38 Rudolf Geigy, *Rural Medical Training at Ifakara. Swiss Help to Tanzania*, in: The Lancet, Vol. 285, No. 7400, 1965, pp. 1385–1387, here: p. 1385.

39 Novartis Firmenarchiv, J. R. Geigy AG, SP 5, Notiz zur Besprechung vom 8. Mai 1961 betreffend Entwicklungshilfe/Tanganjika, pp. 1–2.

40 For a description of the rise of the cooperative movement from the mid-1950s, see: Andrew Coulson, *Tanzania. A Political Economy*, Oxford 1982, pp. 60–69. Geigy himself initiated the creation of a cooperative in Ifakara, including the establishment of a rice-mill, at a total cost of CHF 200,000, to be disbursed by the Basel Foundation – see: Novartis Firmenarchiv CIBA, RE 15.04.11, Basler Stiftung zur Förderung von Entwicklungsländern, Protokolle der Stiftungsratssitzungen 1960–1982, Hilfe an Entwicklungsländer, Besprechung vom 27. April 1960, 10 Uhr, bei der CIBA Aktiengesellschaft, pp. 1–8, here: p. 6.

41 Ibid., Archibald Forbes, Training for Laboratory Work and Spraying, 25 March 1961, pp. 1–3.

small numbers of registered volunteers.[42] Switzerland naturally felt more at home with agriculture. In 1961, members of the DftZ and the pharmaceutical companies met in Bern to discuss a possible contribution by the Swiss government to the training of agricultural field assistants.[43] At this meeting, the Basel Foundation emphasized that it had already invested heavily in building up the RAC, and it was now the turn of the DftZ to cover the costs of training agricultural assistants.[44] An important role in these negotiations – and in the decision of the DftZ to support the scheme – was played by Friedrich Traugott Wahlen, who replaced Max Petitpierre as head of the Department of Foreign Affairs in 1961.

During World War II, Wahlen had been responsible for Swiss agricultural policy – the Wahlen Plan sought to systematically increase agricultural production and thus guarantee Switzerland's self-sufficiency. Before his election to the Swiss government, Wahlen served as Director of the FAO's Agricultural Division and later as its Deputy Director-General. He was familiar with Southern Tanzania. Only four years after the demise of A. T. Culwick's Ulanga Rural Development Scheme in 1951, the region once again came into the focus of colonial development planners – this time, however, with international assistance and imbued with the spirit of what James Scott has called "high modernism".[45] Thus, the discussions of the academic curriculum at the new RAC have to be seen in the broader, international context of foreign aid and socioeconomic changes in Ulanga District.

In 1955, the Tanganyikan government officially requested FAO experts to conduct a preliminary agricultural survey of the Rufiji basin; their report was submitted in 1961.[46] About 180 kilometers inland from the Indian

---

42 BAR, E 2200.83 (A), 1983/26, 3, B. 8.15.1, Experten, Spezialisten, Schweizerärzte, 1962–1963, Erich A. Messmer, Arbeitsmöglichkeiten für Schweizer Ärzte in Tanganyika, 1 May 1962, p. 1.

43 BAR, E 2003–03 (-), 1976/44, 46, t. 912.032, Basler Stiftung zur Förderung von Entwicklungsländern Basel, 1961–1964, Erich Messmer, Aktennotiz über den Besuch der Herren Dr. Wilhelm, Vizepräsident und Delegierter des Verwaltungsrates der CIBA und Dr. O. Niederhauser, stellvertretender Direktor der CIBA am 28. Sept. 1961, 2 October 1961.

44 BAR, E 2003–03 (-), 1976/44, 46, Aktennotiz über den Besuch der Herren Dr. Wilhelm, Vizepräsident und Delegierter des Verwaltungsrates der CIBA und Dr. O. Niederhauser, stellvertretender Direktor der CIBA am 28. Sept. 1961, 2 October 1961, pp. 1–3, here: p. 2.

45 James Scott, *Seeing Like a State. How Certain Schemes to Improve the Human Condition have Failed*, New Haven 1998.

46 FAO (ed.), *The Rufiji Basin Tanganyika. FAO Report to the Government of Tanganyika on the Preliminary Reconnaissance Survey of the Rufiji Basin*, Rome 1961.

Ocean, the Kilombero and Luwegu rivers meet the Great Ruaha to form the Rufiji, Tanzania's largest river. Beginning at Stiegler's Gorge – named after a Swiss hunter who lost his life there in 1907 – the Rufiji meanders through a floodplain (the Lower Rufiji Valley), providing fertile ground for the cultivation of rice, maize and cotton. The FAO team, which included Swiss engineer Max Freimann, recommended large-scale irrigation and flood control measures and the construction of a large dam at Stiegler's Gorge.[47] As historian Heather Hoag has shown, large dam projects – as material symbols of state power and progress – were appealing to African leaders after independence. Many of these projects were inspired by the Tennessee Valley Authority (TVA) model, which provided a blueprint for river basin development planning transferable to different Third World locations.[48] While embracing the transfer of large-scale technology and development planning, the World Bank report's chapters on irrigation and flood control proposed a tentative approach to Tanganyikan development: research and pilot projects were to be used to minimize adverse impacts and to measure success.[49]

Feeling increasingly responsible for what happened in Ulanga District, Rudolf Geigy initiated a pilot project in order to assess the unintended outcomes of such interventions. At the heart of his Lumemo project was the Ihango area, a dry and so far uncultivated strip of land close to Ifakara, consisting of about 2500 acres awaiting improvement.[50] Flood regulation would be guaranteed by the construction of a dam to retain the waters of the Lumemo, a tributary of the Kilombero. Via a large channel and a web of smaller channels, the water would make its way to the emerging cultivation sites under controlled conditions. In September 1962, Max Freimann tested the feasibility of Geigy's proposals, which had strong supporters at the FAO and within the Tanzanian government. Derek Bryceson, then Minister for Agriculture, believed that the creation of a cooperative responsible for the cultivation and marketing of products would fit ideally

47 A. D. Beck, *The Kilombero Valley of South-Central Tanganyika*, in: East African Geographical Review, Vol. 2, 1964, pp. 37–43, here: p. 39.
48 Heather J. Hoag, *Transplanting the TVA? International Contributions to Postwar River Development in Tanzania,* in: Comparative Technology Transfer and Society, Vol. 4, No. 3, 2006, pp. 247–268.
49 International Bank for Reconstruction and Development (ed.), *The Economic Development of Tanganyika*, see especially Chapter 6, pp. 129–140.
50 BAR, E 2003–03 (-), 1976/44, 205, (4), Lumemo-River, Bewässerungsprojekt, 1961–1963, Rudolf Geigy to Hans Keller, 21 May 1962, p. 1.

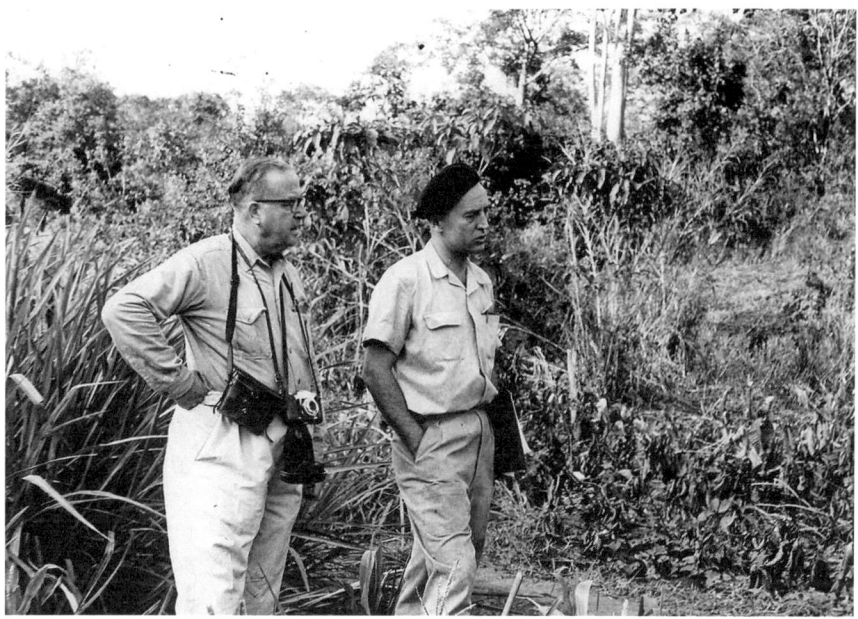

Rudolf Geigy and Max Freimann surveying the Ihango area, 1962, Archive STI

into the government's ideological framework of self-help.[51] After a meeting with Rudolf Geigy and members of the Swiss government in 1962, Bryceson was glad to inform the Tanganyikan public that Switzerland was favorably considering the investment of the GBP 350,000 requested for the development of Kilombero District.[52] Shortly after, Freimann investigated the area and assessed the technical feasibility of the project on the ground. However, rather than treating the selected area as a unit, he preferred a division of the land into three parts: under the overall supervision of a cooperative, one part of the land was to be allocated to individual local (or resettled) farmers; a second part would be used to establish a trial farm, led by Swiss agricultural instructors; and the remaining land was to be

---

51 Ibid., Schenk, Besprechung mit Mr. Bryceson am 20. Juli 1962.
52 BAR, E 2200.83 (A), 1983/26, 3, Agricultural Development (Lumemo), 1962–1963, Press Release. Issued by Tanganyika Information Services. "Mr. Bryceson Returns from Europe with Promises of Aid", 11 May 1962, pp. 1–2, here: p. 1.

taken up by a large farm operating commercially and ensuring the financial sustainability of the whole project.[53]

Before the Tanganyikan government officially requested the DftZ to implement Freimann's proposals, the Swiss project planners were confronted with worrying news issuing from Germany's development offices. Inspired by the World Bank report and the findings of many other expert missions evaluating the development potential of the Rufiji Basin, and especially the Kilombero Valley, the German Technical Assistance agency (GTZ) proposed the establishment of an Agricultural Experimental and Training Center for Water Development and Irrigation and Agricultural Engineering; as well as being geographically close to the Swiss training farm, this scheme was very similar in its intentions. The main difference between the two projects was that the German plans were already more advanced, and the budget of DEM 10 million far exceeded the proposed Swiss contribution.[54]

For Geigy and the DftZ, it was obvious that, with the German ideas taking shape in Ifakara, the Swiss project and the RAC "which was also intended to provide assistance in the agricultural sector" would dwindle away and be reduced to medical courses.[55] On several occasions, Geigy intervened at the Ministry of Agriculture, trying to convince Bryceson that the Lumemo river did not carry enough water for the operation of two farms, and that the local population would find it hard to understand the presence of two nations working at the same location. Understandably, Derek Bryceson was reluctant to reject the generous German offer, even though he had previously stated that "Ifakara and the Lumemo project are 100% Swiss and must remain so" and assured Rudolf Geigy in a letter that he would never allow the Germans "to upset old friends like yourself simply because they have a lot of money to offer us".[56] Now he was inclined to accept the idea that German and Swiss experts could work together.[57] In this situation, Geigy saw two ways out of the impasse: firstly, he proposed to push ahead with the project: "We could start with some families and try to

---

53   Ibid., Max Freimann, Tanganyika. Lumemo-Bewässerungs-Projekt. Provisorischer Vorbericht, 31 October 1962, pp. 9–11.

54   Ibid., German Technical Assistance for the Agriculture of Tanganyika. Report and Expert Opinion by the Delegation, pp. 1–30.

55   Ibid., Rudolf Geigy, Lumemo River Irrigation Project, 9 July 1963, p. 2.

56   Ibid., pp. 2–3.

57   Ibid., Derek Bryceson to August Lindt, 4 October 1963.

grow cotton as a cash crop and rice, maize and soya as food crops."[58] Secondly, he would try to persuade the Swiss ambassador, August Lindt, to pull political strings in Bonn so as to improve coordination of the two projects. Lindt, however, did not share Geigy's opinion that the German project proposal betrayed a lack of local knowledge. Instead, he believed that the plans of the GTZ were more advanced than those of the STI. He concluded:

> Because we are unable to counter the German project with something of equal or even better quality, we believe an intervention in Bonn would not be justified, regrettable though this may be for the development of Swiss efforts in Ifakara. More generally, we have to accept the fact that we have less leverage than other countries in the case of competition in the development sector. [59]

The agricultural experts in Germany viewed Geigy's objections with increasing astonishment. They had always believed that the STI's activities were restricted to the testing of drugs, insecticides and fertilizers, and the training of local personnel. Only the experiments with fertilizers would be likely to overlap with their own plans.[60] They nevertheless decided to determine whether there was any truth in Geigy's belief – defended with such vehemence – that the Lumemo river did not carry enough water for the two planned development projects. When they re-evaluated the site, the German experts could not find any evidence to support Geigy's claims; instead, there was evidence suggesting that the development plans would probably lead to salinization of the whole area. These new findings, together with a proposal that the Swiss could work under German leadership in Ifakara, were enough to put an end to the Swiss initiatives in the Tanganyikan agricultural sector.[61] The abandonment of the Lumemo project foreshadowed the fate of a larger dam project at Stiegler's Gorge which, in the 1970s, was torpedoed by criticism from a politicized Third World movement. The failure of the Lumemo project and the lessons learned about competition in international aid led the STI to shift back from agriculture to medical infrastructure.

58 BAR, E 2003–03 (-), 1976/44, 205, t.941.1 (4), Rolf Wilhelm, Aktennotiz über die Besprechung mit Herrn Prof. Geigy vom 31. Oktober 1963: Lumemo-Projekt, 4 November 1963, pp. 1–2, here: p. 1.
59 Ibid., August Lindt, 27 July 1963.
60 Ibid., Hartmann, Schweizerisch-deutsche Koordination auf dem Gebiet der landwirtschaflichen Entwicklungshilfe, 8 August 1963.
61 BAR, E 2005 (A), 1978/137, 155, t. 311.01, Lumemo-Bewässerungsprojekt, 1964–66, August Lindt to Rudolf Geigy, 16 April 1964.

Development's Pathologies: The Construction of a Pathology Block in Dar es Salaam

With the Swiss agricultural initiatives for Kilombero District in tatters, Geigy and the STI turned to the RAC, which had already been successful in training health personnel. For the STI, the RAC was not a remote outpost, cut off from the latest developments in medical research and training in Dar es Salaam, but firmly anchored within the curriculum of Dar's Medical School. This was largely thanks to Geigy's networking skills: he was a member of the School's Board of Examiners, and the Tanganyikan government's British advisors did not hesitate to involve him in discussions about how best to adjust the medical curriculum to the country's needs. In particular, the Medical School's new principal, Dr. Rankin, was attracted by the training offered at the RAC, with its focus on the study of parasites and the complex modes of disease transmission in a natural setting.[62]

In 1964, negotiations between the STI and the Medical School ended with an agreement that the RAC should have a firm place in the School's curriculum. Originally, the RAC was designed to introduce third-year students to rural health and hygiene and tropical diseases, but given the lack of training in basic health subjects in Dar es Salaam, the RAC was already teaching tropical pathology to second-year students.[63]

The progress made by the Basel Foundation and the STI in the medical sector again opened up a window of opportunity for the DftZ, still struggling to explain Switzerland's retreat from the Lumemo project. Yet, the political climate was favorable for closer Swiss involvement – this, at least, was the view of Peter Wiesmann and Mario Grassi, the two DftZ members who toured the country in September 1965 to identify appropriate new areas of intervention and pave the way for the first legal agreement on technical and scientific cooperation between the two countries, which was signed in October 1966.[64] In their report, Wiesmann and Grassi concluded that, while the political constellation of the Tanzanian republic

---

62   BAR, E 2200.83 (A), 1983/26, 771.1, Rudolf Geigy to R. Schenkel, 23 September 1963.

63   Archive Thierry A. Freyvogel (ATAF), Lettres d'Ifakara (1959–1985), Thierry Freyvogel, 9 August 1964, pp. 1–4, here: pp. 1–2.

64   BAR, E 2005 (A), 1978/137, 155, t. 311-Tanzania – Projekte und Aktionen 1964–1966, Abkommen über die technische und wissenschaftliche Zusammenarbeit zwischen der Schweizerischen Eidgenossenschaft und der Regierung der Vereinigten Republik Tansania, 21 October 1966.

formed by the union of Tanganyika and Zanzibar in 1964 was less pro-West than before, a "swing to the left" was not very likely as long as Nyerere remained in power.[65] During their visit to Ifakara, Wiesmann and Grassi met Rudolf Geigy, who – considering the country's deficiencies in medical training – persuaded them to include the establishment of a Pathology Block in Dar es Salaam in their list of projects worth supporting.

From a Western perspective, a central pathology laboratory facilitating clinical diagnosis of various communicable and chronic diseases would be an ideal starting point in Tanzania's efforts to develop its health sector. The battle against deadly diseases could not be won without proper means of diagnosis and clinical analysis. With the creation of the Medical School in 1963, and later the Faculty of Medicine, Tanganyika had already demonstrated its wish to transcend the legacy of colonial research. But could there be a more vivid symbol of colonial science than the old Ocean Road laboratory, which had been opened by German microbe hunter Robert Koch? Geigy's Pathology Block was to be the realization of various Western development ideals such as knowledge transfer, partnership and self-help – not only because it would employ Tanganyikan staff from the outset, but because it was designed to be handed over to local scientists as soon as this was feasible.[66] The facility the STI had in mind was based on a British model and would cover all the disciplines associated with major university hospitals – pathological anatomy and histology, microbiology, serology and parasitology, as well as clinical chemistry, hematology and a blood transfusion center.[67] In retrospect, it can be said that underlying Geigy's focus on pathology and urban health care was the idea that the RAC should be anchored within Tanzania's rural health system. For Geigy, rural training and research were inextricably interlinked.

But the DftZ was not convinced: far from sharing Geigy's enthusiasm for medical infrastructure, it refused to bear the costs of construction, argu-

65   Ibid., Peter A. Wiesmann, Rapport über die Abklärungsmission in Tanzania 5.–29. September 1965, 10 November 1965, pp. 1–37, here: p. 2.

66   ASTI, Pathologie-Block, Dar es Salaam, Rudolf Geigy, Eingabe der Basler Stiftung zur Förderung von Entwicklungsländern an den Delegierten für technische Zusammenarbeit in Bern, enthaltend einen Vorschlag zur gemeinsamen Finanzierung eines "Pathologie-Blockes", der für die Medizinschule von Tansania auf deren Areal in Dar es Salaam errichtet werden soll, Dezember 1967, pp. 1–12.

67   Ibid., Frédéric Roulet, Bemerkungen zum Vorschlag: Errichtung eines "Central Pathology Laboratory" an der Medical School, Dar-es-Salaam, Tansania, 9 November 1965, pp. 1–3.

ing that the enterprise did not accord with its own development concepts and that it was not clear that a laboratory block designed after a British model would still embody a grain of "Swissness".[68] It was only thanks to his friendship with Lindt – as one DftZ member dryly observed – that Geigy was able to proceed with his plans. On this occasion, Geigy once again demonstrated his ability to forge strong alliances and to mobilize various advocates to champion his cause: one month before the official request was sent to the Swiss government in 1967, the importance of such a pathology block for the Swiss pharmaceutical industry was underlined by the pathologist Frédéric Roulet (who had accompanied Geigy on his first expedition to Africa in 1945) and the physician Otto Gsell;[69] towards the end of the year, Marcel Luy, the Swiss ambassador to Dar es Salaam, also assured Geigy of his "very favorable view of this project, whose realization is strongly desired by the Tanzanian government".[70] The agreement reached in 1967 bore the hallmarks of a compromise: the project would be undertaken as a private initiative led by the Basel Foundation, with the pharmaceutical industry investing CHF 900,000; the Swiss government would contribute CHF 1.2 million to construction costs (50% of the overall budget for Swiss development projects in Tanzania in 1969), while the Tanzanian government would provide over CHF 1 million.[71] Under the agreement signed between the Basel Foundation and the Tanzanian government, the former would provide the head of the Pathology Block for a period of ten years, while the RAC – as an outpost for training and research – would form an integral part of the Pathology Block, "although it remains under the auspices of the Basel Foundation".[72] This formulation was especially im-

68 BAR, E 2005 (A), 1980/82, 243, t. 311-Tanzania – Medical School Dar es Salaam, 1967, Sigismond Marcuard, Notice pour le dossier. Entretien du 28.06.1967 chez le Chef du département avec M. le Prof. Geigy concernant la construction d'un bloc pathologique à Dar es Salaam, 29 June 1967, pp. 1–2, here: p. 1.
69 Novartis Firmenarchiv, CIBA, RE 15.04.1, Basler Stiftung zur Förderung von Entwicklungsländern 1960–1975, Otto Gsell, Frédéric Roulet, Bedeutung eines "Central Pathology Laboratory" (Pathology Block) an der Medical School von Dar-es-Salaam (Tanzania), 16 November 1967.
70 BAR, E 2005 (A), 1980/82, 243, Marcel Luy to Rudolf Geigy, 4. December 1967.
71 BAR, E 2200.83 (B), 1990/26, 10, 771.22.8, Pathologisches Institut Dar es Salaam, R. Dannecker, Projekt Pathologisches Institut Dar-es-Salaam, Zusammenarbeit mit Schweiz. Fachinstituten, 30 July 1971, pp. 1–5, here: p. 1.
72 Novartis Firmenarchiv, CIBA, RE 15.04.11, Protokolle der Stiftungsratssitzungen 1960–1982, E. Stocker, Protokoll der Sitzung des Stiftungsrates vom 23. Oktober 1968, 10.00 Uhr, bei der CIBA Aktiengesellschaft, p. 8; BAR, E 2200.83 (B), 1990/26, 10, Agreement between the Ministry of Health and Housing, Government of the United

portant to the Swiss party and was designed to prevent the RAC being handed over to the Tanzanians after the initial ten-year period.

However, long before the "Africanization" of the Pathology Block could be initiated, the development plans proved to have major weaknesses; as a consequence, responsibility for the whole project was transferred from the Basel Foundation to the DftZ. The problems encountered were of a financial nature. The project planners were initially more concerned with architecture than with the actual operation of the pathology lab. They assumed that scientific equipment from the old Ocean Road lab could be moved to the new building at Muhimbili Hospital. However, this assumption turned out to be wishful thinking. The medical equipment at Ocean Road was so antiquated that it would have been impossible to transfer it to a modern environment. As one of the DftZ developers commented:

> The creation of the pathology laboratory is a prime example of inadequate planning. Construction was started without settling the financial arrangements for laboratory equipment with the Tanzanian partners in advance. Continued use of the older laboratory devices is – with only a few exceptions – out of the question because, as a visit to the former lab revealed, the material is more than 30–40 years old. This fact should have been clear to all of us from the outset. [73]

This situation gave rise to additional costs of about CHF 2.5 million, and new donors had to be found. The DftZ, fearing another development debacle in Tanzania, proposed three possible solutions: firstly, the Basel Foundation would be asked to submit a realistic plan for the project until it could be handed over to the Tanzanians; secondly, the Swiss government would look for a university institute that could continue with the project on behalf of the DftZ; or thirdly, the DftZ would withdraw from the project altogether, since legally the Basel Foundation was still liable for the whole enterprise.[74] In the end, however, it was the Basel Foundation, not the DftZ, that withdrew from the project because of the heavy financial burden and the pharmaceutical companies' lack of interest in the Pathology Block.

Republic of Tanzania (hereinafter referred to as the "Government") of the ONE PART and the Basle Foundation for Aid to Developing Countries (hereinafter referred to as the "Foundation") of the OTHER PART, 23 January 1969.

73 BAR, E2005 (A), 1983/18, 364, t.311.21, Flying Doctor Service in Tanzania 1967–1972, R. Dannecker, Rapport über die Mission nach Tansania – Kenia vom 08.03.1970–29.3.1970, 3 April 1970, pp. 1–36, here: p. 4.

74 Ibid., p. 6.

The DftZ decided to continue the enterprise as a government project and engaged Jacques Rüttner (Director of the Institute of Pathology at Zurich University) to execute it on its behalf.[75] A new donor – the German government – was finally found to finance the scientific equipment.[76] In 1971, the Central Pathology Laboratory was inaugurated, and two years later the Tanzanian J. K. Shaba became the first African head of the lab.

Développement Manqué: The Case of Côte d'Ivoire

A different path into the development decade was taken by Côte d'Ivoire and the CSRS. As we have seen, the immediate aftermath of independence in Tanganyika was marked by continuities and, until 1964, close relations with the country's former colonial master. But while, from the mid-1960s, Nyerere forged new alliances, France remained the point of reference for the Ivorian president Félix Houphouët-Boigny. French institutions in Côte d'Ivoire were scarcely affected by independence. ORSTOM – again – is a case in point. Now positioned as a development agency, the organization became more than ever a strong advocate for the reinvigorated "civilizing mission" and for the application of science and technology. Despite ORSTOM's calm passage into the development decade, three significant changes occurred. Firstly, in a reform introduced in 1960, seven technical committees were created, which led to greater centralization and underscored the monodisciplinary character of scientific research in the postcolony. Secondly, the 1960s saw growing internationalization of research programs, and the pursuit of joint ventures with institutions such as the FAO, UNESCO and the UN. Thirdly, several ORSTOM researchers acted as development planners for ministries of the newly independent country.[77]

ORSTOM's adaptation to the new political constituencies of the postcolony had far-reaching consequences for the CSRS too. The French organization involved Swiss scientists in its research programs more systematically than before. In 1962, for example, ORSTOM allowed the Commission of

75 BAR, E 2200.83 (B), 1990/26, 10, R. Dannecker, Projekt Pathologisches Institut Dar-es-Salaam, 30 July 1971, p. 2.
76 Ibid., R. Dannecker, Aktennotiz. Besuch einer deutschen Delegation für die Diskussion einer deutsch-schweizerischen Zusammenarbeit im Projekt Pathologisches Laboratorium Dar-es-Salaam, 23 November 1970, pp. 1–4.
77 Marie-Lise Sabrié, *Histoire des principes de programmation scientifique*, pp. 227–229.

the CSRS to send the geologist Ruedi Eckert to Adiopodoumé. Eckert's geological investigations were not conducted independently, but as part of a larger ORSTOM program under the leadership of the French geologist Philippe Mangin. The aim was to measure the impact of the climate on soil erosion and sedimentation of the Bandama river.[78] The adoption of a new, ecological research paradigm also increased France's influence over the research agenda of the CSRS. Owing to its diversity, Côte d'Ivoire had long been perceived as an "ecological laboratory".[79] In 1962, the Ecole Normale Supérieure set up a research station 150 kilometers north of Abidjan, which was named "Lamto" after the French scientists Maxime Lamotte and Jean-Luc Tournier. In the attempt to "quantify everything", Lamto became a center for huge collections of specimens. The concept of the ecosystem as being divided up into different, interconnected spheres structured scientific work on the ground, making Lamto a popular research site for scientists from a variety of disciplines – zoologists, botanists, pedologists, meteorologists and geographers.[80] Swiss researchers in Adiopodoumé were not opposed to the new spirit of biological research or the quest for interdisciplinarity. The work of the Swiss scientists Pierre Hunkeler, Peter Vogel and Rodolphe Spichiger was concerned with ecological problems and influenced by charismatic personalities such as the French ecologists Maxime Lamotte and François Bourlière.[81] The "ecological turn" in Adiopodoumé involved a different approach to nature: broadly speaking, nature was no longer conceived as an infinite source of specimens (as it had been a decade before), but as a fragile system deserving conservation and protection from human influence.

---

78 Archives Nationales Fontainebleau (ANF), Archives de l'ORSTOM, 19900236, Art. 57, Philippe Mangin, Etude du couple érosion-sedimentation en Côte d'Ivoire (Opération Mangin). Le point scientifique en novembre 1966, p. 1.
79 Guillaume Lachenal, *L'invention africaine de l'écologie française. Histoire de la station de Lamto (Côte d'Ivoire), 1942–1976*, in: La Revue pour l'histoire du CNRS, Vol. 13, 2005, pp. 1–15.
80 Ibid., p. 6.
81 Interview with Pierre Hunkeler and Peter Vogel, 17 May 2010/11 August 2010. Pierre Hunkeler's wife Claudine published several papers together with François Bourlière in the field of primatology. See: Claudine Hunkeler, François Bourlière, M. Bertrand, *Le comportement social de la mone de Lowe (Cercopithecus campbelli lowei)*, in: Folia primat, Vol. 17, 1972, pp. 218–236; François Bourlière, M. Bertrand, Claudine Hunkeler, *L'écologie de la Mone de Lowe (*Cercopithecus campbelli lowei*) en Côte d'Ivoire*, in: Terre Vie, Vol. 23, 1969, pp. 135–163; François Bourlière, M. Bertrand, Claudine Hunkeler, *Ecology and Behaviour of Lowe's guenon (Cercopithecus campbelli lowei) in the Ivory Coast*, in: J. R. Napier and P.H. Napier (eds.), Old World Monkeys. Evolution, Systematics, and Behavior, New York, London 1970, pp. 297–350.

One consequence of the adoption of ecology as a joint research endeavor was that Swiss CSRS researchers became part of interdisciplinary programs under ORSTOM's umbrella. Among the promoters of closer links between Swiss scientists and French research units was Jacques Miège, who – as we saw in Chapter 1 – was one of the pioneers of French science in Adiopodoumé. In 1964, Miège became Director of the Botanical Gardens and Professor of Botany at the University of Geneva, from where he maintained close ties with ORSTOM in Adiopodoumé.[82] As an honorary member of the SNG and a member of the Commission of the CSRS, Miège constantly supplied the CSRS with young botanical scholars.[83] The emphasis on ecology was of course supported by Jean-Georges Baer, who, since 1958, had served as President of the International Union for the Conservation of Nature (IUCN), with its headquarters at Morges in Western Switzerland.[84]

The dissolution of the boundaries between ORSTOM and the CSRS during the 1960s affected Swiss policymakers' perceptions of the research sites in Côte d'Ivoire and Tanganyika as bulwarks of Swiss development aid in Africa. Honorary consul Wimmer complained about the fact that the CSRS was not fully acknowledged as a bastion of Swiss development efforts in West Africa, and he accused Rudolf Geigy of having focused almost exclusively on Tanganyika in the development race between the two African countries.[85] This accusation was, however, only partly justified. Côte d'Ivoire never escaped Geigy's interest, and indeed Arthur Wilhelm's first development plans included the training of young Ivorian students in medicine, biology and veterinary medicine at the STI.[86] The fact that Swiss development projects were more easily undertaken in East Af-

---

82 Rodolphe Spichiger, *"Jacques Miège" (1914–1993)*, in: Candollea, Vol. 49, No. 1, 1994, pp. 1–22, here: p. 3.

83 Archive Jardin Botanique de Genève (AJBG), Jacques Miège to Jean-Georges Baer, 9 November 1965, p. 1. In the late 1960s and early 1970s, his students Marianne Dugerdil and Rodolphe Spichiger (who succeeded Miège as Director of Geneva's Botanical Gardens in 1987) participated in a multidisciplinary project led by the French geographer Jean Michel Avenard, focusing on contact zones between different ecological milieus such as forests and savannahs; see: ANF, Archives de l'ORSTOM, 19900236, Art. 58, Jean Michel Avenard, Le thème "contact forêt-savane" en Côte d'Ivoire. Motivation, bilan et perspectives, April 1974, pp. 1–46, here: pp. 19–20.

84 Martin Holdgate, *The Green Web. A Union for World Conservation*, London 1999, p. 69.

85 Fonds André Aeschlimann (FAA), Correspondance Côte d'Ivoire 1959–1962, André Aeschlimann to C. Lambert (CIBA), 4 October 1960, pp. 1–2, here: p. 1.

86 Novartis Firmenarchiv, J. R. Geigy AG, SP 5, Wilhelm, Hilfe zugunsten von Entwicklungsländern, p. 10.

rica than in Côte d'Ivoire had more to do with Switzerland's perceptions of French influence over Ivorian politics and with ORSTOM's tutelage of the CSRS, which made the site unattractive for public-private partnerships.

Development – A French Affair

Côte d'Ivoire was one of the African countries which emerged on the radar of Swiss politics on the eve of independence. Good relations with the former French colony seemed unproblematic, as Houphouët enjoyed a reputation in Switzerland shared by few of his African peers – a reliable political partner, a bulwark against the communist waves breaking on the borders of newly independent African nations and an admirer of Switzerland (owning a residence near Geneva). In 1961, Switzerland removed Wimmer as its official representative in Abidjan and opened an embassy headed by Jean Stroehlin, who was responsible for the four countries of the "Conseil d'Entente" (Côte d'Ivoire, Upper Volta, Niger, Dahomey). However, the new embassy owed its existence to a domino effect and a desire to avoid diplomatic resentment. Commenting on the opening of the new Swiss embassy in Conakry (Guinea), Pierre Micheli, the Swiss ambassador to Paris, asked rhetorically:

> Is it advisable – in the circumstances – to leave our post in Abidjan at the vice-consular level? The rivalry between Mr. Houphouët-Boigny (Côte d'Ivoire) and Mr. Sékou Touré (Guinea) is notorious. The promotion of our embassy in Conakry might be received very badly in Abidjan if things remain here as they are now.[87]

In 1962, Switzerland signed a trade agreement with Côte d'Ivoire, covering issues such as investment protection and technical aid, and replacing the agreement of 1955. However, trading volumes between the two countries remained modest, largely as a result of Switzerland remaining outside the European Economic Community (EEC) and operating outside France's sphere of influence. Between 1959 and 1961, Switzerland accounted for CFA 77 million out of a total of CFA 30.24 billion in Ivorian imports, thus

---

87   Cited in: Alioune Dieng, *La Suisse et l'Afrique au lendemain des indépendances. Le cas de la Côte d'Ivoire*, Mémoire de Master en Etudes Internationales (MEI), Histoire et Politique Internationale (HPI), Graduate Institute Geneva, 2010, p. 35.

ranking in sixteenth position, while sharing the modest eighteenth rank with Norway as far as Ivorian exports were concerned.[88]

Equally, technical assistance – now politely called "technical coopera-tion" – never had a chance to take off, even though there was no shortage of suggestions about how best to develop the African country. Advocates of the CSRS, in particular, did not lack creativity in showing how the labo-ratory could now be put at the service of Côte d'Ivoire. In 1961, at the sug-gestion of Eugen Wimmer, Ivorian Minister for Education Joachim Bony visited the DftZ in Bern to officially request that three Swiss teachers be sent to the CSRS, where they could then offer their services to the Ecole Normale de Dabou – a town some 50 miles West of Abidjan.[89] The project, inspired by Wimmer, called for the extension of the CSRS, and Wimmer himself asked the DftZ to provide CHF 100,000 for this purpose.[90] Larger in scope and much more sensitive from a political viewpoint was the idea put forward by Professor Robert-Henri Régamey and his collaborators at Geneva University. They proposed that Switzerland should enter the med-ical sector (as in Tanganyika) by supporting the creation of a medical fac-ulty in Abidjan. This proposal did not come from nowhere: as political re-lations between France and Côte d'Ivoire were being reshaped in the light of the development dogma, Houphouët-Boigny – himself a trained physi-cian – asked the French to invest in the creation of a university in Abidjan.

However, given that similar requests were being made by Léopold Senghor in Dakar, Paris did not enter into negotiations with Houphouët, agreeing only to support the establishment of faculties of law, natural sciences and humanities.[91] In theory, the fact that France turned down Houphouët's request could have facilitated Swiss intervention because the agreement between France and its former colony stated that Côte d'Ivoire could only apply for technical assistance from other nations if France was

---

88 Ibid., p. 61.
89 BAR, E 2200.5 (-), 1979/93, 8, G. 6.61.7, Professeurs pour l'école normale de Dabou, 1961–1962, Centre Suisse de Recherches Scientifiques en Côte d'Ivoire. Aide Tech-nique Suisse pour l'école normale d'instituteurs de Dabou. Exposé, 15 February 1962, pp. 1–4, here: p. 3.
90 Archiv Schweizerische Akademie der Naturwissenschaften, Depot Burgerbibliothek Bern (SCNAT), GA SANW 826, Kommissionen CSRS, Gebäude, Bau und Um-bau-Projekte, Kosten 1951–1973, Eugen Wimmer to Hans Keller, 5 May 1962, pp. 1–3.
91 StABS, ED-REG 42a 2-2-6 (10), Rudolf Geigy, 1960–1972, Eugen Wimmer to Jean Stroehlin, 15 April 1962, pp. 1–2, here: p. 2.

not able or willing to provide it.[92] However, France's monopoly over the course of Ivorian development made it advisable for the DftZ to adopt a cautious approach. The example of Côte d'Ivoire shows that political considerations could be a crucial factor in decisions to grant or refuse development aid. As regards the proposed investment in a medical faculty in Abidjan, Raymond Probst (deputy head of the Department of Foreign Affairs) urged his colleagues not to be too hasty in endorsing the CHF 12 million project, writing that:

> Dr. Keller and myself believe that the project of a medical faculty is not only too ambitious – according to our experience in West Africa, there is hardly any chance of making it a success. Moreover, we are not at all interested in challenging the thin-skinned French in precisely those areas where they help most generously and efficiently.[93]

At the DftZ, more fundamental issues were raised by Roy Preiswerk – later Director of the Graduate Institute of Development Studies in Geneva – in his assessment of possibilities for Swiss technical cooperation in French West Africa:

> All the countries of ex-French West Africa or ex-French Equatorial Africa except Mali and Guinea can be considered as territories where France exerts too much influence for Switzerland to be able to embark on any major projects.[94]

The fear of intruding into what was considered a mainly French affair is again reflected by statistics. Of the CHF 60 million development credit approved by the Swiss parliament in 1961, Côte d'Ivoire received a mere CHF 15,000 for the period 1962–1964. Moreover, no substantial government projects were planned for the coming years.[95] The DftZ approved neither a grant of CHF 100,000 to alleviate the dismal financial situation of

92 BAR, E 2200.5 (-), 1979/93, 8, G. 6.61.5, Faculté de médecine en Côte d'Ivoire, Jean Stroehlin to Hans Keller, 30 November 1962, pp. 1–7, here: p. 3.
93 BAR, E 2200.5 (-), 1979/94, 6, 652.20, 1966/1968, Centre Suisse de Recherches Scientifiques en Côte d'Ivoire, Raymond Probst to Jean Stroehlin, 22 June 1962, pp. 1–2, here: pp. 1–2.
94 BAR, E 2005 (A) 1978/137, 80, t.311-Elfenbeinküste, Projekte und Aktionen 1964–1966, Roy Preiswerk, Possibilités pour la coopération technique suisse en Afrique occidentale d'expression française, 7 May 1964, pp. 1–6, here: p. 2.
95 Ibid., August R. Lindt to Finanzdelegation der Eidgenössischen Räte, 2 March 1964, pp. 1–2, here: p. 1.

the CSRS nor the more substantial grant for a medical faculty in Abidjan. The influence of political perceptions in the offices of the DftZ in Bern is demonstrated by the erratic nature of its development activities and its support for a medically oriented project in Guinea – a country that broke openly with France in the referendum of 1958.

A Medical School for Conakry (Guinea)

The history of Swiss development aid cannot be understood without a global perspective and the acknowledgment that concepts travel from one place to another (after all, what failed in one context might work in another). The decision not to invest time and money in a medical faculty in Abidjan was not a decision to abandon support for medical infrastructure altogether but – in line with Preiswerk's suggestion – to look for another West African country where French influence was less oppressive. The small country of Guinea seemed to fit the bill perfectly. Its relations with France were more or less in tatters after its refusal to join the French Community in 1958, and Swiss aid – so the argument went – could offset the increasing communist influence. In short, helping Guinea would showcase an active policy of neutrality.[96] The interests of the two countries were, however, mutual. In 1960, DftZ collaborator Erich Messmer received a Guinean delegation in Bern, exploring the possibility of Swiss aid. The main item on the agenda was Guinea's wish to stem the flow of students and trainees from Conakry to Paris and to diversify the range of host countries. But in the light of the opening of the Medical School in Dar es Salaam and the rejection of the proposal to support a medical faculty in Abidjan, the idea of medical aid as a possible area of Swiss intervention was never far away. Like many African countries after independence, Guinea envisaged the creation of a medical faculty on its territory and aspired to be self-reliant in crucial policy areas such as health and welfare. The prospect of replicating the Dar es Salaam Medical School in Conakry silenced the more skeptical voices, which included that of Max Joss, the Swiss consul in Conakry, who doubted whether Guinea could ever produce suffi-

---

96 Jérome Schuwey, *La Suisse et la Guinée de Sékou Touré. Les enjeux de la coopération technique au lendemain de l'indépendance 1958–1974*, Mémoire de licence en histoire contemporaine présenté à la Faculté des Lettres de l'Université de Fribourg, Fribourg 2005, p. 43.

cient numbers of students for a medical faculty.[97] However, when Switzerland learned that the project was already underway, with a building over 100 meters high towering into the Guinean sky, the question became simply whether or not Switzerland was willing to provide aid. Rémy Godet summed up the attitude of the DftZ most succinctly: "Fortune favors the bold: given that things have already progressed considerably, Switzerland can only choose between granting or refusing its aid. According to the Political Division … it would be advisable to adopt a positive solution."[98]

During 1964 and 1965, contacts between Switzerland and Guinea over the medical school intensified. In a letter to President Sékou Touré, August Lindt confirmed Switzerland's commitment to the project; two days later, Swiss and Guinean partners met at the STI to discuss the details of possible Swiss support.[99] Representing the STI were Rudolf Geigy and Michel Fernex (a trained physician who would later build up Roche's infectious diseases department). These two men roughly sketched out a new medical curriculum for the school. A few months later, the DftZ decided to reserve CHF 360,000 for the investment in Guinea; all the Guinean requests were to be handled directly in the West African country.[100] While a first Swiss mission comprising Michel Fernex, André Aeschlimann, Robert-Henri Régamey and Otto Gsell was ready to investigate the situation on the ground, the information arriving from consul Joss was still far from encouraging. According to him, collaboration between the Ministry of Health and the Ministry of Education in Conakry left much to be desired as far as this project was concerned. Furthermore, he suspected a misunderstanding on the part of Guinea with regard to the size of the Swiss contribution (indeed, Guinea expected a much larger sum than the DftZ had budgeted for the planning period 1965–1967). Last but not least, Joss reported that Louis Béhanzin, the General Inspector for training at the Ministry of Education, lost no opportunity to remind him that Guinea was ready to exchange Switzerland for a donor country from the communist bloc.[101] Nonetheless, the impressions gathered by the Swiss mission in summer 1965 were consistently pos-

97 BAR, E 2005 (A), 1978/137, 83, t. 311.004, Ecole de médicine Conakry, Bd. 1, 1963–1966, Max Joss, Faculté de médecine en Guinée, 19 December 1963, pp. 1–2.
98 Ibid., Rémy Godet, Création à Conakry d'une Ecole de médecine, pp. 1–2, here: p. 2.
99 Ibid., August Lindt to Sékou Touré, 27.05.1964.
100 Ibid., Notiz an Herrn Lindt. Medizinschule Conakry, Unterlagen für die Besprechung vom 29.10.1964, 26 October 1964, p. 1.
101 Ibid., Max Joss to August Lindt, 4 December 1964, p. 1; Max Joss to DftZ, 5 March 1965, p. 1; Max Joss to DftZ, 12 April 1965, p. 1.

itive. In their report – in line with what they had already learned from Tanzania – the experts stressed that the school could in no way involve a "transfer of European university models" but must be sensitive to the local constituencies.[102] They argued that medical training in Conakry should not be highly specialized, that the physicians should also devote their time to underserved rural areas, and that high priority should be given to preventive medicine in the new medical curriculum.[103] The delegation concluded:

> the DftZ should adopt the project of supporting a medical faculty in Conakry not just for a few but for at least ten years. This positive appraisal is derived from the impression that Guinea meets all the requirements concerning students, medical personnel and medical infrastructure. Furthermore, the costs for Switzerland are tolerable because funding can probably come from various sources.[104]

Not surprisingly, given these favorable accounts, the DftZ envisaged not only designing the school's curriculum but also being responsible for "overall planning", as Lindt wrote enthusiastically in a letter to Otto Gsell.[105] The endorsement of the medical school project by the DftZ was in accordance with the plans and future position of the STI. Its members were sure that the new engagement would markedly enhance the institute's prestige and, with Michel Fernex as the medical school's appointed dean, the STI would have easy access to Guinea's medical sector.[106] On January 20, 1966, a new Swiss delegation went to Guinea to finalize the arrangements. On this occasion, Michel Fernex was accompanied by Rolf Wilhelm and Pierre Nierlé, an architect specializing in medical infrastructure.[107] The visit ended with the signing of an agreement on February 8, 1966, but the encounter with President Sékou Touré took an unexpected turn:

> The president expresses his deep disappointment about the fact that Switzerland is not realizing the entire medical school project. He expected Switzerland to take the lead in the project (construction and training), while granting minor components to

---

102 Ibid., Bd. 2, 1964–1966, Rapport relatif à la création d'une école de médecine à Conakry. Mission des médecins suisses. Eté 1965, pp. 1–25, here: p. 2.
103 Ibid., p. 4.
104 Ibid., Otto Gsell, Robert Régamey, André Aeschlimann, Faculté de médecine à Conakry, Guinée, 26 July 1965, pp. 1–17, here: p. 16.
105 Ibid., August Lindt to Otto Gsell, 22 October 1965, pp. 1–3, here: pp. 1–2.
106 Ibid., Tractanda de la séance qui se tiendra chez Monsieur Lindt, le 15 novembre à 16 heures, 15 November 1965, pp. 1–2, here: p. 1.
107 Ibid., Rolf Wilhelm to Roy Preiswerk, 22 December 1965, pp. 1–2, here: p. 1.

other countries (laboratory equipment). The president is very surprised to learn that Switzerland wants to play a subsidiary role and is not ready to support the project entirely or at least to a very substantial extent. Therefore, the president regards the negotiations as having failed and envisages entering negotiations with another donor country.[108]

Sekou Touré's reaction was a considerable blow to the Swiss plans in the West African country. Though discussions between the two parties were resumed after the memorable meeting with the president, they came to a decisive end with the expulsion of Swiss missionaries from Guinea in 1967.[109]

The experience of Swiss development efforts in Guinea suggests that the possibilities for Swiss development aid in Tanganyika and Côte d'Ivoire were not wholly determined by (imagined or actual) political relations between the colonial powers and the former colonial territories in East and West Africa. Rather, the joint venture between the STI, the pharmaceutical industry and the DftZ in Tanganyika, and the inability of the CSRS to provide a basis for private-public partnerships, suggest that Swiss development aid in the 1960s needed strong private partners to really get off the ground. Private organizations, it would appear, were better positioned within the foreign aid industry than government agencies. They often already had long-established personal connections with the relevant circles in African countries, and they could – if necessary – operate beyond the narrow confines imposed by politics. At a conference in London on the role of philanthropic institutions, Alexander von Muralt (the initiator of the SNSF after World War II) stated:

> It has generally been assumed that private foundations are much better qualified to discover new research domains or other activities, to evaluate their possibilities, and to deliver rapid and efficient aid at an early and critical stage. For government bodies, all projects have to be placed within the limits of the political framework established in advance for each organization.[110]

---

108 Ibid., Rolf Wilhelm, Notes prises au cours des discussions avec les représentants du Gouvernement Guinéen du 21.01 au 14.02.66, pp. 1–13, here: p. 11.
109 Jérome Schuwey, *La Suisse et la Guinée de Sékou Touré*, p. 69.
110 Alexander von Muralt, *Colloque pour le 25e anniversaire de la Fondation Ciba "L'Avenir des Fondations Philanthropiques"*, Londres, 16–19 juin 1974, 18 July 1974, pp. 1–4, here: p. 3.

Von Muralt arrived at this conclusion after serving for many years as President of the Nestlé Foundation, which, in 1967, launched a project to investigate protein-calorie malnutrition in rural Côte d'Ivoire.

The Nestlé Foundation and the Construction of Moderate Protein-Calorie Malnutrition in Côte d'Ivoire

Not many products are as closely linked to Switzerland's national identity as chocolate – the result of an innovative industrial sector in Switzerland which proved highly resilient throughout the nineteenth and twentieth centuries. The history of Swiss chocolate is closely bound up with the economic and social history of West African states in particular. After World War I, companies such as the United Trading Company (UTC), an offshoot of the Basel missionary society, entered the cocoa market in the Gold Coast (now Ghana) and provided Switzerland with the valuable raw material.[111] In the first half of the twentieth century, the Gold Coast was Africa's largest exporter of cocoa, but in the 1970s Côte d'Ivoire outstripped Ghana as the world's largest cocoa producer.

Nestlé's connections with Côte d'Ivoire date back to 1959, when the company established its subsidiary CAPRAL and controlled large cocoa plantations south of Abidjan. Relations between the company and Ivorian political circles were extremely close. Nestlé officials had easy access to the president's offices, and the fruitful collaboration was confirmed by Houphouët-Boigny's many visits to Switzerland. These mutual affinities and the country's vital importance as a market for Nestlé have to be borne in mind when considering Nestlé's decision to promote nutritional research in the West African country. To mark its centenary in 1966, Nestlé announced the creation of the Foundation for the Study of Problems of Nutrition in the World. The Foundation's director was Serge Herzen, who was supported not only by von Muralt but by a series of eminent nutritionists. Indeed, the membership of the Foundation Board reads like a who's who of nutritional science at the time.[112] Of particular importance was Roger

---

111 Andrea Franc, *Wie die Schweiz zur Schokolade kam*.
112 In 1969, it included Emil Mrak (University of California/Davis), Daniel Bovet (University of Sassari/Italy, 1957 Nobel Prize in Physiology), Hugo Aebi (University of Bern) and Norman Wright (who replaced Friedrich T. Wahlen as Deputy Director-General of the FAO in 1959). Additionally, Roger Whitehead and Francis Aylward of-

Whitehead, who in 1968 became director of the Medical Research Council's Child Nutrition Unit at Makerere College Medical School (Kampala, Uganda).[113] The Foundation's first project aimed to study the problem of malnutrition in Côte d'Ivoire. It was intentionally broad in scope and included medical as well as agricultural components. Apart from the country's relevance to the food company, the Foundation's decision in favor of Côte d'Ivoire was facilitated by the presence of the CSRS in Adiopodoumé. Under an agreement negotiated with the SNG, Nestlé was to extend the CSRS with a new laboratory building, which would be transferred to the SNG once the Foundation had finished its research project in 1979.[114]

A "Protein Deficiency"

The history of the Nestlé Foundation in Côte d'Ivoire coincides with an episode in nutritional research extending from the interwar period to the 1970s, which was extremely powerful in explaining Third World hunger in terms of protein deficiency. In the 1930s, the pediatrician Cicely D. Williams – the Gold Coast's first "Woman Medical Officer" – used the local term "kwashiorkor" to designate a nutritional disease the "deposed baby gets when the next one is born".[115] She associated kwashiorkor with a maize diet and reported: "Cases seen very early react well and promptly to an improved diet, rich in accessory substances. Nestlé's sweetened condensed milk with cod-liver oil and malt seemed to be the most successful line of treatment."[116] Williams's protein hypothesis did not stir up nutri-

fered their valuable expertise; see: Fondation Nestlé pour l'étude des problèmes de l'alimentation dans le monde. Rapport annuel 1969.

113 Jennifer Tappan, *The True Fiasco. Efforts to Combat Protein Malnutrition in Uganda and the World 1950–1974*, Background paper for the Mellon Biennial Zuckerman Conference, April 2011, p. 9.

114 SCNAT, GA SANW 829, Convention entre la Commission du Centre Suisse d'Adiopodoumé, représentée par son président, M. le Professeur Jean G. Baer, d'une part, et la Fondation Nestlé pour l'Etude des Problèmes de l'Alimentation dans le Monde, représentée par son président, M. le Professeur Alexandre de Muralt, d'autre part, 21 February 1969, pp. 1–3.

115 Cicely D. Williams, *Kwashiorkor. A Nutritional Disease of Children Associated with a Maize Diet*, in: The Lancet, Vol. 229, 1935, pp. 1151–1152; see also: Michael Worboys, *The Discovery of Colonial Malnutrition between the Wars*, in: David Arnold (ed.), Imperial Medicine and Indigenous Societies, Manchester, New York 1988, pp. 208–225.

116 Cicely D. Williams, *Kwashiorkor*, p. 1151.

tional research very quickly: more than two decades would elapse before the association between kwashiorkor and insufficient protein intake was widely accepted. After World War II, the WHO and FAO paid increasing attention to the disease, and various experts started to investigate the relationship between protein deficiency, kwashiorkor and a number of other nutritional deficiencies.[117] An important event reinforcing the protein dogma and establishing kwashiorkor as an exotic condition confined to the tropics was the publication of a report by J. F. Brock (Professor of Medicine in Cape Town) and Dr. M. Autret (staff member of the FAO) after a field trip to Africa.[118] The authors noted that there was considerable freedom from disease in areas where meat, fish or milk were relatively abundant. They concluded that kwashiorkor could probably be contained by distributing skimmed milk and new protein-rich nutrients.[119] This proposal was taken up by various expert committees such as the Protein Advisory Group (PAG), established in 1955, which advised the WHO, FAO and UNICEF on emerging high-protein (but low-cost) weaning foods.[120]

Not surprisingly, given the importance attached to the introduction of high-protein supplements to various Third World localities, Nestlé's engagement in Côte d'Ivoire was based on the protein deficiency theory. At a scientific symposium held in 1969, Alexander von Muralt reiterated what had become one of the most unassailable dogmas of Western thinking in relation to the Third World:

> The most serious problem in many developing countries is not the supply of calories … but the supply of a sufficient amount of protein in order to overcome the protein-calorie malnutrition. This problem must be considered as the most urgent one among all the other problems in the fight against hunger.[121]

For Nestlé, the innovative element of its research project in Côte d'Ivoire was the attempt to apply the most sophisticated biomedical methods in ru-

117 Monica Kalt, *Tiersmondismus in der Schweiz der 1960er und 1970er Jahre*, p. 420.
118 J. F. Brock and M. Autret, *Kwashiorkor in Africa*, Geneva 1952.
119 Kenneth J. Carpenter, *Protein and Energy. A Study of Changing Ideas in Nutrition*, Cambridge 1994, p. 149.
120 Joshua N. Ruxin, *Hunger, Science, and Politics. WHO, and Unicef Nutrition Policies, 1945–1978*, PhD Study, University College London, London 1996, p. 106.
121 Alexander von Muralt, *Preface*, in: Von Muralt (ed.), Protein-Calorie Malnutrition. A Nestlé Foundation Symposium, Berlin 1969, pp. VII.

ral areas.[122] Nestlé researchers relied on techniques recently developed by Whitehead to detect metabolic changes in the urine of kwashiorkor patients. More eye-catching for rural dwellers, however, was the massive laboratory van that occasionally blew up clouds of dust into the Ivorian sky, a mobile sign of modernity on the doorstep of rural communities. Thus, while the laboratory in Adiopodoumé served as the headquarters for the performance of biochemical assays, Nestlé's attention – in line with the widespread development thinking of the 1960s and 1970s – was focused on more remote areas. One of the most important villages for Nestlé was Kpouébo, chosen as an experimental site by President Houphouët-Boigny himself and located in his native "V Baoulé" region. The President's support facilitated the launching of Nestlé's research projects: political village leaders could not but comply with Nestlé's research plans. However, one of the more fundamental issues facing Nestlé was whether or not rural areas of Côte d'Ivoire were indeed the right place to study the problem of malnutrition. As it turned out, von Muralt was disillusioned after his first scientific exploration of the region. In a report dedicated to Houphouët, he recalled:

> During our [first] talk, I asked you to indicate to me the most suitable area for executing our nutrition project. After thinking about it for a short while, you answered: "The region of the Baoulé's sacred mountain 'Orumbo Boaka'." We therefore established ourselves in Kpouébo, a small village of 1,850 inhabitants located in this region. I make no secret of the fact that, at the beginning of our work, we – as researchers – were a little disappointed to encounter a relatively healthy population in this area, and especially children whose health status seemed fairly good. No kwashiorkor or marasmus.[123]

The absence of any form of protein-calorie malnutrition among the villagers of Kpouébo was confirmed by researchers on the ground. Kurt Schopfer, who, together with his wife, entered the field in 1972 as a young scientist interested in pediatrics, recalled that – far from being characterized by a lack of proteins – the children's diet consisted of chicken, fish and fruit, as well as yams and plantains:

---

122 Archives Historiques Nestlé (AHN), 9564–22, Communication interne, 1967–1970, Alexander von Muralt, Réflexions sur le but et les résultats du voyage en Côte d'Ivoire, 22 October 1970, pp. 1–9, here: p. 1.
123 Archiv Nestlé Foundation, Lausanne, Alexander von Muralt, Introduction, in: Rapport au Gouvernement de la Côte d'Ivoire sur les premiers résultats de notre travail 1970–1972, Lausanne 1972, p. 2.

> The population's diet was well balanced, but the Nestlé Foundation had difficulty in accepting these findings because they were determined to sell their products and open up Côte d'Ivoire as a market.[124]

The Nestlé Foundation and Nestlé urged their researchers on the ground to come up with clear indicators of the prevalence of protein-calorie malnutrition, but children in Kpouébo suffered primarily from malaria and diarrhea rather than protein deficiencies. The proposal to define the people of Kpouébo as suffering from "moderate protein-calorie malnutrition" was more a desperate attempt to gloss over the realities encountered in the field than a sound scientific theory. The ideological tensions between Nestlé, the Foundation and researchers based in Adiopodoumé erupted during the 1970s, when Nestlé's activities in the Third World became the prime targets of a rising solidarity movement in Switzerland and elsewhere.

The Infant Formula Controversy

During the early 1970s, Nestlé's activities in the Third World and, in particular, the policy of propagating milk powder instead of breastfeeding, entered public awareness. Many pediatricians and Third World organizations more or less directly attributed the high levels of infant mortality in Africa to the economic aspirations of food companies such as Nestlé and others. In 1974, the British NGO War on Want published a study entitled "The Baby Killer", in which they pointed out the fatal consequences of bottle-feeding in regions where clean tap water is not necessarily available. The same year, the study was translated into German by the Third World Action Group (AgDW), a Swiss organization. The new title "Nestlé tötet Babys!" (Nestlé Kills Babies) was not only more provocative but unambiguously targeted. Nestlé's response was straightforward: only a few weeks after publication, the company sued AgDW for libel. In 1976, the lawsuit ended with a token fine for AgDW and was thus judged a success for those who accused the company of unethical marketing practices.[125] In

---

124 Interview with Kurt Schopfer, 12 April 2012. In the early 1970s, the Foundation experimented with Fortiran, a protein supplement containing wheat, soya and chickpea produced by Nestlé in Vevey, and Ignasson, a mixture of yams (French "igname") and fish ("poisson") modeled on a similar product marketed in Chad. However, neither of these products went beyond the experimental stage.
125 Monica Kalt, *Tiersmondismus in der Schweiz der 1960er und 1970er Jahre*, p. 427.

the second half of the 1970s, the controversy shifted to the US, where the Infant Formula Action Coalition launched an international boycott against Nestlé, which was not suspended until 1984, ten years after the debate gained public exposure.[126]

The controversy about Third World hunger and multinational corporations' unethical practices was a complex one: concerns about Nestlé's policies in the Third World were raised not only by grass-roots political activists but also by well-known scientists. High-level support for the activists' cause came from Derrick B. Jelliffe of the Caribbean Food & Nutrition Institute and his wife Eleanore F. Patrice Jelliffe, who from the outset emphasized the risks of promoting infant formula for Third World children. In an article published in 1971, Derrick Jelliffe coined the term "commerciogenic malnutrition" to describe the detrimental impact of industry marketing practices on infant health.[127] Patrice Jelliffe was no less outspoken when, at a conference attended by Alexander von Muralt, she declared: "Human milk can in no way be replaced or compared with the standardized formulae manufactured by the alchemists of the food industry, ever anxious to learn the trade secret of the home recipe."[128]

The debates about the characteristics of human milk have to be placed within the broader context of its growing commoditization, which began in the nineteenth century. At this time, the discourse of "natural" breastfeeding and motherhood was challenged by a scientific gaze, which evaluated the nutritional quality of human milk and more generally the role of mothers within society.[129] The transformation of breast milk into a nutritional product had a strong moral component, as the experts' efforts were directed towards improving the living conditions of underprivileged classes. Not surprisingly, the liquid and the associated practices played a vital role within the project of colonialism. Taking the example of the Belgian Congo in the first half of the twentieth century, historian Nancy Hunt showed how the colonial government – driven by fears of population decline – sought to supervise breastfeeding and weaning practices.[130]

126 Ibid., p. 406.
127 Derrick Jelliffe, *Commerciogenic Malnutrition? Time for a Dialogue*, in: Food Tech, Vol. 25, No. 2, 1971, pp. 55–56.
128 E. F. P. Jelliffe, *Maternal Nutrition and Lactation*, in: Breast Feeding and the Mother, pp. 119–139, here: p. 129.
129 Monica Kalt, *Tiersmondismus in der Schweiz der 1960er und 1970er Jahre*, p. 416.
130 Nacy Rose Hunt, *"Le Bébé en Brousse". European Women, African Birth Spacing and Colonial Intervention in Breast Feeding in the Belgian Congo*, in: The International

The postcolony did nothing to alter the European obsession with African breast milk. In the 1970s, however, not only did Western scientists focus on the breastfeeding practices of African women, but the practices of the scientists themselves were subject to a global debate, centering on the interdependency between the First and the Third World. But it should be noted that this debate was not just between two opposed camps, but also between the Nestlé Foundation, with its preconceived ideas about the situation of rural African dwellers, and the scientists whose work in Côte d'Ivoire opened up completely different perceptions.

Unpacking Ideologies: Echoes from the Field

Working in Kpouébo, Nestlé researchers Edgar Lauber and Michael Reinhard soon turned their attention to the composition and quality of breast milk and to the intimate realm of breastfeeding. Unsurprisingly, if inconveniently, they could hardly find fault with the human liquid, and the Annual Report of 1974 stated:

> Observations until now show that the breast milk of all the mothers, even of those who suffer from marginal protein-calorie malnutrition, is excellent compared to Western standards.[131]

The laboratory findings, however, revealed a decrease in protein concentrations over the first semester of lactation – a finding which was, of course, not at all specific to Africa, and the significance of which could not finally be assessed.[132] Not surprisingly, given the heated debates about what was to blame for the poor reception of milk powder in the Third World –unskilled handling and sterilization of bottles, the failure of governments to provide hygienic conditions, or the "ignorance" of mothers – Lauber and Reinhard's assumptions of a "comparatively good quality of breast milk" put a strain on relations between Nestlé and the Foundation. At a meeting between representatives of Nestlé and the Foundation, Alex-

Journal of African Historical Studies, Vol. 21, No. 3, 1988, pp. 401–432.

131 AHN, Rapport Annuel 1974, p. 11.

132 Edgar Lauber, Michael Reinhardt, *Studies on the Quality of Breast Milk During 23 Months of Lactation in a Rural Community of the Ivory Coast*, in: The American Journal of Clinical Nutrition, Vol. 32, 1979, pp. 1159–1173.

ander von Muralt emphasized, in a conciliatory manner, that the two scientists' findings could not be readily extrapolated: having been obtained in Côte d'Ivoire, they were only valid for this West African country.[133] Moreover, the question at issue was not just the protein content of the women's breast milk, but the "brutal" weaning practices whereby children were abruptly exposed to a protein-poor adult diet – which would still justify the distribution of Nestlé's products in Côte d'Ivoire.[134] Von Muralt's balancing act between protecting the work of his scientists in Kpouébo and repudiating what he called the "pseudo-scientific, irresponsible and ill-founded" international accusations did not convince those with clear ideological affinities.[135] John Dobbing, working at the University of Manchester, who subsequently edited the book *Infant Feeding: Anatomy of a Controversy*, could not understand why the Foundation had published the Kpouébo results, thus strengthening Jelliffe's argument about the irreplaceable value of breastfeeding.[136] In a letter to Nestlé's executive board, he wrote: "An openly expressed agreement with the findings of Mrs. Jelliffe (in fact she has none) reads strangely in the present delicate state of your affairs … I know that the Foundation is quite independent, but it is regrettable that its publication was not delayed a few months."[137] Nestlé's response to Dobbing's bewilderment revealed the company's efforts to interpret the results in favor of its general policy. According to Nestlé executive Jacques Paternot, the Kpouébo study confirmed that:

> (a) Ivorian mothers are not … able to produce unlimited amounts of milk for an indefinite period, (b) that the quantity of milk decreases from the 6th month onwards and (c) that the protein content of their breast milk is 30% less than in European mothers. [Taken together the empirical data] show the validity of our position; African mothers just as much as and perhaps more than their European counterparts need our food supplements. We have never said anything else nor done anything but supply our products to all those who need them. Thus, this study strongly supports our position.[138]

---

133 AHN, 9564–1, Administration, 1972–1979, E. Fasel, Visite à la Fondation Nestlé le 20 aout 1976, 23 August 1976, pp. 1–6, here: p. 2.

134 Alexander von Muralt, Dix ans de Fondation Nestlé. Message du Président sortant, in: AHN, Fondation Nestlé, Rapport Annuel 1977, pp. 2–3.

135 AHN, 9564–4, Séances du Conseil, 1973–1975, Serge Herzen, Attaques contre les fabricants d'aliments pour enfants en général, et contre Nestlé en particulier, p. 1.

136 John Dobbing (ed.), *Infant Feeding. Anatomy of a Controversy, 1973–1984*, London 1988.

137 AHN, 9564–1, John Dobbing to M. Gloor, 30 July 1976, p. 1.

138 Ibid., Jacques Paternot to Arthur Fürer, 11 August 1976, p. 1.

Kwashiorkor – An Urban and Social Condition

For others, things were less clear-cut. Facing fierce resistance from the Foundation, Kurt Schopfer finally left Kpouébo to study malnutrition in children with clear symptoms of kwashiorkor at the Hôpital Universitaire de Treichville in Abidjan. Together with Steven Douglas from the Mount Sinai School of Medicine in New York, he published a series of articles exploring host defense mechanisms in patients with kwashiorkor and their susceptibility to infectious disease.[139] Cases of kwashiorkor encountered at the hospital were mainly associated with viral infections such as measles, as well as poor hygienic conditions and poverty, which was the fate of all those forced to live in Abidjan's precarious urban environment: "Malnutrition was closely related to poverty, as experienced in the rapidly growing outskirts of Abidjan, and not at all a rural condition."[140] Convinced about the specific social context of malnutrition, Schopfer, collaborating with W. Page Faulk from the WHO Department of Immunology, once again turned his attention to the countryside. This time, the small village of Syélékaha near the northern town of Korhogo was selected for a nutritional study. The study design was straightforward. After an initial examination, a cohort of children living in the village was divided into two groups. For some months, they were given a daily portion of rice, with only one group additionally receiving a protein supplement. The two groups were then compared, and the immune response to certain vaccinations was measured.[141] The results did not show any significant differences in immune response between the two groups. No signs of malnutrition were found in either group, which is probably one of the reasons why publication of the results was never envisaged by the Nestlé Foundation.[142] The Korhogo study provided further evidence that medical investigation alone was not the right instrument to establish the existence of protein-

---

139 Steven Douglas, Kurt Schopfer, *Phagocyte Function in Protein-Calorie Malnutrition*, in: Clinical & Experimental Immunology, Vol. 17, No. 1, 1974, pp. 121–128; Kurt Schopfer, Steven Douglas, *Neutrophil Function in Children with Kwashiorkor*, in: The Journal of Laboratory and Clinical Medicine, Vol. 88, No. 3, 1976, pp. 450–461; Kurt Schopfer, Steven Douglas, *Fine Structural Studies of Peripheral Blood Leucocytes from Children with Kwashiorkor. Morphological and Functional Properties*, in: British Journal of Haematology, Vol. 32, No. 4, 1976, pp. 573–577.
140 Interview with Kurt Schopfer, 12 April 2012.
141 AHN, Fondation Nestlé, Rapport Annuel 1974, pp. 8–9.
142 Kurt Schopfer, personal communication.

calorie malnutrition in the Ivorian countryside. Consequently, the focus of the Nestlé Foundation's efforts in Côte d'Ivoire shifted from the breast to the brain, with pediatricians being replaced by psychologists.

Malnutrition and the African Brain

On June 28–29, 1971, members of the Nestlé Foundation in Lausanne discussed the nutritional data obtained from three years of intensive research in Côte d'Ivoire. To the experts' surprise, the anthropometric and biochemical findings did not yield a convincing picture of clinical malnutrition. One of the attendees wondered whether the absence of malnutrition could be the result of a genetically acquired adaptation.[143] Another expert conceded that the anthropometric data was within accepted limits but was nevertheless convinced that mental development was affected: "Psychological tests on school children in Kpouébo would certainly show a mental deficiency."[144] In addressing the effects of malnutrition on the brain, the Nestlé Foundation was not just joining in a highly controversial contemporary debate, but focusing on a topic closely connected with colonialism and racial science. Since the beginning of the nineteenth century and the advent of new scientific disciplines such as comparative anatomy, the brain had become *the* epistemic object, whose surface allowed conclusions to be drawn about the nature of man. However, as Nancy Stepan has shown, scientific arguments placing Western civilization on the highest echelons of evolution and explaining differences between "races" in biological terms were not just a nineteenth-century phenomenon. The idea of innate differences between blacks and whites and an understanding of the brain as the "arbiter of all things racial" proved highly tenacious throughout the twentieth century.[145]

While from the mid-1960s onwards, the field of ethnopsychology was challenged by broader accounts of transcultural psychiatry, whose clientele no longer consisted entirely of colonial subjects but included people living on the fringes of Western societies, the question of the intelligence of the underprivileged re-emerged as a prime topic among the world's foremost

---

143 AHN, 9564–4, Minutes of the 7th meeting of the Council, Lausanne 28 and 29 June 1971, pp. 1–28, here: pp. 7–8.

144 Ibid., p. 8.

145 Nancy Stepan, *The Idea of Race in Science. Great Britain 1800–1960*, Oxford 1982, p. 18.

nutritionists in the 1970s.[146] Leading figures in the emerging field of intelligence testing were scientists working in the slums of the burgeoning Latin American cities. A study unprecedented in scope and methodology was the Bogotá research project led by Fredrick J. Stare of the Harvard School of Public Health and partly financed by the Nestlé Foundation.[147] IQ tests involving several siblings were designed to show to what extent genetic and environmental factors could be excluded in explaining the relationship between malnutrition and intelligence. The aim was to determine whether, irrespective of ethnic origin, malnutrition could account for the difference in IQ scores between children in economically deprived settings and their more privileged peers. Certain aspects of this kind of scientific venture were rather controversial. Quite apart from the Eurocentric devices used to measure intelligence, the causal link between malnutrition and impaired mental capacity was more often assumed than scientifically proven.[148] Several experiments with animals suggested a strong relationship between severe protein deficiency and impaired brain growth and organization, but the fundamental question was of course whether this data could be extrapolated to humans. From a physiologist's perspective, Alexander von Muralt had no difficulty in drawing analogies between animal and human experimental models: "For a physiologist the close link between the cellular and biochemical structures and their function is a solid concept. A damage or distortion of structure is always a sign and cause of impairment of function. In the human brain, early malnutrition per se produces distortions similar to those in experimental animals and, therefore, its function must be impaired."[149] Von Muralt admitted that the human brain in early childhood exhibits striking plasticity and an ability to compensate for serious localized lesions, but given the more general detrimental effects of early malnutrition, he doubted whether the brain could compensate for this damage.[150] Thus, while a direct correlation between severe malnutrition and impaired

---

146 For a history of ethnopsychology in a colonial context, see Jock McCulloch, *Colonial Psychiatry and the African Mind*, Cambridge 1995.
147 AHN, Fondation Nestlé, Rapport Annuel 1971, p. 7.
148 Michael C. Latham, *Protein-Calorie Malnutrition in Children and Its Relation to Psychological Development and Behavior*, in: Physiological Reviews, Vol. 54, No. 3, 1974, pp. 541–565.
149 Von Muralt, *Influence of Early Protein-Calorie Malnutrition on the Intellectual Development. The Point of View of a Physiologist*, in: M. A. B. Brazier (ed.), Growth and Development of the Brain. Nutritional, Genetic and Environmental Factors, New York 1974, pp. 307–314, here: p. 311.
150 Ibid.

mental capacity was almost taken for granted, it was still open to debate whether this condition was irreversible and whether statistically significant impairments could also be demonstrated in people suffering from only moderate protein-calorie malnutrition. The latter question was not only of scientific interest but had wide-ranging political implications. Considering the case of Côte d'Ivoire, one of the Nestlé scientists bluntly stated:

> human intelligence depends directly on the quality of nutrition. In Côte d'Ivoire, general intelligence is low – too low to understand the basic rules of let's say hygiene or family planning.[151]

Given these political ramifications, the "moderate malnutrition-intelligence complex" was a popular topic addressed at scientific conferences throughout the 1970s. For example, at the First International Symposium on Brain and Intelligence, held in Miami in 1971, Fernando B. Monckeberg presented his conclusions – based on experiments in rats and humans – about the effects of nutrition on brain growth and intellectual development. In his view, and that of other researchers such as Joaquin Cravioto, there was no reason to doubt that severe malnutrition causes permanent mental deficits.[152] However, in children with subclinical forms of protein-calorie malnutrition, the causal relationship was not as consistent because of many "environmental factors that may negatively influence capacity".[153] This scientific caution was shared by Nestlé scientist Gian Paolo Ravelli when he presented his data from a Côte d'Ivoire study:

> We did not try to establish a relationship between the nutritional status, our findings, and the possible consequences it might have on the mental and intellectual development of the child. We didn't go as far as Dr. Monckeberg did. So, I am afraid that I will perhaps give a kind of flash picture of the nutritional status in this area and that particular village and you have to guess which consequence this situation might have on the development of the children who live there.[154]

---

151 AHN, 9564–1, anon., Visite à la Fondation Nestlé le 20 août 1976, 23 August 1976, pp. 1–6, here: p. 3.
152 Fernando B. Monckeberg, *Effects of Nutrition on Brain Growth and Intellectual Development,* in: Frederick Richardson (ed.), Brain and Intelligence. The Ecology of Child Development, Hyatssville Maryland 1973, pp. 207–228, here: p. 219.
153 Ibid., p. 221.
154 Gian Paolo Ravelli, *Study of Malnutrition among Preschool Children in a Village of the African Bush – Ivory Coast*, in: Richardson (ed.), Brain and Intelligence, pp. 257–265, here: p. 257.

The "flash picture" for which Ravelli apologized was nevertheless the result of selective reporting of scientific data. The children's nutritional status was determined on the basis of anthropometric data (weight/age ratio, chest and head circumference) and biochemical assays (blood/urine). The 72 children living in the small village of Adahou (Toumodi) were then divided into different categories according to weight/age ratio. While none of the biochemical tests revealed any signs of protein-calorie malnutrition, Ravelli found 22 children who could be classified as suffering from "moderately severe protein-calorie malnutrition" – a result that was not entirely supported by the other anthropometric data.[155] Without mentioning the other 50 children (all within the normal range), Ravelli concluded that this moderate protein-calorie malnutrition "may have a profound and lasting effect on the population as a whole … It is therefore essential to change the nutritional pattern for these children by introducing the notion of a special baby meal, to be prepared by the mother aside from the family meal and offered three times a day."[156]

While Ravelli remained in the realm of speculation as far as the relationship between moderate protein-calorie malnutrition and African intelligence was concerned, psychologists working in the tradition of Jean Piaget at the University of Geneva aimed to tackle the issue more thoroughly.[157] Piaget, who studied with Alfred Binet (the father of the IQ test) in Paris, had a complex conception of human intelligence. At the risk of simplification, the basic tenet could be said to be the capacity to adapt to the environment.[158] Piaget proposed an evolutionary four-stage model of cognitive development in children. For the Swiss psychologists, Piaget's model seemed to be worth trying out in an African context, not least because it was claimed to be universally valid. However, as Monckenberg had pointed out, there was a risk that environmental factors could distort the relationship between moderate malnutrition and mental capacity. Once again, Kpouébo was chosen as the study site. For Pierre Dasen, the Geneva

---

155 Gian Paolo Ravelli, *Enquête nutritionnelle en milieu rural africain. Village d'Adahou, S/P de Toumodi, Côte d'Ivoire.* Thèse présentée à la Faculté de Médecine de l'Université de Berne, pour l'obtention du titre de Docteur en Médecine, Berne 1972, p. 39.
156 Gian Paolo Ravelli, *Study of Malnutrition among Preschool Children*, p. 265.
157 Pierre Dasen et al., *Naissance de l'intelligence chez l'enfant Baoulé en Côte d'Ivoire*, Bern 1978.
158 Jean Piaget, *La naissance de l'intelligence chez l'enfant*, Neuchâtel 1959; Pierre Dasen, *The Cross-Cultural Study of Intelligence. Piaget and the Baoulé,* in: International Journal of Psychology, Vol. 19, No. 4/5, 1984, pp. 407–434, here: p. 408.

University researcher who was the principal investigator in Nestlé's psychological study, this village was the ideal location, as it displayed a considerable "cultural and socioeconomic homogeneity" which could mitigate possible interference by environmental factors.[159] In order to measure mental capacity in infants, Dasen applied a standard scale – derived from Piaget's insights and elaborated by Irène Casati and Irène Lézine – which included as markers of intelligence: (a) searching for lost objects, (b) using intermediaries, (c) exploring objects and (d) combining different objects. The study design involved two groups differing in nutritional status, which was previously evaluated using anthropometric data and biochemical assays. The results did not show any major differences in sensorimotor abilities between the two groups, and any correlations existing between moderate protein-calorie malnutrition and impaired intelligence could only be found beyond "narrow statistical criteria".[160] However, the two groups did differ considerably in their ability to experiment with new objects: "This is a very important aspect of intelligence in the sensorimotor stage, as well as in all the following stages. In fact, it is by manipulating objects and the relations between objects that the child constructs its consciousness."[161]

Nestlé's research project was short-lived and did not yield any concrete benefits for the local population. In September 1981, researchers from the Foundation abandoned their scientific station in Kpouébo. This special occasion once again brought together Nestlé representatives, high-ranking politicians from Abidjan and Kpouébo villagers to look back on the decade-long presence of Nestlé researchers in the village and to negotiate the handover of the scientific infrastructure to the local community. One representative of the Ministry of Health proudly addressed the villagers and urged them to continue their collaboration so that Kpouébo could "overcome its lethargy".[162] With the retreat from Kpouébo and other experimental centers in Côte d'Ivoire, the Nestlé Foundation for the Study of Problems of Nutrition in the World ended its commitment to combat hunger in the West African country and directed its attention to other regions of the world.

159 Pierre Dasen et al., *Naissance de l'intelligence*, p. 39.
160 Ibid., p. 270.
161 Ibid., p. 273.
162 Joseph Kouassi, *La Fondation Nestlé quitte définitivement la région*, in: Fraternité Matin, Lundi, 21 September 1981, p. 10.

Variations of Development
and the Power of Phenomenotechnique

In summary, this chapter has suggested that, on the eve of African independence, Switzerland emerged as a key player in the African continent's development aspirations. Development was such a powerful category that it brought together and enrolled various Western and African protagonists in this new field of foreign policy. One of the most prominent players in the landscape of Swiss development at the beginning of the 1960s was the STI and a handful of zoologists who managed to present themselves to the DftZ as indispensable experts for addressing Tanganyikan health problems. The success of the STI in mobilizing the various players was due not just to the close entanglement of science and policy – as "resources for each other", to use Mitchell G. Ash's expression – but also to the specific players' historical trajectories and ways of interpreting their present situation and future strategies.[163]

The ideological undercurrent that held together the various protagonists was the idea that African societies could be improved (i.e. transformed) through Western scientific tools. The Lumemo project is a prime example of this mindset, as well as of the complex interactions between the various Western and African development players. While the Swiss proposals did not survive competition with a more potent political actor, the German proposals suffered a serious setback when a consulate of the German Democratic Republic was accredited to Tanzania, after which West Germany withdrew all its development expenditure from Tanzania.

It was not always possible to undertake large-scale development projects. While Geigy and the pharmaceutical industry entered successful private-public partnerships in Tanganyika, the CSRS – lacking a long-term strategy – was overshadowed by French science and remained largely unattractive for private collaborators. The strong French presence was one of the reasons why a cautious approach was adopted for official Swiss development aid to Côte d'Ivoire, but the absence of the French did not guarantee the success of development aid either. As the example of the medical school in Guinea demonstrated, African politicians and functionaries cunningly

---

163 Mitchell G. Ash, *Wissenschaft und Politik als Ressourcen für einander*, in: Rüdiger vom Bruch and Brigitte Kaderas (eds.), Wissenschaften und Wissenschaftspolitik – Bestandaufnahmen zu Formationen, Brüchen und Kontinuitäten im Deutschland des 20. Jahrhunderts, Stuttgart 2002, pp. 32–51.

capitalized on Western development efforts and took advantage of the di-chotomized world order to play potential donors off against each other.

On the other hand, the strong technoscientific relations forged between France and its former colonies did not deter all Swiss development actors from intervening. Private charities such as the Nestlé Foundation main-tained close relations with the highest levels of Ivorian politics and were warmly welcomed to implement their research plans. The political network was, however, just one side of the coin explaining the power of Nestlé in Côte d'Ivoire. The other side involved Nestlé's capacity to apply modern biochemical methods in rural areas so as to construct a rural pathology – moderate protein-calorie malnutrition – which might then be amenable to Nestlé's own remedies. This capacity, and the efforts to draw general con-clusions about African intelligence, are best captured by the term "phe-nomenotechnique": coined by philosopher of science Gaston Bachelard, it refers to the fact that certain objects of knowledge are not given entities but are created through scientific instruments, which themselves are em-bodiments of scientific knowledge. Science in other words "realizes" its objects.[164] However, this power to realize scientific objects was a source of disapproval on the part of Nestlé scientists themselves. Those working in the field, in particular, were reluctant to reduce kwashiorkor to mere pro-tein deficiency, and interpreted the disease as the outcome of a complex in-terplay of social, environmental, infectious and immunological as well as nutritional factors. In so doing, they shared the view of the many physi-cians and scientists working in Tanzania who went beyond the scope of their own disciplines and embraced the views offered by social medicine.

---

164 Hans-Jörg Rheinberger, *Gaston Bachelard und der Begriff der "Phänomenotechnik"*, in: Marc Schalenberg and Peter Th. Walther (eds.), "… immer im Forschen bleiben." Rüdiger vom Bruch zum 60. Geburtstag, Stuttgart 2004, pp. 297–310, here: p. 304.

Chapter 5
The Empire Retreats: Medical Research, Development and the Rise of Social Medicine

In 1967, Julius Nyerere published the Arusha Declaration, in which he outlined his conception of an African socialism.[1] A reshaped Tanzanian society was to be founded on the concepts of "ujamaa" (brotherhood/socialism) and "kujitegemea" (self-reliance) – two elements of a development strategy designed mainly for rural areas. While socialism involved the creation of ujamaa "vijijini" (villages), serving as social and productive units, self-reliance obliged citizens to contribute their labor and resources to build up the nation.[2] The health sector was a favorite arena for putting socialist ideas into practice. As mentioned earlier, the Five Year Development Plan for 1969–1974 differed from earlier planning efforts in that it put rural health care at the top of the development agenda. More importantly perhaps, it was guided by the conviction that bringing basic health services to the rural masses would require substantial financial investment. In 1972, for the first time, the sums allocated to rural health centers and dispensaries exceeded those for hospital services.[3] The project of restructuring rural livelihoods in political, social and economic terms was partly shaped by foreign influences. One of the countries serving as a model for what could be achieved in rural health was the People's Republic of China, whose barefoot doctors had been heralded as an appropriate solution to Third World health problems, even in the West.[4] In 1968, intrigued by the success of the deprofes-

1   Tanganyika African National Union (ed.), *The Arusha Declaration and TANU's Policy on Socialism and Self-Reliance*, Dar es Salaam 1967; Julius Nyerere, *Freedom and Socialism*, in: Nyerere, Nyerere on Socialism, Dar es Salaam 1969, pp. 27–58.
2   Rebecca Marsland, *Community Participation the Tanzanian Way. Conceptual Contiguity or Power Struggle?,* in: Oxford Development Studies, Vol. 34, No. 1, 2006, pp. 65–79.
3   Ministry of Health (MOH)/Library, Dar es Salaam, Budget Speech by the Minster for Health, Hon. A. H. Mwinyi, MP, for the Year 1972/1973, pp. 1–25, here: p. 4.
4   Ruth Sidel, Victor W. Sidel, *The Health of China. Current Conflicts in Medical and Human Services for One Billion People*, Boston 1982, pp. 35–70; S. M. Hillier, *Preventive Health Work in the People's Republic of China, 1949–1982*, in: Hillier and J. A. Jewell (eds.), Health Care and Traditional Medicine in China, 1800–1982, London 1983, pp. 149–217.

sionalized and decentralized health services arising from the Cultural Revolution, Nyerere invited Chinese medical teams to Tanzania, who then offered their services to rural communities in eight remote districts.[5] The Chinese experience provided the blueprint for the introduction of so-called village medical helpers to ujamaa villages. These individuals, selected and salaried by the villagers themselves, underwent six months' training in a hospital with a view to administering first aid and preventing the most prevalent diseases.[6] This chapter argues that the second half of the 1960s saw a radical shift from former (colonial) health policies, in that the causal link between health and development was reversed. The changing political environment in Tanzania forced Swiss development initiatives to adapt and to embrace new concepts of community medicine and African socialism. However, for the government, health improvement in the context of rural transformation was again one of the major arguments for forcibly moving the rural population into ujamaa villages.

As had been the case in connection with sleeping sickness concentrations in the 1940s, health policy was again in the vanguard of welfarist policies and provided a welcome legitimation for authoritarian intervention by the government in the social fabric of rural populations. In the early 1970s, Tanzanian statism was reinforced as a result of two parallel political processes. Firstly, in 1972, Nyerere announced a government reform aimed at shifting centralized decision-making powers to the regions and districts. As he noted: "It has gradually become obvious that, in order to make a reality of our policies of socialism and self-reliance, the planning and control of development in this country must be exercised at local level to a much greater extent than at present. Our nation is too large for the people at the centre in Dar es Salaam always to understand local problems or to sense their urgency."[7] Contrary to what the political rhetoric might have implied, the policy of decentralization led to the dismantling of local development initiatives and a strengthening of the party within the dual, hierarchically structured system of political representation, extending from the village to district and regional levels.[8] Secondly, the increasing bureaucratization of development policies was accompanied by the more

5   MOH/Library, Dar es Salaam, Budget Speech by the Minister for Health and Social Welfare, L. Nangwanda Sijaona, MP, 1970/1971, Estimates, pp. 1–61, here: pp. 24–25.
6   Walter Bruchhausen, *Medizin zwischen den Welten*, p. 129.
7   Julius Nyerere, *Decentralization*, Dar es Salaam, 1972, pp. 1–12, here: p. 1.
8   Andreas Eckert, *Herrschen und Verwalten*, p. 244.

rigid policy of villagization, which left its mark in the memories of the rural population. In 1973, Nyerere stated that "living in villages has become
an order" and embarked on a more comprehensive villagization program,
with over 5 million Tanzanians being resettled by 1976.[9] It is interesting to
note that, despite the excesses of an authoritarian (albeit weak) state increasingly unable to harmonize the rhetoric of self-reliance on the periphery with the reality of concentration of power in the center, Nyerere's turn
to socialist rural policies did not damage his reputation in the West.[10] In
1967, after the wave of nationalization of banks and foreign companies in
Tanzania, Geigy silenced all those voices in Switzerland who believed that
the socialist regime was now showing its true colors:

> The Tanzanian authorities say that, while … [the nationalizations] were perhaps
> somewhat too brusque an act of force and President Nyerere – as he is himself well
> aware – is prone to such quick and emotional decisions, these measures had to be
> implemented sooner or later. They are nevertheless a far cry from what leftist gov-
> ernments in Europe (Labour in Britain, for instance) understand by the notion of
> "nationalization", where whole business sectors are affected by the process, while
> in Tanzania only a few foreign companies are affected. They assured me that there
> is no communist pressure guiding decisions …[11]

The widespread regard for Nyerere's modesty and his credibility did not
mean, however, that the relationship between foreign NGOs and the Tanzanian state would not be altered in the long run by the rural development
policies and the ideology of ujamaa vijijini. As some scholars have argued,
one of the main characteristics of this relationship was that Nyerere's rural
development ideology was more or less totally embraced by foreign NGOs
working in rural areas. In his history of the British charity Oxfam in Tanzania, Michael Jennings – extending the concept of the "development
front" (Saul and Cliffe) – introduced the term "surrogates of the state" to
indicate the NGO's compliance with Tanzanian government policies in the

---

9   Ibid., p. 253; Leander Schneider, *Freedom and Unfreedom in Rural Development. Ju-
     lius Nyerere, Ujamaa Vijijini, and Villagization*, in: Canadian Journal of African Stud-
     ies, Vol. 38, No. 2, 2004, pp. 344–393.
10 Susan C. Crouch, *Western Responses*.
11 Archive Swiss Tropical and Public Health Institute, Basel (ASTI), Ifakara I, BSFEL
     u.a. Rudolf Geigy, Vorschläge betreffend die zukünftige Gestaltung der Tätigkeit des
     Rural Aid Centres in Ifakara, 1967, pp. 1–6, here: p. 1.

1970s.[12] This line of reasoning is important because similar tendencies towards alignment with Tanzanian policy can also be detected in the Swiss case. Thus, from a historical perspective, Cold War ideologies did not automatically determine the practices of historical actors on the ground. Rather, these actors might or might not exploit these ideologies, depending on their changing interests.[13] As will be shown below, while in the 1960s science and technology had been a promise of modernity and rationality and an instrument of subordination, one decade later this powerful edifice began to crumble. Swiss development work was exposed to pressure from various quarters and drawn into the micropolitics of negotiation and adaptation to a new political environment.

Dismantling the Rural Aid Center – The Road to Preventive Medicine

The new political constituencies laid out in 1967 and the growing importance of health within socialist ideology had repercussions for the content of the training offered by the RAC at Ifakara. Towards the end of the decade, the status of the RAC gradually changed – no longer a foreign donation demanding African gratitude, it became an institution that created a sense of ownership and a strong desire to frame outcomes according to local needs. One of the consequences of the integration of the Medical School into the Faculty of Medicine in Dar es Salaam was that more and more faculty members tried to exert their influence over the RAC and to adapt its overall policy to the perceived needs of the country. Prominent among these was the malariologist Wenceslaus Kilama, who in 1980 would become the first Director General of Tanzania's National Institute of Medical Research (NIMR): "If the Ifakara course is to contribute fully to the development of our students, an integrated programme should be planned and carried out by the members of this faculty. Participation by the Swiss group should be encouraged, but the primary leadership must

---

12 Michael Jennings, *Surrogates of the State. Oxfam and Development in Tanzania, 1961–1979*, London 1998.
13 Lukas Meier, *Die Macht des Empfängers. Gesundheit als Verhandlungsgegenstand zwischen der Schweiz und Tansania, 1970–1980*, in: Itinera, Vol. 35, Basel 2014, pp. 125–144.

stem from the Faculty."[14] Apart from the issue of which party should have a stronger say in the overall policy of the RAC, there was the question of Tanzania's intention to create a new chair of parasitology in Dar es Salaam – which would render the RAC's teaching obsolete – and the more general impression that the RAC's strong focus on biology was out of step with the growing emphasis on social aspects of health care.[15] After discussions between the two parties in 1970, it was concluded that more time should be invested in conducting health surveys and disease control, with less teaching of parasitological topics.[16] However, the dispute about adapting the RAC was not just between the STI and the Dar medical faculty, nor did it concern only its future role within the Tanzanian health system. In the 1970s, the Swiss teaching staff were confronted with a new generation of politically active students, for whom the value of knowledge derived from its capacity to improve society. They wished to "enter more fully into the community … and to give service to the community in a number of ways."[17] The students' criticism was not just aimed at the underlying concepts of health and disease upon which the RAC was built, but touched on the politics of daily life. On one occasion, several of them complained about the low wages paid to the "flyboys" employed to catch tsetse flies and other disease vectors for research purposes. This issue gave rise to heated debate between the Swiss teachers and African employees about the degree of "exploitation" of subaltern staff, but it was finally resolved peacefully. Freyvogel, who chronicled these incidents, commented:

> It is a sign of increasing social awareness, perhaps because of the activities of Mwalimu Nyerere, and that we, who know the country and its inhabitants comparatively well, also have to adjust our attitude and behavior every year. It was interesting to see that in the discussions there was an African and European front opposing each other, even though normally contacts between Swiss and Africans are free of hostilities.[18]

14 ASTI, Ifakara I, BSFEL u.a, Wen Kilama, Some Background Information about the Ifakara Programme, May 1971, p. 2.
15 Archive Thierry A. Freyvogel (ATAF), Lettres d'Ifakara (1959–1985), Thierry Freyvogel, 31 July 1969, pp. 1–3, here: p. 2.
16 ASTI, Unterlagen Antoine Degrémont, RAC, Medical Students' Course 1971, Organisations, Thierry Freyvogel, Medical Students' Course 1971, Working Paper, 29 August 1970, pp. 1–3, here: p. 1.
17 ASTI, Ifakara I, BSFEL u.a, H. Gosling, Some Suggestions Regarding the Course at Ifakara, January 1971, pp. 1–2, here: p. 1.
18 ATAF, Lettres d'Ifakara (1959–1985), Thierry Freyvogel, 26 July 1970, pp. 1–3, here: p. 2.

Adjusting one's attitudes to the new circumstances involved juggling with a term that had different meanings for different historical players – "Africanization". Not surprisingly – given the political and social pressures facing a scientific paradigm as yet unable to bridge the divide between disease etiology and social aspects of health care – the Swiss scientists and philanthropists reflected on the future of their commitment in Tanzania. In the offices of the STI or J. R. Geigy AG, Africanization was seen as a historical process with the ineluctability of a force of nature. Although it was impossible to stem the tide, it was nevertheless worth trying to keep one step ahead and designing strategies to channel the process and "avoid precipitous and crude action".[19]

Opinions as to what Africanization might involve differed among the Swiss protagonists, especially between Victor Umbricht – a member of the Board of Ciba-Geigy AG – and Rudolf Geigy. While Umbricht advocated the complete handover of the development project to the Tanzanian government, Geigy was said to have "done nothing to reduce the Swiss presence in Ifakara".[20] However, both men in one way or another expressed the wish that Switzerland should continue its research activities in Tanzania, and this was more than likely since, in their view, it would take a long time for the Africans to become independent in research matters.[21]

The Medical Assistants Training Center 1973–1978

The Basel Foundation's step-by-step withdrawal from Ifakara was sealed with the decision to transform the RAC into a Medical Assistants Training Center (MATC) in 1973. The extension of training schemes for medical assistants was a high priority for the Ministry of Health in Dar es Salaam. Medical assistants ranked below physicians and assistant medical officers in

19 Novartis Firmenarchiv, CIBA, RE 15.04.1, Viktor Umbricht to Rudolf Geigy, Basler Stiftung zur Förderung von Entwicklungsländern/Ifakara-Projekt, 17 February 1972, pp. 1–3, here: p. 1.
20 Schweizerisches Bundesarchiv Bern (BAR), E 2005 (A), 1983/18, 361, t.311-Tansania 5, Rural Medical Aid Centre Ifakara, 1970–1972, Henri-Philippe Cart, Note de dossier. Entretien de M. Umbricht de Ciba-Geigy avec MJ et CP le 9 mars 1972, 14 March 1972, p. 1.
21 Novartis Firmenarchiv, CIBA, RE 15. 04. 11, Protokolle der Stiftungsratssitzungen 1960–1982, E. Stocker, Protokoll der Sitzung des Stiftungsrats vom 16. Dezember 1970, 10.00 Uhr bei der CIBA-GEIGY AG, pp. 1–7, here: p. 6; ibid., RE 15. 04. 11, Umbricht to Geigy, 17 February 1972, pp. 2–3.

the hierarchy of health personnel and were to perform preventive and curative work in the health centers – the cornerstone of Tanzania's rural health services since the Titmuss report. In 1972, just over 300 medical assistants were employed in government or voluntary agency health services, most of them coming from four schools based at Tanga, Mwanza, Bumbuli and Machame.[22] By 1977, their numbers had risen to about 900.[23] The Swiss and Tanzanian parties agreed that the new MATC should be handed over to the Tanzanian government after a period of six years, during which the Basel Foundation would continuously reduce its support for the project.[24] The new arrangement was not a unilateral imposition. The Ministry of Health successfully avoided all decision-making powers being vested in the hands of the Basel Foundation, arguing for the creation of a board of governors including an equal number of representatives from the Foundation and the Ministry, "with its chairman appointed by our Ministry of Health".[25]

Furthermore, the Tanzanian partners vetoed the original budget plans, which according to them would have transformed the MATC in Ifakara into an institution that was far too sophisticated compared to the other schools for medical assistants.[26] Instead, they proposed that the remaining funds should be invested in the construction of a new health center in Mlimba, around 100 miles southwest of Ifakara, which could serve as a

22 MOH/Library, Dar es Salaam, Budget Speech by the Minister for Health, Hon. A. H. Mwinyi for the Year 1973/74, pp. 1–30, here: pp. 22–23.

23 BAR, E 2005 (A), 1991/16, 400, t.311.Tansania, Allgemeines, 1976–1978, Speech by the Minister for Health Ndugu Leader Stirling, MP for the Financial Year 1977/78, pp. 18–19.

24 The contribution of the Basel Foundation was CHF 800,000, while the missionary society, the Tanzanian government and the Swiss government contributed CHF 200,000, CHF 100,000 and CHF 300,000 respectively; see: Novartis Firmenarchiv, Bestand CIBA, RE 15. 04.11, Basler Stiftung zur Förderung von Entwicklungsländern/Beteiligung des Bundes, 6 April 1973, p. 1.

25 Archiv Novartis Stiftung für Nachhaltige Entwicklung (ANSNE), N. B. Akim to Rudolf Geigy, Proposed Extension of Ifakara Rural Aid Centre into a Medical Assistant School, 20 July 1972, p. 1. Members of the Board of Governors were: B. O. Dendego (TANU Morogoro), Dr. Mgeni (Regional Medical Officer, Morogoro), N. B. Akim (Director of the Health Manpower Development Department, MoH), Dr. Valentin Schuppler (St. Francis Hospital), Bishop Iteka (Diocese Mahenge), Prof. Rudolf Geigy (Basel Foundation); see: Novartis Firmenarchiv, CIBA, RE 15. 04. 11, H. Meyer, Protokoll der Sitzung des Stiftungsrates vom 7. Dezember 1973, 16.00 Uhr, bei der CIBA-GEIGY AG, 7 December 1973, pp. 1–7, here: p. 5.

26 ANSNE Basler Stiftung zur Förderung von Entwicklungsländern (Ifakara), Notiz über die Besprechung von 18. Juli 1972, 18 July 1972, pp. 1.

suitable teaching outpost for the MATC.[27] In marked contrast to the former RAC, the MATC – instead of short-term courses in biology and disease causation – offered three-year courses for 40 students annually; training at Ifakara would thus lose the status of a picturesque episode enhancing the academic careers of Dar es Salaam students and become the basis for a long-term engagement. The school was placed under the direction of St. Francis Hospital, with the Swiss physician Oscar Appert serving both as Medical Superintendent of St. Francis and as Principal of the MATC.[28] While STI staff still taught tropical parasitology at Ifakara, the teaching responsibilities were largely shouldered by the overburdened Swiss hospital physicians. Perhaps paradoxically, while the development project was designed to shift the emphasis from curative to preventive medicine, the new commitments for St. Francis fueled its demands for further increases in the number of Swiss physicians in Ifakara.[29]

The most important innovation, however, was the inclusion of community and public health topics in the MATC's curriculum. The students' long-term engagement in Ifakara made it feasible to change the outmoded policy of "raising the rural community's awareness of the unhygienic conditions they live in", without actively seeking to improve these conditions.[30] In their second year, MATC students were occasionally sent to selected districts of Ifakara, where – in joint efforts with the local community – they built latrines and wells and passed on their knowledge of adequate nutrition, hygiene and the prevention of communicable diseases.[31] This community work was in close alignment with official Tanzanian health policy. In 1972, the country launched a campaign under the heading "Mtu ni Afya" (Man is health), spreading messages through various media to remote households.

This was not the first Tanzanian health campaign, but what was new about "Mtu ni Afya" was that, rather than being considered as passive recipients of health messages, the population was organized into groups and asked to contribute actively to the improvement of their health status: "This time, each group was to build some sort of health monument, some

27   Ibid., Akim to Geigy, 20 July 1972, p. 1.
28   In 1975, the physician Valentin Schuppler became Principal of the MATC.
29   ANSNE, C. A. Steiner, Rapport d'activités 1975–1976, December 1976, pp. 1–8, here: p. 7.
30   ASTI, Korrespondenz Appert, Eichenberger, Schuppler, Ifakara, Thierry Freyvogel to Gerhard Eichenberger, 31 October 1973, p. 1.
31   ASTI, Courses 1966–1971, Oscar Appert, 1972, pp. 1–3, here: pp. 2–3.

physical evidence of environmental change resulting directly from the campaign."[32] As Budd Hall noted, clearing vegetation around houses and building new latrines were the two favorite activities, far ahead of other interventions such as boiling water or avoiding group use of drinking containers and cigarettes.[33] In response to these developments, the STI – for the first time since the era of Thierry Freyvogel and Fritz Haerdi – sent a biologist on a long-term contract to Ifakara. Gerhard Eichenberger, a former PhD student of Rudolf Geigy, had dual responsibilities, which were not easy to reconcile: on the one hand, he was expected to revitalize the field laboratory and thus promote scientific research in the tropics; on the other, he was to support the social medicine and community health efforts initiated by the Tanzanian state – which was where Eichenberger's inclinations lay. Apart from teaching at the MATC, he spent a great deal of time

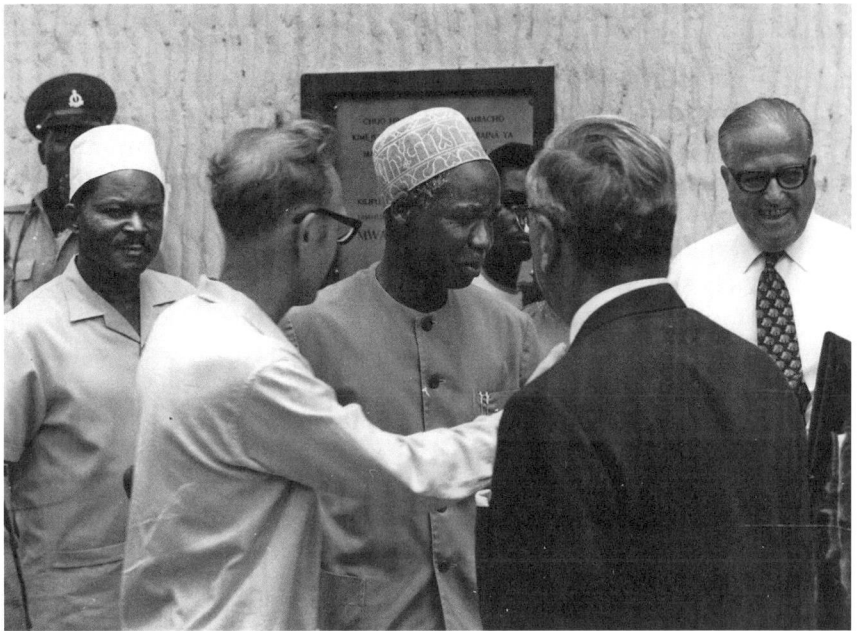

Tanzania's president, Julius Nyerere, inaugurates the MATC, 1973, Archive STI

32 Budd L. Hall, *Mtu ni Afya – Man is Health. Tanzania's Health Campaign*, Washington 1978, p. 45.
33 Ibid., p. 46.

preparing and executing a public health project aimed at sanitizing a district of Ifakara and sensitizing the local community to the health education provided by MATC students. As well as health information, which it was not always easy to comply with given the privations of daily life, the project involved more practical efforts. Eichenberger encouraged the construction of pit latrines, and – with the help of the mission and patients from the leprosy asylum – concrete top covers were produced and traded locally. However, the idea of establishing latrines was not wholeheartedly embraced by the community. Eichenberger recalled: "The problem with development work is that you never know what you'll achieve. The success or failure of development projects can only be assessed retrospectively."[34] But Eichenberger's public health campaign was never evaluated, nor was it continued after he left Ifakara in 1976.

What was demonstrated by these initial public health ventures – albeit without a scientific component – was the close alignment of Swiss scientists and physicians with Tanzanian health policy and the co-production of health and socialist superstructure. The argument that socialist ideologies and health were mutually reinforcing is based on the fact that health was de-individualized. Community health in the 1970s differed from public health efforts in colonial times in that the promotion of hygiene – nicely captured in the latrine fetish – did not spring from Western experts' fear of "disease dealing natives".[35] The strategy employed was not isolation of those already sick but promotion of behavior change among those not yet affected, for the benefit of all. As Eichenberger recalled, the message delivered in the 1970s was that general cleanliness and hygiene benefited the wider community, as did the establishment of latrines to reduce hookworm infection.[36] Conversely, noncompliance with these principles would have been interpreted as a threat to other community members and a blow to the concept of biological citizenship.[37]

Policy entered the MATC at other points too. In 1975, answering the call of the Ministry of Health, most of the country's school principals gathered in Kibaha, where they were informed that, as a self-reliance strategy,

34   Interview with Gerhard Eichenberger, 31 October 2008.
35   Warwick Anderson, *Colonial Pathologies. American Tropical Medicine, Race, and Hygiene in the Philippines*, Durham, London 2006, p. 87.
36   Interview with Gerhard Eichenberger, 31 October 2008.
37   Nikolas Rose, Carlos Novas, *Biological Citizenship*, in: Aihwa Ong and Stephen J. Collier (eds.), Global Assemblages. Technology, Politics, and Ethics as Anthropological Problems, Malden 2008, pp. 439–463.

all schools would have to cover 25% of their running costs through farming and animal husbandry.[38] Moreover, within a period of four years, the government reserved the right to withdraw all funding provided to the medical assistants schools. In order to increase its own contribution, the MATC in Ifakara was allotted an area of one hectare, where students regularly planted and harvested maize, onions and rice.[39] Despite the increasing demands placed on the medical schools, Oscar Appert supported the official policy: "The MATC complies fully with the official health policies and I want to add that I still agree with them in principle."[40] Thus, it would be wrong to interpret the MATC as a mere bulwark of Western biomedicine in Africa. Rather, it became a powerful instrument for planting the seeds of socialist policies in rural areas on behalf of the Tanzanian government at the height of its resettlement efforts. Swiss researchers' and physicians' vision of the content and effects of these policies was somewhat selective. While highlighting idealistic aspects such as equality and prevention of exploitation, they tended to disregard the increasing violence of resettlement sweeping across the countryside. While the notion of a "biomedicalization" of the African countryside by Western NGOs in the 1970s does not stand up to historical scrutiny, the idea of a stealthy process of "Tanzanization" of development circles in Switzerland seems more fruitful. It can be argued that the experiences of various Swiss development workers in Tanzania contributed substantially to the re-emergence of social medicine in Switzerland.

The Rise of Social Medicine in Switzerland

The shift in negotiating power between Tanzanian and Swiss players in the 1970s – as far as Swiss-initiated development projects were concerned – and Swiss researchers' close alignment with Tanzanian development policy is just one side of the coin. The other side involves the argument that the re-emergence of social medicine in Switzerland is closely tied to experiences in Tanzania. From the 1970s onwards, new nongovernmental actors entering the public health scene in Switzerland were able to place health high up on the Swiss government's development agenda. Worth mentioning in this regard is Medicus Mundi Switzerland (MMS), a branch of Medicus

---

38   ANSNE, Oscar Appert, 28 November 1975, pp. 1–3, here: p. 2.
39   Ibid., p. 2.
40   ASTI, Courses 1966–1971, Oscar Appert [undated], pp. 1–3, here: p. 3.

Mundi International founded in 1973. MMS is an umbrella organization fa-cilitating coordination of the heterogeneous development activities of vari-ous groups. More specifically, it has played an active role in recruiting and preparing candidates ready to dedicate part of their medical careers to ser-vice in a Third World country.[41] A key member of MMS was the physician Edgar Widmer (nephew of Edgar Maranta), who was familiar with the Tan-zanian health sector from his work at St. Francis Hospital in Ifakara – an ex-perience Widmer shared with several other members of MMS.[42] Though it focused on the medical system of developing countries, and the impact of its physicians' activities was generally confined to the hospital setting, MMS was important in spreading a new concept of health and questioning con-ventional development strategies. At a conference held at Rüschlikon (Zu-rich) in 1975, an MMS working group concluded that the "new target has to be primary health care for all; that means focusing on comprehensive med-icine which sees human beings within their specific cultural and socioeco-nomic environments and which is geared towards preventive measures for the healthy instead of only curative actions for the ill."[43]

It was decided at the outset that the MMS secretariat should be placed under the auspices of the STI and led by Antoine Degrémont (later Direc-tor of the STI). Degrémont, who held a medical degree, was largely re-sponsible for a shift within the STI from a biological towards a more pub-lic health-oriented approach.[44] This shift was triggered by the retirement of Rudolf Geigy, his replacement as Director by Thierry Freyvogel in 1972 and the emergence of a new group of politically perceptive individuals at the STI. Like Geigy, this new generation of development-minded physi-cians and biologists was extremely powerful in influencing the develop-

---

41   Archiv Medicus Mundi Schweiz (AMMS), DEH, Documents base, 1967–1981, Edgar Widmer to Thomas Raeber, 21 June 1972, pp. 1–2, here: p. 1.
42   Widmer published a dissertation in the field of medical history; see: Edgar Widmer, *Zur Geschichte der schweizerischen ärztlichen Mission in Afrika unter besonderer Be-rücksichtigung des medizinischen Zentrums von Ifakara*, Tanganyika, Basel 1963.
43   BAR, E 2005 (A), 1985/101, 11, t.024.04, Arbeitsgruppe Bevölkerungsprobleme und medizinische Entwicklungszusammenarbeit, Karl Appert, Neues Konzept für interna-tionale medizinische Entwicklungshilfe, in: Pressedienst der Schweizer Ärzte-Infor-mation, 26 May 1975, p. 1.
44   ASTI, Antoine Degrémont, Jean-Pierre Gontard, Aperçu global de la coopération Suisse au développement dans le domaine de la santé [typescript 1994]. Gontard ar-gued that 1973 marked a turning point in Swiss medical aid; see: Jean-Pierre Gontard, *Aperçu global de la coopération Suisse au développement dans le domaine de la santé, 1960–1993*, in: Jahrbuch Schweiz-Dritte Welt, 1994, pp. 169–184.

ment strategies of the DftZ. The fact that the new international health orientation did not emerge from the center of Swiss development aid but grew slowly from the periphery is illustrated by the contribution of the Working Group Health (WGH), a consultative body convened in 1974 to assist the DftZ in the area of medical development.

The Working Group Health

As well as Antoine Degrémont and Thierry Freyvogel, the members of the WGH included scientists, physicians and government actors, most of whom had experience of working in Tanzania.[45] The group's function was to advise the DftZ on its overall health policy, which was be more tailored to the needs of developing countries, and to define criteria for the assessment of new project proposals.[46] The new developments in the Tanzanian health sector, which fed back to the DftZ, were vital in framing new policies. But what made the lessons drawn from Tanzania's socialist health interventions so attractive for Swiss development planners? The answers to this question are multidimensional and have to be seen in the context of the history of Switzerland's experience with other countries' health sectors. First and foremost, Tanzania served as a model of a developing country testing homegrown solutions for its health problems, while deploying a rhetoric of self-reliance and equity in the health sector that was a perfect match for the new development discourses arising in Switzerland at the beginning of the 1970s. New conceptions of development work emerged when it became evident that many development efforts of the 1960s – inspired by the theory of modernization and notions of large-scale technological fixes – had ultimately failed. This can be described as a turning-away from the simplistic picture of a division of labor between the West, providing technical solutions, and the "underdeveloped" country, welcoming all these blessings in order to catch up in the march towards modernity. Instead, the new discourse reflected the West's own role in the generation of global inequalities, while still not being able to escape the

---

45 Apart from Degrémont and Freyvogel, this was true of Noa Zanolli (SDC), Jacques Rüttner (University of Zurich), Per Schellenberg (MMS) and Klaus Gyr (University of Basel).
46 Noa Zanolli, *Aus der Praxis lernen. Über die Aufgaben der Arbeitsgruppe Gesundheit*, in: Antenne, Vol. 2, 1976, pp. 5–6.

discursive dichotomies of "developed/underdeveloped", "traditional/modern", "industrial and scientific progress/stagnation" and so forth.[47]

Secondly, the DftZ's espousal of Tanzania's "demedicalized" and low-cost health care for the rural masses and the close connection between development and health has to be interpreted not just against the backdrop of general dissatisfaction with the previous course of Swiss development and political pressure on the official organs of Swiss development aid, but also in the light of the DftZ's recent experiences with improving Third World health. In a project led by the University of Bern, CHF 5 million had been granted by the Swiss government to the massive Duke of Harar Hospital in Addis Ababa. In 1974/75, however, the Swiss partners had to withdraw because of a decision by the Ethiopian military regime to shift attention from urban development planning to rural health care.[48] The adoption of a new health concept by the DftZ in the early 1970s was thus due to three factors – the Tanzanian experience of being the sorcerer's apprentice in one's own development laboratory, a new Swiss approach to development and, at an international level (as discussed below), a range of historical experiences resonating into the present.

The discussion papers drafted by the WGH provide evidence of the attempt to demedicalize health care and to link health and development – the chicken-and-egg phenomenon.[49] As the WGH's first paper stated: "Development aid in the realm of medicine has to be seen in the context of the socioeconomic conditions of developing countries in general and of the target

47 Manuel Schär, *Wie entwickeln wir die "Dritte Welt"? Kontinuitäten und Brüche im Entwicklungsverständnis um 1968 in der Schweiz*, in: Janick Marina Schaufelbuehl (ed.), 1968–1978. Ein bewegtes Jahrzehnt in der Schweiz. Unter Mitarbeit von Nuno Pereira und Renate Schär, Zurich 2009, pp. 99–111, here: p. 108.

48 Noa Zanolli, *Gesundheitliche Entwicklungszusammenarbeit des Bundes. Anfänge, Erfahrungen und die Projekte heute*, in: Sozial und Präventivmedizin, Vol. 24, 1979, pp. 192–194, here: p. 192; BAR, E 2005 (A), 1985/101, 688, t. 751–339, Medicus Mundi Basel, 1973–1975, Per Schellenberg, in: Bulletin Medicus Mundi Schweiz, Vol. 2, 1975, pp. 1–8, here: p. 4.

49 As Rolf Wilhelm wrote: "If the health of the impoverished masses in developing countries can be substantially improved in this way, an important goal of development cooperation is thus also fulfilled: a crucial basic human need is satisfied. This in turn will affect other areas of human life. As is well known, healthy people are better workers. But they also have a different attitude to the problems of their own future. And only then are they in a position to really help themselves." See: Rolf Wilhelm, *Auch die Gesundheit gehört zur Entwicklungsarbeit,* in: Antenne, Vol. 2, 1976, pp. 1–2, here: p. 2.

country or region in particular."[50] However, the new health and development discourse – with its emphasis on equal access to health care ("creation of basic health care services"), preventive rather than curative medicine and a focus on specific risk groups ("medicine in developing countries is to a large extent pediatrics, especially in a prophylactic sense"[51]) – was slow to establish itself and was not entirely free of contradictions.

Among the points about which members of the WGH were uncertain was whether or not disease prevention could be successfully applied in Third World countries. One of the major obstacles, it was felt, was that the outcome of preventive measures could not be as readily measured or counted as the numbers of surgical interventions or patients waiting in hospital outpatient departments. The success of prevention was a distant prospect:

> Although a major priority in principle, preventive medicine faces major constraints in Third World contexts. The time span in which the successes of preventive medicine become evident is the most important factor. During this period, which can extend over two generations, curative medicine will be crucial as a precursor of preventive concepts.[52]

It was therefore concluded that: (a) preventive medicine should be integrated into the existing system of curative services, (b) preventive medicine had the potential to trigger new curative services and (c) it was curative medicine that provided the mutual trust necessary for the launching of preventive measures.[53]

The uncertainties about the basic tenets of Switzerland's new approach to Third World health were not just inherent in the discourse but reflected in daily practice. However, this is not to say that the WGH was reluctant to prevent certain projects from being executed. In 1975, for instance, Degrémont and Freyvogel turned down a project aimed at improving cardiovascular surgery in Senegal on the grounds that it did not correspond to the basic principles of Swiss medical aid.[54] But such isolated events should not obscure the

---

50 ASTI, DEH/DDA, Arbeitsgruppe Gesundheit, Diskussionsgrundlage Medizinische Entwicklungszusammenarbeit: Grundlagen, Ziele und Mittel, 28 August 1974, p. 1.

51 BAR, E 2005 (A), 1985/101, 11, Franz Perabo, Zusammenfassung der Besprechung über Medizinische Entwicklungshilfe, 20 September 1974, p. 1.

52 ASTI, DEH/DDA, Arbeitsgruppe Gesundheit, Medizinische Entwicklungszusammenarbeit: Grundlagen, Ziele und Mittel, 3. Fassung, 29 October 1974, p. 4.

53 Ibid.

54 BAR, E 2005 (A), 1985/101, 11, Thierry Freyvogel, Antoine Degrémont to Rolf Wilhelm, 5 September 1975, pp. 1–2, here: p. 2.

fact that the approved funds were mainly allocated to multilateral coopera-tion projects and invested in vertical (and highly technical) health interven-tions focusing on specific diseases. A case in point was the large-scale multi-lateral Onchocerciasis Control Program (OCP) in West Africa, initiated by the World Bank President Robert McNamara and launched in 1973.[55] Swit-zerland's contribution to this program was by far its most substantial invest-ment directed to the health sector in developing countries at the time.[56]

The debates during the 1970s about the best strategies to apply in de-veloping countries and the appropriateness of the preventive approach cul-minated in the International Conference on Primary Health Care (PHC) at Alma-Ata, which came to symbolize these efforts.

Alma-Ata, Primary Health Care and the Counterrevolution

At the international level, the 1978 Alma-Ata Conference was crucial in bringing together the individual elements of Switzerland's early-1970s health discourse into a more coherent whole. At Alma-Ata – partly in re-sponse to experiences in Tanzania – the WHO adopted a new approach to health and the provision of health care. In contrast to the short-term, dis-ease-specific interventions that had characterized earlier WHO efforts, the Alma-Ata Declaration and Director-General Halfdan Mahler's slogan of "Health for All by the Year 2000" called for an intersectoral and multifac-eted approach. The PHC strategy emphasized the use of "practical, scien-tifically sound and socially acceptable methods and technology", commu-nity participation and the importance of health as a tool for socioeconomic development.[57] The Declaration reflects diverging opinions within the WHO, as well as broader political changes at the global level.[58] The Peo-

---

55 Thierry Freyvogel, *Flussblindheit und ihre Bekämpfung in Westafrika*, in: Bulletin Medicus Mundi Schweiz, Vol. 49/50, 1992, pp. 37–45, here: p. 37.

56 Peter Wiesmann of the SDC spoke of a total amount of CHF 12–24 million over a pe-riod of six years; see: ASTI, DEH/DDA, Arbeitsgruppe Gesundheit, Dokumente allge-mein, II, 1979/80, Peter Wiesmann, Bundesbeitrag an den Fonds zur Bekämpfung der Onchozerkose in Westafrika (OMS-Programm), 15 May 1979, pp. 1–9, here: p. 1. Be-tween 1980 and 1992, Thierry Freyvogel was a member of the OCP Expert Advisory Committee (including five years as its president).

57 Theodore Brown, Marcos Cueto, Elizabeth Fee, *The World Health Organization*, p. 67.

58 For a detailed history written from a WHO perspective, see Socrates Litsios, *The Long and Difficult Road to Alma-Ata. A Personal Reflection*, in: International Journal of

ple's Republic of China and the Soviet Union, in particular, played a significant role in the WHO's adoption of the new PHC ideology. While China provided the blueprint, with its barefoot doctor model, it was "the Soviets that led WHO to create a new rhetoric at Alma Ata, which eschewed the former goal of diffusing Western techniques around the world in favour of a strident, politicised advocacy of primary health care."[59] In theory – though this is largely forgotten today – the Alma-Ata Declaration and PHC was not just a strategy geared towards low-cost health care for the rural masses in Third World countries but also a standard for public health services in affluent industrial nations. In his report on the Alma-Ata Conference, Ulrich Frey, Director of the Federal Health Office and head of the Swiss delegation, reflected on the applicability of PHC for Switzerland, whose health system, in his view, shared many characteristics of those in developing countries: it was highly specialized and medically oriented, and large disparities and gaps in provision remained between the urban centers and underserved mountainous regions.[60]

According to Frey, the recommendations concerning the integration of PHC into a national health system, the links between health and other sectors (agriculture, education, public services, nutrition), and systematic health education were especially worthy of consideration, and he proposed the establishment of an ad hoc working group to explore the application of the PHC concept to Switzerland.[61] In 1982, however, a proposed federal law on preventive medicine elaborated under Frey's leadership failed to pass the consultation stage. The cantons in particular – traditionally the main actors in Switzerland's federal health system – were opposed to the transfer of decision-making powers to central government. Resistance came also from industry groups, who argued that in a liberal society, prevention was the responsibility of rational individuals rather than the state.[62]

Health Services, Vol. 32, 2002, pp. 709–732; Marcos Cueto, *The Origins of Primary Health Care and Selective Primary Health Care*, in: American Journal of Public Health, Vol. 94, No. 11, 2004, pp. 1864–1874.

59 Lee Sung, *WHO and the Developing World. The Contest for Ideology*, in: Andrew Cunningham and Bridie Andrews (eds.), Western Medicine as Contested Knowledge, Manchester 1997, pp. 24–45, here: p. 33.

60 ASTI, DEH/DDA, Arbeitsgruppe Gesundheit, Ulrich Frey, Bericht über die internationale Konferenz über primäre Gesundheitsversorgung (Soins de santé primaires) Alma Ata (USSR) 6.–12. September 1978, pp. 1–25, here: p. 21.

61 Ibid., p. 25.

62 BAR, E 6100 (C), 1998/106, 1, 660.6, Antrag auf Einsetzung einer nichtständigen Expertenkommission zur Erarbeitung von Grundlagen für ein BG über Krankheitsvor-

198 The Empire Retreats

Thus, the prospects for prevention and comprehensive PHC were poor, both in Switzerland and internationally. The Bellagio Conference, organized by the Rockefeller Foundation a year after the seminal Alma-Ata meeting, concluded that the comprehensive PHC model and the goal of "Health for All by the Year 2000" was too idealistic and too unspecific from a methodological viewpoint to be successful in practice. The publication on which the conference was based – written by Julia Walsh and Kenneth Warren (Director of Health Science at the Rockefeller Foundation) – proposed "selective PHC" as an interim and more cost-effective strategy.[63] Selective PHC prioritized certain diseases on the basis of prevalence, morbidity and mortality, and the feasibility, effectiveness and cost of control measures.[64] While Warren emphasized that he considered selective PHC simply as a realistic approach within the broader PHC framework, proponents of the comprehensive approach argued that the two concepts are in fact irreconcilable.[65] In 1982, the streamlined version of PHC was endorsed by UNICEF, which proposed a program known as GOBI-FF, focusing on children and pregnant women.[66]

Despite this counterrevolution, spearheaded by powerful actors such as UNICEF and the Rockefeller Foundation, the comprehensive PHC vision served as a catalyst for the reorientation of Swiss development policy. In 1979/80, in the ideological wake of Alma-Ata, the DftZ once again revised its guidelines for Third World health and development strategies.

Compared with earlier drafts, the new documents were unambiguous as regards the direction of development initiatives: health was understood holistically and prevention was strongly prioritized over curative medicine.[67]

beugung, Auswertung der Vernehmlassung zum Präventivbericht, pp. 1–16.

63   Julia Walsh, Kenneth Warren, *Selective Primary Health Care. An Interim Strategy for Disease Control in Developing Countries*, in: New England Journal of Medicine, Vol. 301, 1979, pp. 967–974.

64   Debabar Banerji, *Primary Health Care. Selective or Comprehensive*, in: World Health Forum, Vol. 5, No. 4, 1984, pp. 312–315, here: p. 312.

65   Susan Rifkin, Gill Walt, *Why Health Improves. Defining the Issues Concerning "Comprehensive Primary Health Care" and "Selective Primary Health Care"*, in: Social Science and Medicine, Vol. 23, 1986, pp. 559–566, here: p. 560.

66   The acronym "GOBI-FF" stands for Growth monitoring, Oral rehydration therapy, Breastfeeding, Immunization (against measles, diphtheria, pertussis, tetanus, tuberculosis and poliomyelitis), Family planning and Food supplements (for pregnant women and young children).

67   ASTI, DEH/DDA, Arbeitsgruppe Gesundheit, Dokumente allgemein, II, CZ, VT, aux membres du Groupe de Travail "Santé." Séance du 09.02.1979, projet de révision des directives en matière de santé, 30 January 1979, pp. 1–19, here: p. 14.

New strategies to improve deficient health systems ranged from education to the improvement of sanitation and hygiene, family planning, community involvement, and control of specific diseases. Most importantly, applied research was assumed to be an effective tool for promoting health in developing countries.[68] Not surprisingly given the close relationship between health and development, it was argued that health-related initiatives should be given more weight within the Swiss development agency.[69]

Decolonizing Swiss Medical Research in Tanzania

The new emphasis on health and development issues was paralleled by institutional changes in Swiss medical aid in Tanzania. As had been agreed in 1973, the Basel Foundation handed over the MATC to the Tanzanian state on April 1, 1978. The new acting principal, appointed by the MOH, was Boniface Bembeleza, who – as a former teacher – was familiar with the school's daily activities. One of the most pressing questions arising from the Basel Foundation's withdrawal from development work in Tanzania concerned the future of the STI's scientific activities and the fate of the field laboratory. With the chemical industry turning its back on Tanzania, funding for the field laboratory was drying up. On November 26, 1979, the Basel Foundation and the STI agreed that the field laboratory and staff housing should be made over to the latter, which meant that the STI now had to cover the full expenses of its scientific outpost.[70] This new situation, caused by the withdrawal of a key Swiss development actor, destabilized the governance structure that had been in place since the 1960s and initiated an ambivalent and multifaceted process of "decolonization" of Swiss biomedical research in Tanzania.

Firstly, in 1982, what is now the Swiss Agency for Development and Cooperation (SDC) became the major supporter of the STIFL in Tanza-

---

68 Ibid., p. 10.
69 Ibid., p. 18.
70 BAR, E 2025 (A), 1991/168, 812, t.751–014, Schweizerisches Tropeninstitut, Bde I–II, 1979–1981, Schenkungsvertrag zwischen der Basler Stiftung zur Förderung von Entwicklungsländern, in Basel (im folgenden "Stiftung" genannt) und dem Schweizerischen Tropeninstitut, in Basel (im folgenden "Tropeninstitut" genannt), 26 November 1979.

nia.[71] This meant that medical research was no longer to be conducted solely for its own sake but should reach out into society and serve humanitarian goals. Applied research within a PHC context was seen as a vehicle for promoting development and tackling local priorities, and it was to be carried out in collaboration with local partners: "Tanzanian health authorities want to be informed about what kind of scientific problems are tackled [at the field laboratory] and they insist on having a say in these matters."[72] However, the extent to which they had a say was determined by the Swiss partners. STI scientists were aware of the importance of the field laboratory for the institute in Switzerland and were not keen to compromise this position. As was stated in 1977:

> Seen from a Swiss perspective, the STIFL should not be downgraded to a mere service center for the Tanzanian health authorities but should still be able to work for the Swiss Tropical Institute (which does not, of course, exclude close collaboration with Tanzanian bodies). In the future, the laboratories should also increasingly execute projects and mandates that the Tropical Institute receives from the WHO. The field lab will thus maintain its vital role for the Swiss Tropical Institute.[73]

Secondly, in the 1980s, the STIFL maintained close relations not only with the SDC and the Tanzanian health authorities but also with a number of African scientists, who from the 1980s onwards started to apply for jobs at the field laboratory.[74] The professional status of these researchers and field assistants went far beyond that of "mere" collectors of specimens or laboratory sweepers. The newly appointed men (and, much later, women) acted as cultural brokers, who found themselves in the delicate position of translating biomedical messages from the "technoscientific world" (David Turnbull) of the STIFL to rural village life and back again. At the very

71 From 1976, the DftZ was known as the Directorate for Development Cooperation and Humanitarian Aid (DCHA) and from 1996, as the Swiss Agency for Development and Cooperation (SDC).
72 Novartis Firmenarchiv CIBA, RE 15.04.11, H. Meyer, Protokoll der Sitzung des Stiftungsrates vom 16. 12. 1977, bei der CIBA-GEIGY AG, 16 December 1977, pp. 1–6, here: p. 3.
73 Ibid., p. 4.
74 In 1981, the STIFL had 9 full-time staff members; 10 years later the number had risen to 88. See: Marcel Tanner, Andrew Kitua, Antoine Degrémont, *Developing Health Research Capability in Tanzania. From a Swiss Tropical Institute Field Laboratory to the Ifakara Centre of the Tanzanian National Institute of Medical Research*, in: Acta Tropica, Vol. 57, 1994, pp. 153–173, here: p. 162.

center of all these changes and developments, however, were ruptures in the epistemic structure of science itself. Essentially, the 1980s saw the rise of a new understanding of disease causation. Diseases were no longer conceived solely as the result of invasion of the human body by pathogens, but placed within a complex, interrelated system involving human bodies, microorganisms and socioeconomic factors. This is not to say that a reductionist concept of etiology prevailed before the 1980s, but that systematic and applied field studies investigating more complex patterns of health and disease were only undertaken by the STIFL from the 1980s onwards. This new approach was summarized by an STI scientist as follows:

> Everyone acknowledges the importance of integration at all levels of the applied domain: integration within development in general, integration of preventive and curative medicine, integration of the different control mechanisms. It seems logical to us to try to do the same in applied research, which means considering the largest number of possible factors contributing to one's well-being and studying their interrelations.[75]

Thirdly, with the conception of health and disease as outcomes of the interaction of human behavior, economic structures, epidemiological and environmental conditions, a new emphasis was placed on previously neglected diseases such as schistosomiasis (bilharzia). This disease is caused by parasitic worms of the genus *Schistosoma*, transmitted by freshwater snails acting as intermediate hosts. Sufferers contract urinary or intestinal schistosomiasis in pools of stagnant water scattered across the rural landscape. Public health experts' growing interest in this condition can be explained by its close association with the transformations undergone by the African countryside during the development decade. The links between irrigation projects or the improvement of communication networks and the spread of bilharzia have contributed to its reputation as a "disease of development".[76] In fact, the STI's involvement in bilharzia research dates back to the 1970s. In 1973, Health Minister Leader Stirling assured Thierry Freyvogel during an informal meeting that Swiss researchers were still

---

75 BAR, E 2200.83 (B), 1999/351, 10, 771.22.18, Schweizerisches Tropeninstitut 1982-1984, anonymized, Développement d'un programme de recherches appliquées au Swiss Tropical Institute Field Laboratory (STIFL) Ifakara, Tanzania, pp. 1–14, here: p. 8.

76 Steven Feierman, *Struggles for Control. The Social Roots of Health and Healing in Modern Africa*, in: African Studies Review, Vol. 28, No. 2/3, 1985, pp. 73–147, here: p. 96.

welcome in Tanzania provided that they put bilharzia at the top of their research agenda.[77] In 1977, Adrian Zumstein (head of the field laboratory) began investigating possible factors influencing the epidemiology of urinary schistosomiasis in the district.[78] During the first half of the 1980s, bilharzia remained the focus of the STIFL in the area. Apart from the disease's close association with processes of development and modernization, there was a more mundane reason for the continued research efforts – the STIFL's research options were restricted by the NIMR's insistence that malaria studies should only be carried out at its own research centers.[79]

Fourthly, the ambivalence of the process whereby Swiss medical research was decolonized lay not only in the need to share responsibility for research activities more broadly with Tanzanian actors while still exploiting the field site for the STI in Basel. More generally, and from a local perspective, decolonization entailed an increase in scientific activity and an intensification of knowledge production within Tanzanian society. This is in accordance with the observations made in the 1940s and 1950s that decolonization is associated with intense scientific activity. While the former field laboratory was expanded into society at large, the new modes of knowledge production should not be too hastily interpreted as the all-encompassing deus ex machina, analyzing, cataloguing and venturing into the unknown landscapes of foreign bodies, as postcolonial theorists such as David Arnold would have it. Rather, the translation from the lab to the field opened up spaces for negotiation between scientists and Tanzanian villagers as to which diseases should be placed on the research agenda and what paths towards development should be followed.

The Death of the Clinic

When he arrived in Ifakara in the early 1980s, one of Marcel Tanner's foremost concerns as Director of the STIFL was to place its scientific activities on a firm footing: at the district level, this collaborative strategy involved joining forces with Dr. Wolfram Moll (Medical Superintendent of St. Fran-

77   Interview with Thierry Freyvogel, 1 December 2008.
78   Adrian Zumstein, *A Study of Some Factors Influencing the Epidemiology of Urinary Schistosomiasis at Ifakara (Kilombero District, Morogoro Region, Tanzania)*, in: Acta Tropica, Vol. 40, No. 3, 1983, pp. 187–204.
79   Interview with Marcel Tanner, 3 February 2012.

cis Hospital), teachers at the MATC and Sarvato Tayari (District Medical Officer responsible for Kilombero). In a joint brainstorming process, the researchers, physicians and officials singled out four health topics for future investigation. Two of the projects were hospital-based: physicians at St. Francis Hospital were eager to study the hepatic disorders frequently encountered in their patients and the phenomenon of fevers of unexplained origin.[80] The latter, especially, was perceived as an urgent problem because so far, owing to a lack of adequate diagnostic tools, most of the various fevers recorded at St. Francis were interpreted and treated as cases of malaria. This practice probably had an impact on the degree of chloroquine resistance found among malaria sufferers – a problem that had emerged at the beginning of the 1970s and was attributed to the dispensary staff's "hopeless faith in injections".[81] The other two projects were inspired more by community medicine insights. The nutrition rehabilitation project was especially revealing for the public health experts, as it demonstrated the limits of medical care and prevention within the hospital or dispensary setting: what is the use of fortifying undernourished children at the dispensary or explaining to mothers how to prepare appropriate food, when the prevailing socioeconomic conditions preclude a more balanced diet? As Marcel Tanner concluded, "You simply cannot show people how to prepare a chicken at the hospital when there is no money to buy chicken!"[82] What was required was not an approach that removes patients from their everyday surroundings and confines them within the walls of a dispensary, but a sound analysis of the various factors influencing health and illnesses in rural village life. The last of the four projects, ambitiously if not surprisingly, aimed to study the relationships between nutrition, infection, immunity and environment (NIIE) within rural communities.

The extension of biomedical activities into people's homes called for a new knowledge of everyday life. In the eyes of the Swiss researchers, St. Francis Hospital was not a reliable partner for the provision of such

---

80 ASTI, Ifakara, 1980–1982 (vor DEH), Marcel Tanner, Priorities for a project on applied field research at the Swiss Tropical Institute Field Laboratory (STIFL) in Ifakara as pointed out by the District Medical Officer and by the responsible physicians of the St. Francis Hospital and the Medical Assistants Training Centre (MATC), May 1981, pp. 1–2, here: p. 1.
81 BAR, E 2025 (A), 1993/130, 456, t.311-Tansania.45, Recherches médicales au Swiss Tropical Institute Field Lab à Ifakara, Bde. I–II, 1981–1984, anonymized, letter to Rolf Wilhelm (SDC), 23 May 1982, pp. 1–2, here: p. 1.
82 Interview with Marcel Tanner, 30 May 2009.

data. This, at least, was the impression of Eric Burnier, a STIFL physician who assisted hospital staff in their daily duties and for whom "the future of St. Francis was a major concern".[83] Reviewing the work of St. Francis Hospital's dispensaries in the area, Burnier complained about the lack of adequate statistics, patient histories and working procedures:

> The activities of the 17 dispensaries dependent on St. Francis Hospital are a difficult issue: Dr. Moll did not want to or could not provide me with a single document. I also spent many hours delving into Sister Sarah's folder where all the papers concerning the dispensaries are kept but without avail. To be honest, all this is completely useless … there is nothing that would give you an idea about how these dispensaries functioned. Nothing but short notes written in all possible languages or travel reports where every author proposes different things year after year in his own manner. No statistics about staff, the number of diseases encountered, or birth rates that would be really useful.[84]

The intention here is not to assess the performance of particular dispensaries or even to consider more generally the history of health delivery services in Kilombero District; for this, readers are referred to another study.[85] The point to note is that, with the STIFL assuming a greater role in the field of medicine in Kilombero District, the concepts of "health", "disease" and "patients" were given different meanings and subjected to a different set of practices. Burnier's insistence on statistics about staff, the distribution of diseases and birth rates is important because it indicates a shifting of attention from the clinic to the population. In twentieth-century Tanzania – in analogy to Michel Foucault's observations on eighteenth-century France – the STIFL sought to move away from the prevalent model of treating individuals within clearly defined institutions towards a model concerned with the distribution and prevention of pathologies within larger societal systems. While the former model focused on the interpretation and treatment of specific symptoms, the paradigm shift issuing from systems theory gave rise to new biomedical practices, including (most notably) operational research. This type of research originated during World War II, when scientists developed cybernetic and mathematical models to optimize the

---

83 ASTI, Swiss Tropical Institute Field Laboratory (STIFL), Correspondence, 1981–1987, Eric Burnier to Antoine Degrémont, 4 May 1983, pp. 1–5, here: p. 1. Between 1982 and 1985, Burnier was paid by the STI in Basel, and later by the NGO SolidarMed. In 1988, he returned to Switzerland.
84 Ibid., Eric Burnier to Antoine Degrémont, 1 March 1983, p. 1.
85 Marcel Dreier, *Health Care, Welfare, and Development in Rural Africa.*

use of scarce resources in line with overall political and military objectives.[86] After the war and especially in the 1960s, operational research was applied to other public and corporate sectors, and it is now more generally referred to as the science of decision-making in complex social systems.[87] STIFL researchers themselves defined operational research as the "systematic study, by observation and experiment, of the working of a system with a view to improvement".[88] A good illustration of how operational research worked in practice is the above-mentioned NIIE project, which studied the impact of different variables (nutrition, infection, immunity, environment) on the health status of children living in the village of Kikwawila.

Practicing Social Medicine on the Ground: Experiences in Kikwawila

Kikwawila, a small village some 14 kilometers north of Ifakara, comprises three main areas – Kikwawila, Kilama and Kapolo. Unlike many other villages in the district, Kikwawila did not emerge artificially as a result of Nyerere's resettlement program during the 1970s. It therefore lacked most of the political structures typical of a "normal" ujamaa village.[89] Notable characteristics of the village were its rural economy (based on maize, rice and cassava cultivation), its ethnic heterogeneity and the lack of even the most basic health infrastructure. Kikwawila was a suitable site for long-term scientific studies because most of its characteristics were said to be representative of other valley communities too. Spread over a large area, extending from the Udekwa mountains in the north to the Kilombero river

86 Maurice W. Kirby, *Operational Research in War and Peace. The British Experience from the 1930s to 1970*, London, Birmingham 2003; Robert Lilienfeld, *The Rise of Systems Theory. An Ideological Analysis*, New York, Chichester, Brisbane, Toronto 1978, p. 103.

87 Martin Lengwiler, *Risikopolitik im Sozialstaat. Die schweizerische Unfallversicherung 1870-1970*, Köln 2006, p. 315.

88 ASTI, STIFL, Kilombero Health and Research Project (KIHERE), Administration 1986, Kilombero Health and Research Programme. Working Paper for the Programme Proposal of Phase II. July 1985–June 1988, November 1984, pp. 1–14, here: p. 4.

89 ASTI, STIFL, NIIE/KIK, Annemarie Schär, Kikwawila – Ein Dorf in Südosttansania. Aspekte der Detribalisierung und Integration, 20 February 1985, p. 4.

plain in the south, it offered a "cross section" of the Kilombero valley.[90] However, what distinguishes Kikwawila from most other nearby villages today is the pipe that supplies villagers with clean water. This pipe, dating back to the 1980s, is the result of collaboration between the SDC and the Swiss NGO Helvetas, after years of field research conducted by STIFL scientists.

The pipe is probably the most obvious remaining trace of the STI's research activities in Kikwawila. Others are more subtle, residing in villagers' memories. Mzee Limo, for instance, a former ten-cell leader[91], still vividly recalls the days when Dr. Tanner and other researchers from the STIFL and St. Francis Hospital used to visit the village on a regular basis. He pointed out to me where the researchers' table had stood, with lines of people queuing up to donate blood and other samples.[92] On a visit to Kikwawila-Kilama in 2010, I met Twaibu Likumi, a STIFL-trained village health worker. After the interview, Likumi took a pen and wrote down on a small piece of paper the amounts of cement, bricks, tubes and other building materials that would be required for a pipe to supply his house with running water. Clearly, he expected Dr. Tanner and the STI scientists to work towards the fulfillment of his personal desires.[93]

In the early 1980s, contacts between villagers and public health specialists became almost routine. In an effort to establish a sound "community diagnosis" that would facilitate the evaluation of "PHC implementation, selective population chemotherapy, health education, sanitation and schistosomiasis transmission control", the STIFL sent numerous experts to the village, many with backgrounds in more than one discipline.[94] For example, the tropical agriculturalist Andreas Zehnder, in collaboration with the STIFL and the Tanzanian Food and Nutrition Center (TFNC), employed a community-based approach to strengthen agricultural production, with the ultimate aim of mitigating nutritional problems. Stephan Biro, a Swiss

---

90   Marcel Tanner et al., *Longitudinal Study on the Health Status of Children in Kikwawila Village, Tanzania. Study Area and Design*, in: Acta Tropica, Vol. 44, 1987, pp. 119–136, here: p. 123.
91   A ten cell is an administrative unit consisting of ten households and supervised by a ten-cell leader.
92   Interview with Mzee Limo, 8 February 2009. I am very grateful to Zachary Likopa for his assistance during the interviews conducted in Kikwawila.
93   Interview with Twaibu Likumi, 4 April 2010.
94   Marcel Tanner, Don De Savigny, *Monitoring Community Health Status. Experience from a Case Study in Tanzania*, in: Acta Tropica, Vol. 44, 1987, pp. 260–270, here: p. 262.

doctoral student, focused on the identification of anopheline vectors and the distribution of larvae and adults throughout the area, while George Lwihula approached the problem of schistosomiasis transmission from a sociological perspective and Reto Suter tested the impact of a local plant molluscicide on disease vectors.[95] In 1982, these longitudinal field activities were brought under the umbrella of the SDC-financed Kilombero Health and Research (KIHERE) project, which – in various stages between 1982 and 1991 – combined research on specific diseases (malaria, bilharzia), health systems research (HSR) and PHC components.[96] However, these new ways of looking at rural communities – focusing on the interrelations between disease, nature and culture so as to counteract the STIFL's reputation as a "benevolent bush-lab which imposes its own culture onto others" – are only one side of the coin.[97] On the other side is the

95 ASTI, Korrespondenz Thierry Freyvogel, 1972–1987, Andreas Zehnder et al., Proposal for a Community-Based Approach to Strengthen Agricultural Production and, thus to Contribute to the Control of Nutritional Problems in the Kilombero District, September 1984, pp. 1–3; Andreas Zehnder, *Agricultural Production in Kikwawila Village, Southeastern Tanzania*, in: Acta Tropica, Vol. 44, 1987, pp. 245–260; Marcel Tanner, Zohra Lukmanji, *Food Consumption Patterns in a Rural Tanzanian Community (Kikwawila Village, Kilombero District, Morogoro Region) during Lean and Post-Harvest Season*, Tanzania Food and Nutrition Centre Report No. 940, 1985; Stephan Biro, *Investigations on the Bionomics of Anopheline Vectors in the Ifakara Area (Kilombero District, Tanzania)*, Inaugural-Dissertation zur Erlangung der Würde eines Doktors der Philosophie vorgelegt der Philosophisch-Naturwissenschaftlichen Fakultät der Universität Basel, Basel 1987; George Lwihula, *Human Behaviour and Social Factors Influencing* S. haematobium *transmission in Kikwawila (Kilombero District, Morogoro Region) Tanzania*, London 1985; Reto Suter, *The Plant Molluscicide* Swartzia madagascariensis *and its Application in Transmission Control Measures Against* Schistosoma haematobium. *Experience from Kikwawila (Kilombero District, Tanzania),* Inaugural-Dissertation zur Erlangung der Würde eines Doktors der Philosophie vorgelegt der Philosophisch-Naturwissenschaftlichen Fakultät der Universität Basel, Basel 1986.

96 BAR, E 2025 (A), 1997/200, 642, t.311-Tansania.45, Recherches médicales au Swiss Tropical Institute Field Lab à Ifakara, vols. 1–2, 1985–1987, Tansania: Programme de recherches médicales appliquées au laboratoire de terrain de l'Institut Tropical Suisse à Ifakara, pp. 1–14. The organization of the KIHERE project – with the SDC as funder, the STI as executing agency and the STIFL responsible for operations on the ground – revealed the fragile foundations of the new development arrangements. With each new phase (1982/1985/1987/1989), the STI had to apply to the Swiss government for funding on behalf of the STIFL, without ever knowing what would be allocated. See: ASTI, STIFL, Evolution/Integration, 1988–1994, The Evolution of Ifakara Center – STIFL and its future perspective [no date], p. 1.

97 Don De Savigny, paraphrased in: ASTI, STIFL 1.2. General, Policy, Evaluation, Ulrich Schmid (sda), Tropeninstitut Ifakara. Praxisorientierte Feldforschung, pp. 1–4,

question how the villagers of Kikwawila received the presence of the Western researchers and their preventive health care messages, which undercut the conventional understanding of Western biomedicine as symbolized by St. Francis Hospital in Ifakara. In other words, what form did interactions between the biomedical experts and villagers take when whole segments of the population – sick or healthy – came under scientific scrutiny? Working within rural communities, STIFL scientists now had to explain and legitimize their presence, and to offer manifest benefits in return for scientific specimens: what they established was a barter economy, where body tissues and fluids were exchanged for water pipes and pit latrines. How are these changes to be understood, and how were they interpreted in the light of the different cultural and historical experiences of the biomedical protagonists and the rural farmers?

Negotiating Primary Health Care

Answers to this question were provided by Charles Mayombana in an interview in 2011. Mayombana left his home in the Kagera Region of northern Tanzania in 1977 to enroll at the MATC in Ifakara. At the end of his studies, he met Marcel Tanner, who was just about to take over from Adrian Zumstein as head of the STIFL. There were informal talks between Tanner and Mayombana about future work for the STI in Kilombero District, but at the time Tanner was unable to make any firm promises. Mayombana returned to the Kagera Region, where he found employment in the regional hospital. In 1983, when the STIFL turned to applied and operational field studies, he was called back to Ifakara to become the institute's first Tanzanian senior staff member, liaising between the STIFL and rural communities. For him, the difference between his hospital work in Kagera and his new position could not have been more pronounced:

> That is really the difference. In the clinic you are sitting there and you are waiting for patients to come. They tell you their problem, you treat them and they pay much more attention to you because they came to seek health. With my second job, which was more in the village improving public health, it was different because you talk about malaria, you talk about bilharzia, you talk about what the district health system should do to improve the health of the people – all this kind of things. Sometimes it is not their problem … We were supposed to be doing that be-

here: p. 2.

cause in the training we were also taught how to do, for example, community diagnosis, yes? Before patients come, you look through the window to see where they live and what makes them sick, yes, various factors from family to the individual. So this is the difference. So now, when you walk from the hospital and go there to see them and talk about what normally they suffer from, this is fine, but when you come to ask "Can I take your blood?", "Can I check your stool?", "Can I check your urine?", then the viewpoint is different because – "Why are you interested in looking at me when I am not sick?"[98]

The only legitimate reason for working within communities and approaching farming societies was PHC. In 1983, a PHC program was officially adopted, and Tanzania embarked on a village health worker (VHW) scheme in five pilot regions.[99] However, implementation of the various PHC efforts rested mainly in the hands of foreign NGOs. From a Western science perspective, PHC – and the question "Why are you interested in looking at me when I am not sick?" – called for a new approach, going beyond interventions based on epidemiological data. However, such data is important in understanding how biomedical interactions altered with the advent of PHC. In 1982, the STIFL set up its own VHW program, training and deploying VHWs in the three areas of Kikwawila and organizing the provision of essential drugs.[100] The men and women selected by their respective communities were responsible for curative as well as preventive health care.[101] One of their duties was to report in detail why sufferers sought advice at their village health posts. The headache/fever complex (malaria) was by far the most serious health problem in the village, followed by other ailments such as respiratory tract infections, gastroenteritis, and eye or skin diseases.[102] In 1982, schistosomiasis was not mentioned at all, but from 1983 and 1984 onwards, it began to be reported as a health problem,

98 Interview with Charles Mayombana, 9 February 2011.
99 Ministry of Health (ed.), *National Guidelines for the Implementation of the Primary Health Care Program in Tanzania*, Dar es Salaam 1983; Tanzania National Archive (TNA), 450/HEH/30/7, Primary Health Care, Flavian Magari, Julius Sepeku, Country Paper on Organization and Implementation of Primary Health Care in Tanzania. Presented at the South-East Asia Regional Conference on PHC 7–16 September, 1983, Pyongyang, The Democratic People's Republic of Korea, pp. 1–12.
100 ASTI, STIFL, PHC, 3. 2 (P.1), Working Document No. 1, Collaborative Primary Health Care Project in Kilombero District, Tanzania, September 1989, pp. 1–22.
101 Marcel Tanner et al., *Longitudinal Study of the Health Status of Children in Kikwawila Village*, p. 133.
102 Antoine Degrémont et al., *Longitudinal Study of the Health Status of Children in a Rural Tanzanian Community. Comparison of Community-Based Clinical Examinations,*

especially among children. The difference in perceptions of malaria and schistosomiasis may be due to the course of the two diseases: while malaria often kills very rapidly, schistosomiasis is a chronic condition and, even though parasitological data might be unequivocal, it was often interpreted by villagers as general fatigue and indisposition.[103] The important point here is that, with a conventional approach, morbidity and mortality patterns would have been noted, and vertical health interventions would have been used to tackle these specific diseases. In contrast, with the PHC approach, researchers and villagers came together to discuss public health and development priorities. What the STIFL scientists had to learn was that public health problems did not rank very high among the Kikwawilans' concerns. More pressing for them was fulfillment of the promises of the villagization campaign, which had fallen short of their expectations as regards the improvement of village infrastructure. It was therefore agreed that, as part of a schistosomiasis control program, the STIFL would collaborate with the SDC and other NGOs on improving the water supply system, thereby guaranteeing villagers' support for further health interventions. As Marcel Tanner noted: "The implementation of a water supply scheme is the spearhead of the ongoing and future actions: it assures community participation. At the same time it prepares the ground for the initiation of latrine campaigns."[104] Thus, for the researchers, the water pipe was the starting point for all subsequent PHC projects, but for the villagers it was also the end product shaping all present interactions. According to Antoine Degrémont, this was apparent during the research process: "For the standard questionnaires and the household interview, people were also influenced in their answers, particularly those concerning schistosomiasis, by the interest and activities of health professionals they were aware of behind the interviewers."[105] In short, while schistosomiasis was a biological entity encountered through the lenses of Western microscopes, its pres-

---

the Diseases Seen at Village Health Posts and the Perception of Health Problems by the Population, in: Acta Tropica, Vol. 44, 1987, pp. 175–190, here: p. 179.

103 This is not to say that there is no need for schistosomiasis control. Taken together with other neglected tropical diseases, it is associated with higher mortality than malaria, and its disappearance from today's public health agenda is to be regretted.

104 Marcel Tanner et al., *Community Participation within a Primary Health Care Programme*, in: Tropical Medicine and Parasitology, Vol. 37, 1986, pp. 164–167, here: p. 167.

105 Antoine Degrémont et al., *Longitudinal Study of the Health Status of Children in a Rural Tanzanian Community*, p. 187.

ence in the village was due to culturally shaped interactions and expectations. In retrospect, the STIFL's selection of schistosomiasis as one of its main targets could not be explained by the wish for infrastructural improvement. In an interview, a former VHW was asked to explain the emphasis placed by Swiss scientists on schistosomiasis control:

> Why then did the STIFL decide to tackle bilharzia and not malaria?
>
> I don't know why they selected bilharzia because at that time most children were dying from malaria. They sat together with the village authorities and they saw that bilharzia affected more people, especially the children who went to the river.
>
> Would you have preferred an intervention that addressed malaria instead of bilharzia?
>
> You see, malaria we could prevent, but bilharzia at that time we could not prevent.[106]

However, Kikwawila was never a place that allowed for unconstrained, nonhierarchical exchanges between scientists and villagers; on the contrary, power struggles at various levels became more pronounced. It became evident that the agreement to exchange water pipes for body fluids and individual compliance had ended. On several occasions, STIFL scientists complained about the villagers' reluctance to fully embrace latrine construction, and the village leaders started to fine the laggards. The work of the VHWs – some of whom confused their appointment with a "government position rather than a community worker"[107] – also involved strong elements of social control. A former VHW in Kikwawila remembered hiding behind a tree close to the river to record who was using it, when and for what purpose, and thus causing widespread unease among the villagers.[108] Historian Rebecca Marsland discerns competing understandings of the term "participation" in the context of Tanzanian local development. That proposed by Western development experts involves notions of "empowerment" and "involvement", while the other – more deeply embedded in Tanzanian history – is informed by the notion of "self-reliance" (kujitegemea), where citizens are obliged to contribute their labor and resources in a community effort to "build the nation".[109] Marsland concludes

---

106 Interview with JM, Kikwawila 2009.
107 Archive Ifakara Health Institute, Ifakara (AIHI), unlabeled, Charles Mayombana, Village Health Workers in Kilombero District. Training, Performance and Supervision, p. 4.
108 Interview with TJ, Kikwawila, 4 April 2010.
109 Rebecca Marsland, *Community Participation the Tanzanian Way*, p. 66.

that participation was such a popular concept in Tanzania because it invoked kujitegemea and allowed the state to "retain control over its citizens".[110] Under the Ujamaa Village Act, introduced in 1976, village governments were allowed to pass "appropriate" by-laws for health promotion purposes. The areas deserving special attention ranged from the construction of "adequate" houses to sanitation, personal hygiene and the suppression of "harmful cultural practices".[111] This legal framework was still shaping the relationship between village leadership and villagers when the STIFL started its community-based health projects. With regard to the mixed success of latrine promotion, one of the scientists commented:

> Sometimes you have to push development, especially those kind of developments that people would not really see as necessary, like latrines – you know, there are many bushes in Kikwawila.[112]

Swiss and Tanzanian scientists were the first to acknowledge that "Development is very political in Tanzania."[113] Comparison with the STIFL-led VHW program conducted in Namawala is especially instructive as regards how public health interventions are affected by the "political anatomy" of villages.[114] Unlike Kikwawila, Namawala emerged during the 1970s villagization campaign and was administered by an effective leadership which was always ready to contribute to the salaries of VHWs in order to enhance their commitment. Comparing Namawala and Kikwawila, Charles Mayombana observed:

> Whereas there is quite a good integration of the village health workers in one village, where even remuneration and support from the community has been achieved, the lack of leadership in the other villages makes the implementation of Primary Health Care difficult. It is worthwhile to mention that the request to have village health workers came from the community in the first village and that this community might be better motivated to support their village health workers than

110 Ibid., p. 70.
111 Ministry of Health (ed.), *National Guidelines for the Implementation*, p. 53.
112 Anonymized, Interview held in Dar es Salaam, 2011.
113 Michael Jennings, *"Development is Very Political in Tanzania." Oxfam & the Chunya Integrated Development Programme, 1972–1976*, in: Ondine Barrow and Michael Jennings (eds.), The Charitable Impulse. NGO's and Development in East and North-East Africa, Oxford, Bloomfield CT 2001, pp. 109–132.
114 Marcel Tanner, *From the Bench to the Field. Control of Parasitic Infections within Primary Health Care*, in: Parasitology, Vol. 99, 1989, pp. 81–92, here: p. 84.

the latter. The strong leadership in the first village contributed to the successful running of a village health post.[115]

But the success or failure of PHC programs did not depend only on the political organization of the villages concerned. In the 1980s, partly because of the STIFL's activities, Kilombero District became a popular site for interventions of other powerful health actors, who favored a more vertical approach to PHC. This was true of UNICEF which, according to STIFL scientists Don DeSavigny and Christoph Hatz, operated as the "second or parallel Ministry of Health in Tanzania" and which, from 1987 onwards, embarked on a large-scale PHC/nutrition program in Morogoro Region.[116] The STIFL was eager to foster close links with UNICEF, not least because such collaboration facilitated the exchange of relevant biomedical data which might not have been available from the Tanzanian Ministry of Health.[117] While it must be acknowledged that serious efforts were made to integrate activities into district structures, the performance of powerful health actors such as UNICEF and the STIFL raises questions about the sustainability of PHC projects. In most cases, the Kilombero District health authorities were not in a position to continue the health interventions that were initiated. Apart from the creation of dual health structures, which in the case of UNICEF left Tanzanian agencies with a minor role in the health sector, the District's weaknesses were largely due to the fact that the shifting of power from the administrative center to the periphery remained mere rhetoric, thus "leaving pilot projects alone, drifting on one or the other side of the road to 'health for all' but not on that to community development".[118] Consequently, Western health protagonists often tried to sustain interventions artificially. Although all PHC activities were supposed to be handed over to Kilombero's PHC coordinator, Cletus Makero, in 1986, two years later the STIFL was still covering most of the costs for VHWs and for the running of the Village Essential Drug Program for Kilombero District, thus addressing the District's complaints about financial

115 AIHI, unlabeled, Mayombana, Village Health Workers in Kilombero District, p. 3.
116 ASTI, KIHERE Letters, 1985–1988, Don De Savigny, Christoph Hatz, 7 March 1986, pp. 1–15, here: p. 7.
117 Marcel Tanner, *Monitoring of Community Health Status. Experience from a Case Study in Tanzania*, in: Acta Tropica, Vol. 44, 1987, pp. 260–270, here: p. 268.
118 ASTI, KIHERE Letters, 1985–1988, Marcel Tanner to Christoph Hatz and Calum Macpherson, 29 May 1988, p. 4.

constraints.[119] From the perspective of the Western biomedical organizations, the health system was only functional when it was activated and sustained through ongoing commitments.

Bringing Science Back in: The Emergence of a New Dispositive

This last remark reflects the sobering end of a decade that had begun with so much verve and development optimism. At the end of the 1960s, Tanzania was considered a model in exchanging curative for preventive medicine and actively involving rural communities in the new (or re-emerging) health regime. By reversing the causal link between health and development, the East African country influenced development policies in Switzerland's corridors of power, as well as practices in Kilombero District. New financial modalities within Swiss development work and the new policy context of socialism and decentralization in Tanzania gave rise to a new scientific "dispositive" in Kilombero – understood by Foucault as a heterogeneous entity comprising discourses, institutions, scientific doctrines, laws and so on.[120] The new formation had its new pathologies (bilharzia), its renewed scientific paradigms (PHC) and its new practices. A prominent locus was the laboratory and scientific research revitalized by close links with development ideology. In practice, however, the laboratory lost many of its former constituencies. Instead of science being practiced within laboratory walls, the local community around Ifakara became actively involved in the research process. This translation of the laboratory to the field made the former boundaries between lab and society increasingly indistinct. STIFL scientists started to immerse themselves in African society, collecting the health-related data required as a basis for the evaluation of new interventions. What they brought with them was a new mode of knowledge generation that followed an experimental logic: rather than new approaches being tested within the laboratory for later application to society, the formerly separate activities of research and application co-

---

119 Ibid., Letter to Don De Savigny, 21 February 1986, pp. 1–13, here: p. 8; ASTI, KI-HERE File 1988, Jan bis Juni, B. Chahali (District Executive Director) to Christoph Hatz (STIFL), REF: Village Health Workers in Kilombero, 18 January 1988, pp. 1–2 and Christoph Hatz's reply, 23 February 1988, pp. 1–2.
120 Deleuze argued for a dynamic understanding of Foucault's term, see: Gilles Deleuze, *Was ist ein Dispositiv?*, in: François Ewald and Bernhard Waldenfels (eds.), Spiele der Wahrheit. Michel Foucaults Denken, Frankfurt am Main 1991, pp. 153–162.

alesced within rural communities.[121] What can be observed, however, is not just a process of scientification of African communities, but a reverse process of society "speaking back" to Western and Tanzanian scientists. The premise of "participatory development" required new, socially acceptable strategies and research outcomes. As the example of Kikwawila has shown, this involved not only negotiations about which disease to tackle but also engagement in material improvements, which in turn was to guarantee villagers' compliance with public health projects. However, the Western concepts of "participation", "development" and "local empowerment" could not be readily transferred to Kikwawila and other sites because of the multilayered and even contradictory meanings of the term "participation", as well as different understandings of what, and for whose benefit, "development" should be. Anthropologist Maia Green once argued that Ulanga's rural inhabitants have a very different understanding of development than that brought in by Western development agencies: instead of relating the term "maendeleo" (development) to the "forthcoming" of entire communities, they emphasize individual achievement. Above all, development means "development of a person by themselves".[122] This does not, of course, mean that individuals did not benefit from Western development projects. For a short time at least, the VHWs of Kikwawila assumed a new role in their communities, climbing up the ladder of social mobility. But what people in Kikwawila long for, as shown by the list handed to me by Twaibu Likumi, is a form of development that does not follow Western ideals of community participation and progress. Far from being just ephemeral episodes in the course of a PhD study, the two water pipes – real and envisioned – are the material signs of improvement and the immaterial "expectations of modernity" that capture the changes in the organization and practices of scientific research in Kilombero District at the beginning of the 1980s.[123]

121 Richard Rottenburg, *Social and Public Experiments and New Figurations of Science and Politics in Postcolonial Africa*, in: Postcolonial Studies, Vol. 12, No. 4, 2009, pp. 423–440.

122 Maia Green, *Participatory Development and the Appropriation of Agency in Southern Tanzania*, in: Critique of Anthropology, Vol. 20, No. 1, 2000, pp. 67–89, here: p. 81.

123 James Ferguson, *Expectations of Modernity. Myths and Meanings of Urban Life on the Zambian Copperbelt*, Berkeley 1999.

Chapter 6
The Transformation of Swiss Science in the Era of Structural Adjustment

The belief in a causal link between development and health, and the idea that community participation would contribute to Western notions of emancipation and empowerment, were rather short-lived. The ideals formulated at Alma-Ata evaporated as African economies underwent drastic changes under structural adjustment regimes.[1] Both Côte d'Ivoire and Tanzania were seriously affected by the 1973 oil crisis, and a chain reaction ensued. In Côte d'Ivoire, this marked the end of a period of political stability and economic performance unmatched in sub-Saharan Africa. At the end of the 1970s, the collapse of world market prices for cocoa and coffee led to what Bruno Losch has called a "double déclassement" (double downgrading) of Côte d'Ivoire. Economically, the new situation put an end to the successful Ivorian marketing system based on a strong alliance between the government and French Lebanese traders, as well as planters, and politically, the country was no longer the focus of France's attention as one of Africa's most geostrategically important territories.[2]

Tanzania, too, was seriously affected by the new economic realities. As Deborah Bryceson noted, higher oil prices led to rising international shipping costs, which in turn increased domestic transport costs for export crops.[3] Inadequate rainfall in 1973–1975, combined with the upheaval of Nyerere's villagization program, brought several rural areas of Tanzania to the brink of a serious hunger crisis. Although the country's economy recovered slightly in 1976 and 1977, the war against Idi Amin's Uganda – triggered by the October 1978 invasion – consumed the lion's share of

1   Nicholas van de Walle, *African Economies and the Politics of Permanent Crisis, 1979–1999*, Cambridge 2001.
2   Bruno Losch, *Libéralisation économique et crise politique en Côte d'Ivoire*, in: Critique Internationale, Vol. 19, No. 2, 2003, pp. 48–60; Bruno Losch, *Côte d'Ivoire, la tentation ethnonationaliste*, in: Politique Africaine, Vol. 78, 2000, pp. 5–25, here: p. 10.
3   Deborah F. Bryceson, *Agrarian Fundamentalism or Foresight? Revisiting Nyerere's Vision for Rural Tanzania*, in: Kjell Havnevik and Aida C. Isinika (eds.), Tanzania in Transition. From Nyerere to Mkapa, Dar es Salaam 2010, pp. 71–98, here: p. 76.

Tanzania's scarce resources.[4] After a further economic crisis in 1979, a period of economic reform began in 1980, with the IMF and the World Bank calling for liberalization of markets and public services.[5] The IMF's use of conditionality left African governments with no possibility of influencing vital policy areas such as health care provision.[6]

Even though Paul Nugent cautions against drawing a direct line from foreign-imposed structural adjustment programs (SAPs) to possible adverse effects, the impacts of SAPs in the realm of health care were deeply ingrained in the memories of STI researchers working in Tanzania, as well as the Tanzanian population.[7] Writing from Ifakara, STI scientists Christoph Hatz and Don DeSavigny reported:

> The major event is the first budget of [Ali Hassan] Mwinyi ... which moves substantially towards the IMF requirements and is resulting in rapid devaluation of the shilling. Prices have jumped another 50% just in the last week and will entail more hardship for the Tanzanians since there is no immediate provision to increase wages.[8]

4   Ibid.
5   In 1991, Tanzania abandoned its socialist health policy and introduced measures to privatize the health sector. Cost sharing was introduced through user fees in the public health care system; see, for instance: Aili M. Tripp, *Changing the Rules. The Politics of Liberalization and the Urban Informal Economy in Tanzania*, Berkeley 1997.
6   Among the burgeoning literature, see, for instance: Meredeth Turshen*, Privatizing Health Services in Africa*, New Brunswick, New Jersey 1999; Angwara D. Kiwara, *Health and Health Care in Structurally Adjusting Tanzania*, in: Lucian Msambichaka, Humphrey P.B. Moshi and Fidelis P. Mtatifikolo (eds.), Development Challenges and Strategies for Tanzania. An Agenda for the 21st Century, Dar es Salaam 1994, pp. 296–290; Andrew Kiondo, *Structural Adjustment and Non-Governmental Organizations in Tanzania. A Case Study*, in: Peter Gibbon (ed.), Social Change and Economic Reform in Africa, Uppsala 1993, pp. 161–183; N. J. Spalding, *State-Society Relations in Africa. An Exploration of the Tanzanian Experience*, in: Polity, Vol. 29, 1996, pp. 65–96.
7   Paul Nugent, *Africa Since Independence*, Basingstoke 2004, p. 334; Vinay Kamat, *"This Is Not Our Culture!" Discourses of Nostalgia and Narratives of Health Concerns in Post-Socialist Tanzania*, in: Africa, Vol. 78, No. 3, 2008, pp. 359–383; Margunn M. Bech*, Changing Policies and their Influence on the Interaction between Health Workers and Patients. A Government Health Worker Perspective from Rural Mbulu District, Tanzania*, paper presented at the international conference "The History of Health Care in Africa. Actors, Experiences, and Perspectives in the 20th Century," Basel, 12–14 September 2011.
8   Archive Swiss Tropical and Public Health Institute, Basel (ASTI), KIHERE Letters, 1985–1988, Christoph Hatz, Don DeSavigny, 4 July 1986, pp. 1–8, here: p. 1. Under Ali Hassan Mwinyi's presidency (1985–1995), the country relaxed its socialist policies and moved towards a more liberal market economy.

In addition to skyrocketing fuel and food prices, Kilombero District suffered extensive flooding in the first half of 1986, leaving many people without homes or crops.[9] The district's economic foundations were shaped not only by the policies of structural adjustment but perhaps more fundamentally by large-scale development efforts dating back to the 1970s. In particular, the construction of the Chinese-sponsored TAZARA (Tanzania-Zambia Railway Authority) railway, which zigzagged through Kilombero District to connect Dar es Salaam with the Zambian Copperbelt, acted as a magnet for laborers from the Mbeya, Iringa and Ruvuma regions.[10] In her subtle account of the history of the "Freedom Railway", Jamie Monson emphasizes not only the connection between its construction and Nyerere's resettlement policies, but also its symbolic significance as a pan-African development project. Equally important, the TAZARA railway brought new economic opportunities especially for small-scale traders, who in the era of structural adjustment were no longer forced to sell their products to government cooperatives but could exchange their crops directly in local and regional markets.[11]

Notwithstanding the many local initiatives, the hollowing-out of government structures during the period of structural adjustment had a strong impact on Swiss development policies in Tanzania and Côte d'Ivoire. While in the case studies presented in earlier chapters the differences outweighed the similarities, the economic experiences led to a convergence of the two countries' trajectories. In international development policy, the new situation gave rise to a bewildering variety of concepts and actors. Against this background, this chapter describes a period of transition for the two laboratories, at the end of which Swiss science emerged with the dual strengths of being locally embedded and more international at the same time. The paradoxes of this transition – whereby Swiss science became at once more African and more global – are best understood by reviewing the redistribution of power and exploring its effects on processes at the microlevel, such as institutional integration, administrative reforms and staff development, or the struggles among the various actors in the field of Swiss development aid. When considering Switzerland's late de-

---

9   Ibid., Don DeSavigny, 8 April 1986, pp. 1–2, here: p. 1.
10 Rudolf Peter Mayombo, *Economic Structural Changes and Population Migration in Kilombero Valley*, PhD Study University of Dar es Salaam, Dar es Salaam 1990, p. 94.
11 Jamie Monson, *Africa's Freedom Railway. How a Chinese Development Project Changed Lives and Livelihoods in Tanzania*, Bloomington, Indiana 2009, p. 103.

colonization, it is useful first to recognize the disillusionment about past development efforts which set in among politicians, development workers and the wider public during the 1980s.

Development's Hangover and the Failure of Primary Health Care

The beginning of the 1980s was a time of sobering self-reflection for Swiss development aid. The enthusiasm of the 1960s and 1970s – when development meant a transfer of Western technology to Third World countries – evaporated with the realization that, despite countless initiatives, development indicators still showed no signs of improvement. At home, the policy and practice of development aid faced an increasing number of critics from civil society and from the political arena, interpreting these efforts either as a neoimperialist strategy for cementing global inequalities or – more prosaically – as a waste of taxpayers' money. In other words, development aid in the 1980s was highly contested.[12] In 1983, Federal Councillor Pierre Aubert justified budget cuts for development aid as follows:

> The government's appreciation of the needs of Third World countries has not changed. However, the Confederation's financial policy – and in particular the parliament's motion to regain financial stability – means it is no longer possible to sustain the growth in public aid seen in recent years. The financial policy priorities set by the Swiss parliament mean that any increase in public development spending must be in line with the growth of Switzerland's own resources.[13]

Past health interventions undertaken in the name of development aid were also subject to critical reflection. As indicated in the previous chapter, the idea of comprehensive PHC was subverted from the outset. However, in many development agencies the principles of PHC remained unchallenged, especially in discussions about the most valuable approaches to health in tropical countries. The SDC's health policy for the Third World changed little during the 1980s. Even though, from the mid-1980s, SDC policymakers placed more emphasis on the implementation of health poli-

---

12   Konrad Kuhn, *Entwicklungspolitische Solidarität*, p. 24.
13   ASTI, DEH/DDA, Arbeitsgruppe Gesundheit, Korrespondenz allgemein, Pierre Aubert, 31 January 1983, pp. 1–2, here: p. 2.

cies or focused more on certain aspects of health within the overarching health systems framework, the key messages of Alma-Ata still reverberated strongly in Swiss medical aid.[14] However, one of the consequences of budgetary constraints was the idea that development outputs, outcomes and impacts could be measured according to predefined categories. This gave rise to a series of evaluations, which not only consumed much of the time previously invested in project work but started to reveal serious cracks in the edifice of PHC. In particular, it became the received wisdom that the ideas and promises of PHC did not easily bear fruit in the context of economic constraints. A key document conveying this message was the second SDC-commissioned evaluation of medical activities in Tanzania, published in 1986.[15] Brian Cooksey, the main author of the study, recommended that Switzerland continue its involvement in the Tanzanian health sector until 2000, albeit with a stronger emphasis on planning, monitoring and evaluation as core activities, as well as a concentration of efforts within the politico-administrative boundaries of Kilombero District.[16] More thought-provoking, however, was his assessment of the efforts undertaken so far in the area of PHC:

14   ASTI, DEH/DDA, Arbeitsgruppe Gesundheit, Dokumente allgemein, III, Immita Cornaz, Summary. Health Policy of Swiss Development Cooperation (SDC), 21 July 1986, SDC Health Policy. Possible New Developments, 25 July 1986; Immita Cornaz, *Santé et Développement*. Exposé à l'Association Suisse de Médecine Tropicale et de Parasitologie, 18 November 1988, in: Bulletin Medicus Mundi Schweiz, Vol. 45, 1990, pp. 5–15.

15   Archive Ifakara Health Institute, Ifakara (AIHI), P. 40, Brian Cooksey et al., Evaluation of Swiss-Funded Health Projects in Tanzania. A Report for Swiss Development Cooperation, November 1986, pp. 1–69. In 1977, an independent expert group had scrutinized the working and impact of five DftZ-supported health projects, including the Central Pathology Laboratory (CPL) in Dar es Salaam, the MATC and St. Francis Hospital in Ifakara. While the impact of the CPL on rural health care and PHC was never much debated, the evaluation of the MATC was more sensitive because its efforts to strengthen PHC in Kilombero had always seemed to be exaggerated. In the eyes of WHO expert Daniel Flahault, the closeness of the MATC to St. Francis Hospital made it difficult for the training center to embrace preventive approaches. As he notes, "it seems that not enough emphasis has been given in the past to preventive services, and this may be due to the fact that the St. Francis hospital is very much oriented towards curative services, most of the teachers are clinically oriented and because diagnosing and treating are more immediately rewarding." See: ASTI, Klaus Gyr, Swiss-Tanzanian Joint Evaluation of Swiss Cooperation to Tanzanian Health Projects, May 1977, and ASTI, Daniel Flahault, Swiss-Tanzanian Joint Evaluation of Swiss Cooperation to Tanzanian Health Projects. Sectorial Report on Education and Training in the Field of Health, April 1977, p. 16.

16   AIHI, P. 40, Cooksey et al., Evaluation, p. 6.

We have seen that in practice the implementation of PHC policy in Tanzania has been severely limited by the inertia of the existing health system with its established urban/curative bias. Despite the significant progress made to date, the primary health component does not yet constitute the core element of the national health system, either in terms of services or support activities. Substantial donor, including Swiss, support goes to the maintenance of the "non-PHC" elements of the system.[17]

It is striking that the failures of PHC in practice were never associated with the mismatch between the utopia of PHC and the logic of development projects seeking fast and measurable results, but with a changing socioeconomic context that inhibited meaningful development work. The conclusions drawn from the assessment of Switzerland's involvement touch on some of the most striking paradoxes of (however well-intentioned) Western support for the Tanzanian health system: Tanzania's increasing dependence on Western aid and the economic remedies prescribed by the IMF and the World Bank led to dysfunctional health systems and probably also to a certain alienation from biomedicine.[18] According to the observers, the fact that medical aid did not reach those most in need was, however, not due to contradictory donor strategies, but to the fact that "the authorities do not have the … capacity to plan the integration of health aid into the national health-care system".[19] In other words, the blame for the failures of PHC was placed on the Africans themselves, rather than on the international aid system.

The economic downturn, decreasing standards of living in Kilombero District and continued enthusiasm for PHC provide the context for two political processes that will be discussed below. One concerns the attempts to integrate STIFL into the Tanzanian health system, the other the reconfiguration of development aid in Kilombero District following discussions between the SDC and the STI about whether or not biomedical research offers a suitable framework for raising standards of living and increasing self-reliance in Tanzania.

17   Ibid., p. 13.
18   Maia Green argued that the "decline in utilisation of public health services, particularly among the poor, is not simply due to perceptions of increased costs, although these are significant, but to an emerging national culture of distrust of state medical provision." See: Maia Green, *Public Reform and the Privatisation of Poverty. Some Institutional Determinants of Health Seeking Behaviour in Southern Tanzania*, in: Culture, Medicine and Psychiatry, Vol. 24, 2000, pp. 403–430, here: p. 405.
19   AIHI, Cooksey et al., Evaluation, p. 21.

Integrating the Swiss Tropical Institute Field Laboratory into Tanzanian Health Structures

In 1984, having opened up new venues for scientific research in Tanzania, the outgoing head of STIFL Marcel Tanner formulated various strategies for the future direction of the laboratory.[20] On the basis of past experience and his extensive work in Kilombero District, he realized that "in the long run, STIFL has to be integrated into Tanzanian health structures, led by Tanzanians and thus answer their priorities as well as their possibilities".[21]

Even though Tanner had previously sketched similar plans before leaving for the field, the need for transformation became more pressing with the SDC taking over financial responsibility for STIFL in 1982. Indeed, the integration of the field laboratory into Tanzanian health structures and the associated issues of power were discussed by the SDC and the STI throughout the 1980s. The wish for integration was based not only on the STI's sense of moral obligation but on the fact that, with the SDC assuming responsibility, the STIFL now had to be transformed into a local institution and the role of the STI limited to "one of an implementing, executing agency, with involvement, of course, in all important issues and steps".[22] The complexity of the matter arose from the need to accommodate STIFL's research tradition to that of possible Tanzanian partner institutions, while not losing influence over the Tanzanian health sector altogether.[23] As it turned out, the STIFL's three main activities – training, research and service provision – did not easily fit into one of the existing Tanzanian institutions. In 1988, the most likely candidates were the National Institute of Medical Research (NIMR), the Ministry of Health (MOH) and the Tanzanian Public Health Association (TPHA), a largely Canadian-funded NGO.[24] The NIMR was a parastatal organization created

20 ASTI, STIFL, Correspondence, 1981–1987, Marcel Tanner, Concept pour le laboratoire de terrain du STI à Ifakara. Draft, January 1984, pp. 1–6.
21 Ibid., p. 1.
22 ASTI, STIFL, Evolution/Integration, 1988–1994, P. Fellay (SDC) to Antoine Degrémont, Forthcoming Mission of Messrs. Degrémont and Tanner to Tanzania to Prepare Integration of STIFL, 4 January 1988, pp. 1–2, here: p. 1.
23 Ibid., Marcel Tanner, Antoine Degrémont, Mission Report: Integration of the Swiss Tropical Institute Field Laboratory (STIFL), Ifakara, into Tanzanian Structures. SDC Mission, 15 January – 2 February 1988, p. 56.
24 ASTI, KIHERE Letters, 1989-, Marcel Tanner to Calum Macpherson and Thomas Teuscher, 10 February 1989, p. 1.

by an act of parliament in 1979 with a mandate to take responsibility for the country's research institutes, which – until the dissolution of the East African Community in 1977 – had been in the hands of the East African Medical Research Council. The colonial inheritance left the NIMR with a research tradition very much geared towards vector control. This was just one of the reasons why the NIMR's first director, Wenceslaus Kilama, was reluctant to embrace the idea of assuming responsibility for the STIFL. In addition, the NIMR lacked not only the necessary manpower but also a vision for the future role of the laboratory within the Tanzanian health system.[25] The NIMR's reluctance was not unwelcome to all of the STI's scientists. As one can imagine, the institutional decolonization process was not uniformly supported, and there were differences of opinion between those working in Switzerland and the scientists in the field. Writing from Ifakara, leading STIFL staff members Christoph Hatz and Calum Macpherson called for restraint:

> As Prof. Kilama is cautious concerning the future of STIFL we think that it is not necessary for STI/STIFL to push the handing-over but to work hard on a strong and integrated center in Ifakara.[26]

The MOH was not considered a suitable candidate either. Only in the area of operational research was there an overlap with the STIFL's activities, and in the eyes of the STI the government body's decision-making mechanisms were too sluggish to move medical research in the country forward. The TPHA option was also problematic: within the socialist framework of Tanzania, integration through an NGO was hardly feasible. Wenceslaus Kilama recalls: "We were still looking at government to do everything. NGOs, including TPHA, were still suspect, although there was nothing wrong with them."[27] The STI and the SDC were thus inclined to pursue the NIMR solution, which was acceptable to the latter, given the substantial infrastructure and manpower support provided by the Swiss government. In 1991, although the STIFL was not formally integrated into the NIMR institutions, it became an "affiliate" and was renamed the Ifakara Center

---

25 Schweizerisches Bundesarchiv Bern (BAR), E 2025 (A), 1997/200, 642, t.311-Tansania.45, anonymized, MEMO: Betrifft: Nouvel dénomination pour le "Swiss Tropical Institute Field Laboratory" (STIFL) d'Ifakara, 30 December 1987, p. 1.
26 ASTI, KIHERE Letters, 1985–1988, Christoph Hatz, Calum MacPherson, 7 November 1987, pp. 1–4, here: p. 2.
27 Interview with Wenceslaus Kilama, 9 February 2011 in Dar es Salaam.

(IC). Five years later, the name was changed once again to the Ifakara Health Research and Development Center (IHRDC), and it was registered as a trust, with Tanzanian partners today holding a majority of seats on the Board of Governors.

Thus – in contrast to the Africanization of the CSRS in Côte d'Ivoire discussed later in this chapter – the integration of the STIFL into Tanzanian structures was not so much a moral as a highly technical issue. For the Swiss party, integration meant including various stakeholders in the research process without, however, losing track of its own research interests. One of the major obstacles was the fact that the research institutions in Tanzania were considered to be either weak (in the case of the NIMR) or not a suitable partner (the MOH). The STIFL's transition from an STI research center to an NIMR affiliate needs to be seen against the background of the wider political changes in Tanzania which followed the retirement of Julius Nyerere in 1985, leading to a multiparty system and market liberalization in the 1990s. Marcel Tanner's view, expressed in 1984, that the STIFL had to be integrated into Tanzanian health structures, led by Tanzanians and respond to their needs, gave way to the partnership culture, which, since the 1990s, has been widely recognized as the most promising approach to development problems. The Ifakara Health Institute (IHI, as the STIFL is called today) occupies a privileged position within the Tanzanian health sector. According to the MOH, it is the second leading institution (after the NIMR) to which the Ministry turns when research mandates are to be assigned. But public-private partnerships are naturally also composed of stronger and weaker players. According to Salim Abdulla, Director of the IHI, the Tanzanian MOH still plays a minor role within the IHI's policymaking.[28] The complex power relations associated with the attempt to integrate Western biomedical research into Tanzanian institutions are apparent from the discussions surrounding the role and responsibilities of the first Tanzanian director.

Administrative Reforms

In the midst of discussions about how to integrate the STIFL into Tanzanian structures and the best possible channels for collaboration with Tanzanian counterparts, the institution's links with the STI were reaffirmed by

28   Interview with Salim Abdulla, 12 February 2009 in Dar es Salaam.

an administrative reform introduced in 1990. This does not mean that the STIFL and the STI were not working towards the inclusion of various institutions at the district, regional and national level. Rather, the suggestion is that the ongoing transformation of the STIFL into a Tanzanian-based NGO went hand in hand with increased (administrative) control of the STI over the STIFL's fate. In 1990, the numerous complaints about administrative overload at the field lab were finally resolved by the division of tasks between a scientific and an administrative director. While the former served as chief scientist and project leader, the latter was responsible for providing the administrative basis for research practices, as well as managing the transition of the IC into the NIMR network.[29] In many cases, the new key positions were still held by expatriates. After the resignation of Calum Macpherson as STIFL head in March 1990, his former deputy Thomas Teuscher agreed to take over and to take responsibility for the KIHERE program, while Stefan Mörgeli and Inez Azevedo served as administrative director and research assistant respectively.[30] The SDC monitored these changes carefully and with a certain amount of mistrust for, as one SDC member stated, the "entire staff development is one of the crucial elements of transition/integration into Tanzanian structures".[31] As far as the new position of administrative director was concerned, the SDC agreed to cover the costs provided that the assignment was for a limited term and "with the explicit objective of training and nurturing a Tanzanian administrative officer by the end of these 2 years".[32] More problematic, however, was the issue of familiarizing a Tanzanian scientific director with the subtleties of leading a scientific research institution in a rural African setting. The NIMR stipulated that the future director should have a PhD in biology or another relevant discipline. A promising candidate was Tanzanian-born

---

29 ASTI, KIHERE Letters, 1989–, Agreement between the Swiss Federal Council and the Government of the United Republic of Tanzania concerning Kilombero Health Research Centre – Project. First Draft, 8 August 1991, pp. 8–9.

30 ASTI, Kihere File 1990, January-June, Marcel Tanner to Erwin Bänteli, RE: KIHERE Health Research Programme; Changes in Management Structure, 15 March 1990, pp. 1–3, here: p. 1: The post of research assistant was shared between Dominique Morona and Inez Azevedo from 1 April 1990 onwards.

31 BAR, E 2025 (A), 2000/138, 753, t.311-Tansania.45, Recherches médicales au Swiss Tropical Institute Field Lab. à Ifakara, Bd. 1–2, 1988–1989, anonymized, Subject: Ifakara Centre Project: staff developments – external evaluation, pp. 1–5, here: p. 1.

32 ASTI, Kihere File 1990, January-June, Erwin Bänteli to Marcel Tanner, KIHERE Health Research Programme; Changes in Management Structure, 4 April 1990, pp. 1–2, here: p. 1.

Andrew Kitua, who was a recognized expert in the field of public health. After training at the WHO and the London School of Hygiene and Tropical Medicine, he had been working for the MOH in the Seychelles. Despite his extensive experience, Kitua did not yet hold a doctoral degree. He was, however, selected as the most suitable candidate and, in 1992, was offered the opportunity to become the first Tanzanian director of the institute, starting in mid-1994. In 1992, Thomas Teuscher decided to step down, although he remained in Ifakara until mid-1993 to "devote more time to the public health and scientific issues".[33] It was arranged that Kitua would come to Ifakara to serve as a senior community health officer/public health specialist from October 1, 1992 to June 30, 1994, while working on a doctoral thesis in the context of a vaccine trial conducted in the district; in the meantime, the post of scientific director was to be filled by the Swiss physician Thomas Schick. Compared to Kitua, Schick had little experience in the field of tropical health, but he was "familiar with the approaches" of the STIFL and the STI.[34] This constellation of two Swiss scientists assessing the suitability of an African prospective scientific director over a two-year period raised some eyebrows among SDC staff: "The two-year evaluation (in his position as senior community health officer) and the supervision (in his position as scientific director) of Mr. Kitua through Teuscher/Schick has a somewhat paternalist-colonial taste to me."[35] In a later interview, Kitua commented on the situation as follows:

When you came to Ifakara in 1992, you spent two years being evaluated by Thomas Teuscher and Thomas Schick. How did you feel at that time?

I was not so happy with the future in Seychelles because I did not see my future there, as the health situation was quite good and I felt guilty because I was not working where the problem was … so I did really want to work in Tanzania, and coming back I was not aware about the long evaluation process. I took it because I wanted to be in Tanzania and just thought, well, I will go through, and in the beginning I was appointed as supervisor of the vaccine trial, of the persons outside … and at that moment I thought, how best can I also benefit in the process, and that is when I requested to do my PhD through the project as well. That was accepted, so here I was of course having a supervisor as a student which was Marcel Tanner, but also looking at the position, taking over the position as director.

---

33   BAR, E 2025 (A), 2000/138, 753, anonymized, RE: Ifakara – NIMR-Kihere-Project; follow-up Steering Comittee Meeting 1 July and some specific future priority issues, 5 July 1992, pp. 1–5, here: p. 3.
34   Ibid.
35   Ibid., Ifakara-NIMR-Kihere-Project, 24 July 1992, pp. 1–2, here: p. 1.

So you were in a quite ambivalent position, being a PhD student and scientific director at the same time?

Yes, an ambivalent position, yes.[36]

Even after he became scientific director, Kitua did not have much room for maneuver on the policy and administrative level. He acknowledged that all the core funding came from Switzerland – either from the SDC or the STI (the latter helping to alleviate the dismal financial situation). The STI also used its networking skills and finalized applications to global health organizations and national governments so as to diversify financial contributions. In the 1990s, there were no Tanzanian institutions that would have funded scientific research in Tanzania. It was only recently that Tanzania's president agreed to allocate 1% of GDP to scientific research, and the Commission for Science and Technology (COSTECH) started to issue calls for proposals in order to stimulate scientific research.[37] While decision-making within the integration process remained in the hands of Switzerland, there were nevertheless changes at the microlevel (scientific planning and execution). According to Kitua, the process of defining research priorities was no longer solely the Swiss partners' responsibility but was shared among the Swiss and Tanzanian stakeholders and conducted in an atmosphere of trust and mutual collaboration.[38]

These staff development policies and handover processes coincided with changes in aid modalities at the international level. At issue was the redistribution of responsibilities between the SDC and the STI/IC as regards their respective contributions to Kilombero's development.

Remodeling Development: The Micropolitics of Development Aid in the Post-Alma-Ata Era

The period of the structural adjustment regime in Tanzania and the development hangover in Swiss and other European development agencies saw two significant tendencies within the international aid community. The first was increased transnationalization of the aid sector via a process described

---

36   Interview with Andrew Kitua, 22 January 2011 in Geneva.
37   Ibid.
38   Ibid.

by James Ferguson and Akhil Gupta as "outsourcing of the functions of the state to NGOs and other ostensibly non-state agencies" and exemplified by the appearance of the International Development Association (IDA)/World Bank on the African health stage.[39] The other was a decisive shift away from the experience of the 1960s and 1970s – when health was viewed within the political and symbolic boundaries of the nation – towards a focus on district health systems, which became the main locus of foreign intervention. Transnational collaboration and subnational intervention are evident in the case of Swiss development aid to Tanzania. At the beginning of the 1990s, the SDC became a strong partner of the IDA/World Bank in the Dar es Salaam Urban Health Project (DUHP), executed by the STI, as well as in the overall process of health sector reform, which involved decentralization of financial and administrative power, comprehensive district health plans and a diversification of funding sources.[40] The focus on Kilombero District as the major point of reference for Swiss development aid led to a redistribution of responsibilities between the SDC and the STI/IC, and to a disentanglement of research and health service provision.

Overcoming the Past – Reinventing the Future: The Redistribution of the Development Burden within Kilombero District

The attempts to concentrate Switzerland's health development efforts in Kilombero District, and to work out more integrated approaches, led to a redistribution of responsibilities between the Swiss development institutions working in the district and to closer scrutiny of the activities of the former field laboratory and its KIHERE project. At issue here were such questions as: which of the two institutions enjoying long-term SDC support – St. Francis Hospital or the IC – was better suited to work towards improving the health status of the local population? Which had the capacity to

---

39   James Ferguson, Akhil Gupta, *Spatializing States*, p. 990.
40   BAR, E 2200.83 (B), 2000/281, 8, 771.20.0, Technische Zusammenarbeit Schweiz-Tansania, allgemeines, Max Honegger et al., Jahresbericht 1990 – Jahresprogramm 1991, Januar 1991, pp. 1–12, here: p. 2; AIHI, D.M.O (Kilombero) and R.M.O. (Ulanga), Correspondence, Health Sector Reforms in Tanzania. Origin, Contents and Experience, pp. 1–5, here: pp. 3–4; Gaspar K. Munishi, *Intervening to Address Constraints through Health Sector Reforms in Tanzania. Some Gains and the Unfinished Business*, in: Journal of International Development, Vol. 15, No. 1, 2003, pp. 115–131.

elaborate a comprehensive, realistic health plan with the district authorities, which could then be put into practice? And what kind of exploitable results would be left after the scientific machinery set in motion by the IC came to a halt? The 1993 evaluation of the IC's contributions was influenced by the SDC's general doubts as to whether scientific research – basic, applied or operational – was compatible with their development ideals. The prevalent view was summarized by one of the SDC members involved:

> After years of cohabitation between the renowned and sophisticated Ifakara Center and the oversized St. Francis Hospital … it is important that Kilombero District should benefit from measurable development impulses. In my opinion, one should be open for solutions which could be different from those stipulated at the moment; for instance, working towards a real district development project with a strong community component and with a leading NGO … which is not so much on the biomedical side as is the case with the Swiss Tropical Institute.[41]

Overall, the evaluation identified two fundamental weaknesses of biomedical science as conducted by the IC in the Kilombero District. The first had to do with scientific practices within a context of poverty. While Swiss and Tanzanian researchers might indeed have cooperated closely with district or regional authorities, amassing data and information and making this available to the authorities, the crucial point, according to the evaluators, was that the District Health Management Teams (DHMT) lacked the means to translate the information into tangible improvements: "Of what use is research if the results cannot be applied in practice for lack of funds and sustained cooperation?"[42] The second point mentioned was the unequal power relations between the STI/IC and the Tanzanian partners in their quest for better health policies. Imbalances existed not only between these parties but also between the STI and the IC, with the former controlling "the whole planning, financing, implementation and monitoring of research undertaken at Ifakara".[43] The STI's strong position in the Tanzanian health sector derived partly from its early presence in the district and the strategic alliances forged with various partners over the years, and also from the fact that Tan-

41   BAR, E 2025 (A), 2002/145, 802, t.311-Tansania.45, Recherches médicales au Swiss Tropical Institute Field Lab. à Ifakara, Bd. 5–7, 1992–1993, anonymized, Bericht Dienstreise nach Tansania vom 15.10–27.10.1992, pp. 1–2, here: p. 2.

42   Ibid., External Evaluation of the Kilombero Health Research and Support Project. Mandated by: SDC, East Africa Section, Berne, Switzerland. Draft, Dar es Salaam April 1993, pp. 1–52, here: pp. 17–18.

43   Ibid., p. 25.

zania inherited only a rudimentary research infrastructure from British colonialism. However, as the evaluation pointed out, the SDC contributed a
great deal towards strengthening the STI vis-à-vis Tanzanian research bodies. A telling example is the STIFL's affiliation to the NIMR, discussed
above. On the one hand, the SDC mandated the STI to administer Swiss
support to the NIMR; on the other, the STI's former field station was to be
integrated into the still weak NIMR research structure. This complex relationship between the STI and the NIMR would lead to a "double-bind"
which was "difficult to live with".[44] As a useful strategy for the future, the
authors proposed more "demand driven" scientific research, as well as a
stronger focus on health systems research rather than on specific diseases.

New Ideologies, New Actors, New Instruments: Essential Na-
tional Health Research and the Research User Fund

The point of dwelling on this evaluation report is not to answer the question whether or not criticisms of the work of the IC were justified. In fact,
as we have seen, from the early 1980s onwards, Swiss researchers intensified collaboration with district and regional health authorities. Tanzanian
national health policymaking was significantly influenced by the field laboratory's efforts in the training of village health workers and investigating
chloroquine resistance. The point to note here is that the report marked a
watershed in the relationship between the SDC – which favored a development approach aimed at improving conditions for rural dwellers – and a
biomedical research institution which, though indeed concerned with
strengthening the district health system, also had to meet the expectations
of a more diverse clientele. This is clear from the response of STI Director
Antoine Degrémont to the evaluation:

> We are especially disappointed that the evaluators only considered the center's im-
> pact on the population and on the district's health services; this is in our opinion
> not relevant because we are talking about a research center and therefore the eval-
> uator's focus only reveals half the truth at best.[45]

44   Ibid.
45   Documents Marcel Tanner (DMT), SDC-TZ, Antoine Degrémont to Erwin Bänteli
     (SDC), Concerne: External Evaluation of the Kilombero Health Research and Support
     Project. Final Report of June 1993, 27 August 1993, pp. 1–2, here: p. 2. For other re-
     sponses to the external evaluation, see: ASTI, unlabeled, Cyril Pervilhac to Michel

Even though the SDC always emphasized that the evaluation did not represent its own views, many of its members welcomed it as a trigger for a fundamental reframing of Swiss development activities in the district.[46] The changes initiated at the institutional, conceptual and policy level were of paramount importance for the future of the IC in the context of Swiss decolonization. The SDC's chief impression about the research activities undertaken so far was that Swiss scientists largely monopolized priority-setting, as well as actual scientific efforts in the district. In order to address this situation and to promote demand- rather than supply-driven biomedical research, the SDC advocated the establishment of a research user fund, in which "policymakers as well as implementers should have more say on types of research to be undertaken".[47] The research user fund was supposed to minimize the gap between research and implementation. The idea was that policymakers themselves would come up with research proposals, which would then be addressed by the scientists. Former NIMR Director Kilama gave a concrete example:

> You may say, OK, a woman goes to a hospital or to a health center and they say, ah, you are coming to deliver, so give us money to buy gloves, give us money to get clean water – well maybe not clean water, but you know … things of that nature. So the hospital says, we are not charging them, so it was thought that policymakers would come up with areas of policy they would like to be addressed in the research. It was thought that decision makers could come up with problems – they say, OK, I am a decision maker, it has something to do with money, maybe it has something to do with personnel, and how to allocate them and so on, there are problems here. You sit and then you come up with a proposal made by the decision maker sitting with researchers … and both are now going to be researchers.[48]

Mordasini (SDC), REF. External Evaluation of the Kilombero Health Research and Support Project, 14 August 1993, pp. 1–5 and ASTI, Kihere File 1993, August-October, Phase V, Marcel Tanner, Comments on: Final Report of the External Evaluation of the Kilombero Health Research and Support Project (KHRSP), 20 August 1993, pp. 1–8.

46 BAR, E 2025 (A), 2002/145, 803, t.311-Tansania.45, Recherches médicales au Swiss Tropical Institute Field Lab. à Ifakara, Bd. 8, 1993, anonymized, Planning for Calendar Year 1994, KOBU Tanzania: Health Sector, 15 October 1993, pp. 1–2, here: pp. 1–2.

47 BAR, E 2025 (A), 2002/145, 802, anonymized, Position on Key Issues Concerning Future Planning Exercise for the KHRSP as per the Evaluation Report, 3 November 1993, pp. 1–3, here: p. 2.

48 Interview with Wenceslaus Kilama, 9 February 2011.

Organizationally, the research user fund was placed within the NIMR structure and fed by various donors, whose contributions were administered by a board. As a consequence of this new instrument, the SDC progressively withdrew its core funding from the IC and channeled support to the NIMR-based research user fund, which meant that the IC had to diversify its range of donors.[49] In the eyes of the SDC, this new arrangement was not only meant to distribute decision-making procedures for scientific research more democratically among different stakeholders; it was also assumed that it would help Tanzania move towards what was known as Essential National Health Research (ENHR). In a highly influential report produced in 1990 by the Commission on Health Research for Development, ENHR was proposed as a strategy for relieving the burden of disease in developing countries.[50] The Commission had been set up in 1987 as an independent international initiative, with two thirds of its members coming from developing countries.[51] Its findings were presented without any mention of the complexities, achievements or failures of earlier research initiatives in sub-Saharan Africa or other regions. Scholars such as Debabar Banerji interpreted the report as "another effort to obscure the message of self-reliance contained in the Alma-Ata Declaration on Primary Health

49 DMT, SDC-TZ, Swiss-Tanzanian Development Cooperation – Annual Programme 1995, p. 1; AIHI, unlabeled, Minutes of the Consultation Meeting Between SDC and Ministry of Health on Policy Key Issues Regarding the Future Planning of the Kilombero Health Research and Support Project (KHRSP) held on 3 December 1993, pp. 1–7, here: p. 3. The Ifakara Centre was able to attract new donors in Spain (Spanish Ministry of Foreign Affairs, Catalan Government, Medicus Mundi Catalunya and the Hospital Clínic i Provincial de Barcelona) and to engage in long-term scientific collaboration, especially in the fields of malaria vaccine and health systems research; see: ASTI, KIHERE File 1994, 15. Dezember–20. März, Phase V, Pedro Alonso, Constanza Alberti, Contribution of Spanish Institutions to the Ifakara Centre, 8 March 1994, pp. 1–11; BAR, E 2025 (A), 2002/145, 803, Bd. 8, Kilombero Health Research and Support Project, Minutes of the 4th Steering Committee Meeting of 22nd September 1993, in Dar-es-Salaam, 26 October 1993, pp. 1–38, here: p. 8; AIHI, unlabeled, Ifakara Centre Health and Research Support Project, Phase VI (July 1 1994 – June 30 1997), Project Document Version of 21 February 1994, prepared by Ifakara Centre, p. 6.
50 Commission on Health Research for Development (ed.), *Health Research. Essential Link to Equity in Development*, New York 1990. For the burden of disease approach, see: Christopher Murray, Alan Lopez (eds.), *The Global Burden of Disease. A Comprehensive Assessment of Mortality and Disability from Diseases, Injuries and Risk Factors in 1990 and Projected to 2020*, Cambridge 1996.
51 Debabar Banerji, *Report of the Commission on Health Research for Development and the Countries of the South*, in: International Journal of Health Services, Vol. 22, No. 1, 1992, pp. 169–177, here: p. 170.

Care".[52] It may at least be said that ENHR was not born out of revolutionary zeal. On the one hand, the report stressed the importance of collaboration by scientists, policymakers and local communities in addressing country-specific health issues and stated that: "Many aspects of global health research must be carried out in the field conditions of developing countries, such as trials of new vaccines for tropical diseases and tests of nutritional supplements such as vitamin A."[53] On the other hand, the authors argued that developing countries should also contribute to research on what they called global health problems: "studies of the rapidly growing problems of diabetes, coronary heart disease, hypertension, and cancer in selected populations in developing countries could provide unique insight into the determinants of these chronic diseases and lead to preventive measures of benefit worldwide."[54]

In adopting a concept that could conceal neither its political interests nor its lack of historical foundations, the SDC at least partly undermined its support for health systems research, which was central to the 1993 evaluation.[55] ENHR did not prioritize one research approach over another, and programs focusing on biomedical investigations were very much in line with ENHR ideology. For the history of health research and health care provision in Kilombero District, Switzerland's propagation of ENHR – together with the reallocation of SDC funding from the IC to the NIMR – was important because it led to a division of labor between the SDC and the IC, and to a tectonic shift in the institutional setting of health promotion in Kilombero District. The 3rd Steering Committee meeting held in Dar es Salaam in spring 1993 thus concluded that the activities of the IC "will probably continue under more biomedical oriented research … and the strengthening of District Health Services [will be] more Health Systems Research oriented, and more SDC supported."[56]

The SDC's attempt to reinvent district collaboration and to curtail the IC's political influence on the district authorities was known as the Kilombero District Health Support (KDHS) project, which replaced the KI-

---

52   Ibid., p. 169.
53   *Health Research. Essential Link to Equity in Development*, p. 85.
54   Ibid., p. 21.
55   BAR, E 2025 (A), 2002/145, 803, Position on Key Issues, pp. 2–3.
56   BAR, E 2025 (A), 2002/145, 802, Minutes of the 3rd Steering Committee Meeting. Dar-es-Salaam, May 5th 1993, Draft May 29th, 1993 Version, pp. 1–12, here: p. 5.

HERE project in 1991.[57] The executing agency selected by the SDC because of its in-depth knowledge was the Schweizerischer Katholischer Missionsärztlicher Verein (known since 1987 as SolidarMed). SolidarMed's contribution to Kilombero's health services to date had been restricted to the recruitment of Swiss physicians for St. Francis Hospital, and the organization had no experience whatsoever of conducting health projects. Nonetheless, SolidarMed's new tasks were ambitious. Among other things, it was to assist the district in drawing up and implementing a district health plan, as well as establishing close links to the community, while the IC would act "as a collaborator that provides assistance through action research and health systems research".[58] The new arrangements were put to the test in 1994, when the various Swiss and Tanzanian institutions sought to establish a district health plan. Considerable time was invested in assessing the performance of the district's health system for "the DHMT did not have a clear and up to date picture regarding the various components of the health care delivery system at each of the health facilities in the district".[59] The baseline assessment report offered a familiar bleak picture: the community health situation was considered as generally poor, with communicable diseases and poor sanitation, and the health facilities lacked the most basic drugs. Accordingly, the community had a "negative image of the health services provided by the health facilities in the district".[60] However, the question now was whether the organizational changes made to Swiss development aid in 1993 would make a difference to health care provision in Kilombero District, and whether SolidarMed could in fact develop into a district support institution. In mid-1995, some SDC staff had considerable doubts as to the wisdom of the decision to replace the STI/IC's public health expertise with SolidarMed, whose members had traditionally been more active in the field of curative medicine. It is worth quoting one member of the SDC in full:

57 AIHI, SDC, Agreement between the Swiss Federal Council and the Government of the United Republic of Tanzania concerning Kilombero Health Research and Support-Project, Draft, 25 September 1991, pp. 1–15.

58 ASTI, KIHERE File 1994, 21. März-30. Juni, Phase V, Markus Frei, Vera Kücholl, Draft. Kilombero District Health Support (KDHS) Vision 2000, 9 June 1994, pp. 1–5, here: p. 3.

59 BAR, E 2026 (A), 2005/9, 861, t.311-Tansania.69, Kilombero District Health Support (KDHS), Bd. 1, 1993–1994, Planning Process for the Proposed Kilombero District Health Plan, p. 1.

60 Ibid., Bd. 2, 1994, Kilombero District, District Health System, Baseline Assessment Report, September 1994, p. 3.

The Ifakara Center (STI) has clearly expressed its willingness to play a new role. The DHMT however is somewhat disconcerted because it does not know what will replace the Ifakara Center's support – support that has been experienced as ambivalent (benefits of close supervision, which in turn involves strong dependence). SolidarMed considers itself as the institution which will support the DHMT in the future, but during the workshop it did not leave the impression that it is able to do so. The informal gatherings after the workshop showed that SolidarMed still lacks a conceptual framework. The changes in the relationship between the Ifakara Center and the DHMT – from assistance to a relationship where the DHMT appears as the principal – requires that the DHMT articulates its needs, formulates clear instructions and is able to monitor execution. It is, however, clear that considering the existing capacities it would still need assistance. From an organizational point of view, it is reasonable that this assistance is no longer provided by the Ifakara Center. SolidarMed would be a suitable institution to do so (knowledge of the environment, integration of St. Francis) … The workshop and the meetings with SolidarMed, however, raised some questions as to whether SolidarMed is really aware of this situation and whether it can provide the necessary input.[61]

Apart from SolidarMed lacking a conceptual framework, there were major inconsistencies between the development concepts of the DHMT and those of the Swiss protagonists. According to SolidarMed, community participation was a concept "not very well understood" and even "objected to" by the DHMT. Furthermore, "when it became clear that more cars and allowances for the DHMT … were not a priority of the KDHS, enthusiasm dropped even more."[62] However, the DHMT's wish list – on which the procurement of vehicles and the electrification or renovation of health centers featured prominently – is not a sign of "misconceived" development, but a reflection of the precarious macroeconomic situation with which the district and the entire country had to contend. Thus, while the institutional setting for Swiss development aid changed fundamentally during the late 1980s and early 1990s, the sustainability of projects was still threatened by the economic situation. In 1995, one project document thus stated that "the macro-economic situation in Tanzania makes it difficult to achieve sustainability particularly in the health sector."[63]

61 Ibid., Bd. 1, anonymized, Kilombero District Health Support Workshop. Ifakara 26.-28. Januar 1994 (Ergänzung zum Missions-Bericht (Vertraulich), pp. 1–2, here: p. 2.
62 Ibid., Bd. 2, 1994, anonymized, Letter SolidarMed to SDC, 6 November 1994, pp. 1–2, here: p. 1.
63 BAR, E 2025 (A), 2000/253, 9, t.311-Tansania.69, Abk. CH/Tansania betr. "The Kilombero District Health Support" – Phase I, 1994–1997, Kilombero District Health Support. Phase 1, 1 July 1995 – 30 June 1997. Project Document. Final Version, 31 May 1995, pp. 1–21, here: p. 2.

The End of the "Pacte Colonial": Scientific Disconnects and the Africanization of the CSRS in Côte d'Ivoire

The period of structural adjustment was a watershed in the history of the CSRS too. Nestlé had left the CSRS with a bitter-sweet legacy – on the one hand, a new laboratory building and new prospects of nutritional research, increasingly undertaken in collaboration with the ETH Zurich, and on the other, the sense that Africans should somehow participate in the scientific activities of the CSRS. "Nestlé has transformed the CSRS too quickly into a big enterprise," one CSRS member complained.[64] The "Ivorisation" of the CSRS became the major issue at the beginning of the 1980s, and rather than being conducted in terms of the professionalization and scientific competence of Africans, the debate assumed overtly moral tones. The question of "how Africans digested the legacies of colonialism" was, of course, not specific to the CSRS, but part of a much broader process transforming social and public life in Côte d'Ivoire during the 1970s and 1980s.[65] By the end of the 1980s, the higher levels of the civil service were staffed by Ivorians or other Africans, leaving only a handful of French technical advisors in key ministries.[66] In contrast to the STIFL in Tanzania, members of the CSRS were never able to take an active role in positioning the center within a changing political and scientific landscape. In analogy to what has been shown in previous chapters, the fate of the CSRS was closely tied to the history of ORSTOM, which ended abruptly with the expulsion of all scientific staff from the site in 1988. These external shocks – which the CSRS could only react to – forced Swiss science to collaborate more closely with Ivorian institutions. But first, it is important to briefly recall the character of the Franco-Ivorian scientific complex as it emerged in the 1970s.

---

64 Archiv Schweizerische Akademie der Naturwissenschaften, Depot Burgerbibliothek Bern (SCNAT), GA SANW 825, Sitzungen der Kommission CSRS, 1951–1990, Hansjörg Huggel, Protokoll – Kommissionssitzung vom 22. Februar 1986, 20 March 1986, pp. 1–5, here: pp. 3–4.

65 Patrick Chabal, *Power in Africa. An Essay in Political Interpretation*, London 1992, p. 201.

66 Richard C. Crook, *Politics, the Cocoa Crisis, and Administration in Côte d'Ivoire*, in: The Journal of Modern African Studies, Vol. 28, No. 4, 1990, pp. 649–669, here: p. 652.

Shifting Alliances: The Breakup of the Franco-Ivorian Scientific Complex

In 1974, ORSTOM-trained botanist Guédé Lorougnon was named head of the Ministry of Scientific Research, which had been established in 1971. During their first years in office, Lorougnon and his staff aimed not only to define a sound science policy for the country, but to shift decision-making powers from the various French research institutions to the new ministry.[67] In certain respects, the country's scientific system was exceptional, as it rested on a "système de programmation", which ensured the exchange of information, the coordination of research within a wider national policy context (and especially with Planning Ministry development initiatives) and the definition of national research priorities. Notwithstanding all the new vigor, Ivorian scientific aspirations in the 1970s remained agriculturally biased, seriously underfunded and highly influenced by French experts. For instance, through its centers, ORSTOM participated in all of the more than 30 program committees that existed in 1975 and coordinated 3 of them.[68] The execution of French scientific projects was scarcely restricted, not least because French science fell under the general agreement on development aid signed in April 1962. The valuable impact of French science on Ivorian development was thus undisputed. Ongoing dependence found its clearest expression in financial matters. In 1973, the two parties agreed that scientific activities motivated largely by French interests would be covered by France, expenditures on programs of joint interest were to be shared between France and Côte d'Ivoire, and the Ivorian government would raise funds for programs which it asked France to pursue.[69] Prior to the framework agreement of 1984, most of the French budget went to ORSTOM and the Research Group for Development of Tropical Agronomy (GERDAT), with national research institutes benefiting only very haphazardly.[70] As a consequence, Ivorian policymakers faced

67 Archive Ministère de la Recherche Scientifique Côte d'Ivoire (AMRSCI), Balla Keita, 5 February 1975, pp. 1–33, here: p. 4.
68 Ibid., Bernard Pouyaud et al., Rapport sur les activités, la situation matérielle et sociale et les relations extérieures de l'ORSTOM en Côte d'Ivoire, établi à la demande de Monsieur le Ministre de la Recherche Scientifique [undated], pp. 1–12, here: p. 7.
69 Ibid., Commission Mixte Ivoiro-Française de concertation en matière de recherche scientifique et technique, Abidjan, 29–31 May 1973, pp. 1–7, here: p. 6.
70 Ibid., Dixième Commission mixte Franco-Ivoirienne en matière de recherche scientifique et technique, Abidjan, 7–9 March 1983, pp. 1–4, here: p. 3.

severe constraints in building up a national scientific infrastructure. Apart from financial matters, the legacies of French colonialism were most apparent in the area of Ivorization. The extent to which young Ivorian scholars could work within French research institutes was a question that dominated negotiations between the two parties throughout the 1970s and 1980s. The Ivorian government did not necessarily pursue a policy of replacing French scientists with African personnel. Rather, the idea was that promising scholars should be trained by senior French scientists under specific programs, so that "their former comrades (in colonial times) now become their friends".[71] As far as ORSTOM was concerned, France never wholeheartedly embraced this form of friendship. In response to labor market pressures, ORSTOM's director in Côte d'Ivoire, J. P. Tonnier, suggested that the institute should create a legal "parallel structure" as soon as possible, in order to prevent Ivorian scientists – considered as mere "technicians" – from using the ORSTOM label.[72] This proposal met with the approval of ORSTOM's director general, Guy Camus, who, in a letter to Tonnier in 1978, insisted on the small but significant distinction between "encadrement" (training) and "insertion" (integration): while training of a limited number of Ivorians was politically unavoidable, permanent integration was to be avoided at all costs.[73] Not surprisingly, the recruitment of Ivorian scientists by ORSTOM remained far below Ivorian expectations.[74] The fragile bonds of friendship implied by the term "Ivorization" were torn apart in the latter half of the 1980s. The most important event in this regard was the signing of the 1984 framework agreement concerning "Ivorian sovereignty over and ownership of the real estate and property of all French research facilities in Côte d'Ivoire".[75] France subsequently withdrew its financial contributions to scientific research in the country, and – in analogy to what happened in Tanzania in the mid-1960s – the Ivorian government vigorously pursued new relationships with potential donor

---

71 (ANF), Archives de l'ORSTOM, 19900236, Art. 57, M. Gleizes, [untitled and undated], pp. 1–9, here: p. 7.

72 Ibid., J. P. Tonnier, Principaux problèmes en suspens. Note remise à M. Gleizes à l'occasion de sa mission en Côte d'Ivoire, 15 May 1975, pp. 1–4, here: p. 3.

73 (ANF), Archives de l'ORSTOM, 19910536, Art. 8, Côte d'Ivoire, 1971–1978, Guy Camus, "personnelle et confidentielle", 8 May 1978, pp. 1–3, here: p. 1.

74 In 1980, there was only one Ivorian researcher working for ORSTOM; see: AMRSCI, Bernard Pouyaud et al., Rapport, p. 3.

75 AMRSCI, Accord Cadre relatif à l'aide et à la coopération en matière de recherche scientifique entre le Gouvernement de la République de Côte d'Ivoire et le Gouvernement de la République Française, 25 April 1984, p. 2.

countries.[76] The strains in scientific relations – first detectable in the framework agreement and culminating in the unceremonious expulsion of all ORSTOM personnel in 1988 – gave rise to new possibilities for the CSRS. It was clear from the framework agreement that other countries' scientific bodies were not affected by the nationalization process:

> Foreign, non-French scientific facilities were outside the scope of the assumption of control of French institutions by Côte d'Ivoire. For instance, the Centre Suisse de Recherches Scientifiques (CSRS) … was not affected when ORSTOM in Adiopodoumé and the specialized centers of the CIRAD [Agricultural Research Center for International Development] … were placed under the control of the Ivorian government.[77]

Stepping out from under the Colonial Shadow: The CSRS and the Quest for Africanization

Even though Switzerland was not subject to the historical sensitivities pervading the negotiations between France and Côte d'Ivoire, the reappropriation of ORSTOM's property had direct consequences for the CSRS, as it also affected the land on which the center was built.[78] Thus, while the CSRS had operated for over 30 years under the political shadow of its powerful French neighbor, Switzerland was now for the first time brought into direct contact with the Ivorian government. In 1978, in the face of financial constraints and new political realities, a Swiss delegation consisting of members of the Swiss Society of Natural Sciences (SNG) and the Swiss National Science Foundation had gone to Abidjan to discuss the future of the research site and find out whether the Ivorian government was in favor of Swiss research in the country. Most importantly, the delegation met with the Scientific Research Minister, Lorougnon, who assured them that he would regret the CSRS closing down. Indeed, he asked the Swiss

---

76   Ibid., Traore Kassoum, *Histoire de la Recherche Scientifique en Côte d'Ivoire*, p. 31.
77   Ibid., Hubert Oulaye et al., Etats Généraux de la Recherche: Rapport de la Commission "Cadre Juridique et Institutionnel", 1999, p. 14.
78   ASTI, CSRS, Adresses, Commission, Principes, Centre Suisse de Recherches Scientifiques en Côte d'Ivoire (CSRS), Wichtige Beschlüsse des Senats der SANW, welche das Zentrum an der Elfenbeinküste betreffen und Auszüge aus den dem Senat vorgelegten Berichten über das Centre, pp. 1–7, here: p. 3.

party to play a stronger role in Ivorian research policy, thus establishing a counterweight to France's predominance.[79] Given Lorougnon's favorable opinion and the many research possibilities offered by the country, the delegation proposed that the research station should continue to operate for three years (until the end of 1982), but with a shifting of priorities. Rather than mainly serving Swiss interests, it should now also address national and regional research priorities, as well as training African researchers.

In addition, Swiss research was no longer to be determined by the interests of individual Swiss scientists, but was to be conducted within agreed research programs matching local priorities, such as parasitology, botany or ethology (primatology). In 1979, the delegation's proposals for the continuation of activities in Adiopodoumé were accepted by the Senate of the SNG. As in the case of the STIFL in Tanzania, CSRS policymakers also requested funds from the SDC, which similarly brought a new dynamic into Swiss-Ivorian relations. The funds released by the SDC for 1979–1982 were intended to foster scientific collaboration with the Third World and to help build up an independent scientific infrastructure. Furthermore, these resources were to allow the CSRS to explore possibilities for closer collaboration with the Research Ministry and university institutes. In particular, the CSRS was to investigate how African researchers could be involved in its research activities.[80] One year after the agreement between the SNG and the SDC, Christian George, a Lausanne University zoologist, was sent to Côte d'Ivoire to explore the prospects for closer links with young Ivorian researchers. The results were very modest: a parasitological student proposed by the new Research Minister Balla Keita could not be integrated into the CSRS because no parasitologists were currently working there, and a planned research visit to Switzerland could not take place after the candidate in question obtained disappointing grades in his final examinations.[81]

One of the first to propose a comprehensive plan for the Ivorization of the CSRS was Marc Bachmann, a nutritionist based at the ETH Zurich and

79 SCNAT, GA SANW 448, Senat, 1977–1984, Bericht der Delegation SNG/Nationalfonds (SNF) über den Besuch am Centre Suisse de Recherches Scientifiques (CSRS) in Adiopodoumé (Elfenbeinküste) vom 23.-25.11.1978, p. 71.

80 SCNAT, GA SANW 448, Senat, E. Niggli, Senatsprotokoll der 75. Senats-Sitzung der Schweizerischen Naturforschenden Gesellschaft, pp. 1–85, here: p. 30.

81 BAR, E 2200.5 (-), 1998/4, 13, 652.2, Associations et institutions scientifiques, 1985–1988, Rapport sur l'enquête effectuée en Côte d'Ivoire par le Dr. Ch. George (resumé des activités), pp. 1–4, here: p. 3.

President of the CSRS Commission. Bachmann envisaged a long-term strategy ultimately leading to complete Ivorization. As a first step, the Ivorian government was to be persuaded to contribute to the running costs of the CSRS, and a number of scientists were to be offered the opportunity to participate in current research projects. In a second phase, the government's financial contribution was to be increased and the first Ivorian projects initiated. Under Bachmann's plans, this phase would also see the appointment of a "suitable Ivorian" as co-director of the CSRS, with responsibility for internal affairs. In a third and final phase, overall leadership of the CSRS would be handed over to Côte d'Ivoire, with Switzerland still providing limited financial contributions.[82]

Not surprisingly, Bachmann's proposals encountered fierce resistance from other members of the Commission. Most agreed that political pressures made total opposition to broader Ivorian participation impossible. As Aeschlimann put it, "If we don't make the first step ourselves, the Ivorians will make a big one, which could be definitive."[83] But agreeing to train African students was still a long way from the complete Ivorization envisaged by Bachmann. More than anything, the question of Ivorization was one of scale. At a meeting held on February 16, 1985, the Commission agreed that they would oppose (a) the appointment of an Ivorian co-director, (b) losing their academic freedom, (c) the pursuit of Ivorization without a clear plan, (d) a financial disaster and (e) 100% Ivorization.[84] The debate on Ivorization thus focused on what should be prevented, rather than the direction to be pursued. Furthermore, the discussion had moral undertones. While the term "Tanzanization" was eschewed in favor of the more technical and seemingly apolitical notion of integration, the persons responsible for the CSRS did not hesitate to consider the adverse effects of African influence on the quality of Swiss knowledge generated in Côte d'Ivoire. Reflecting on new forms of collaboration, Eugen Wimmer – the driving force behind the CSRS since its humble beginnings – alluded to the specific way of life and "anti-individualism" which were likely to undermine the lab's financial independence: "In general, he [the African] lives together with his parents, and if he finds himself in a position to

---

82 SCNAT, GA SANW 830, Marc Bachmann, Gedanken zu einer eventuellen Mitbeteiligung ivorianischer Forscher an den Arbeiten des Centre Suisse, pp. 1–2.
83 Ibid., André Aeschlimann to Marc Bachmann, 22 February 1985, p. 1.
84 SCNAT, GA SANW 825, Hansjörg Huggel, Procès-Verbal de la Commission du CSRS du 16.2.1985, pp. 1–7, here: p. 6.

support them, he will certainly do so. This attitude could be called 'family parasitism'."[85] Leaving aside the issue of what was perceived as corruption, others interpreted the prospect of Ivorization more generally as the decay of scientific infrastructure or as a process spelling the end of a glorious past. One of the former directors of the CSRS evoked the familiar trope of once thriving research sites becoming an archaeologist's paradise:

> The prospect of complete Ivorization saddens me. In Niger, Burkina Faso and Mali, I saw the remains of totally run-down scientific facilities that had been enthusiastically built up. Former Nestlé scientists who returned to the village of Kpouébo – their experimental site – told me about the total failure of their development programs. Obviously even the involvement of sociologists and psychologists was to no avail. In September 1985, I visited the former French research station of Lamto, which is now administered by the University of Abidjan. The formerly flourishing station is almost completely abandoned today. It was desperate! That is why Ivorization should not be a goal but should be delayed as much as possible.[86]

However, given the pace of external changes, the delaying of Africanization could not be an appropriate strategy. In the latter half of the 1980s, the fate of ORSTOM continued to concern CSRS managers. At the second Francophonie Summit, held in Quebec in September 1987, delegates decided on the transformation of ORSTOM Adiopodoumé into the "Institut International de Recherche Scientifique pour le Développement d'Adiopodoumé" (IIRSDA). Heralded as the first international francophone research institute south of the Sahara, the IIRSDA was to focus on agricultural and biomedical research. As is often the case when research structures are reconfigured, certain elements are more likely to change than others. Exemplifying the latter was the decision to nominate the former ORSTOM director Bernard Boccas as new director general of the IIRSDA, albeit with an Ivorian co-director.[87] Responsibility for decision-making rested with a Governing Board (made up of delegates from different countries) and a Donors Committee, where nonstate actors could also exert an influence over the scientific programs. The Canadian, French and Ivorian gov-

---

85 SCNAT, GA SANW 830, Eugen Wimmer, Ivoirisation du Centre Suisse, [undated] p. 1.
86 Ibid., anonymized, 03.1985, pp. 1–4, here: p. 2.
87 ASTI, CSRS, Adresses, Commission, Principes, Beat Sitter, André Aeschlimann, Bericht, Vereinbarung zwischen der Regierung der Republik Elfenbeinküste und der SANW betreffend das Centre Suisse de Recherches Scientifiques en Côte d'Ivoire (CSRS), 24 August 1988, pp. 1–9, here: p. 8.

ernments who currently constituted the IIRSDA were of course eager to draw in as many new donor countries as possible. Not surprisingly from a linguistic, financial and historical viewpoint, Switzerland was one of their prime targets.

Observing the gradual internationalization of France's once giant scientific machinery, the SNG had to maneuver carefully between the political pressures exerted by France and Côte d'Ivoire and negotiate its own legal status, which had been in limbo since 1985. In 1988, the SNG signed a draft agreement with the Ivorian government, containing both rights and obligations. Future scientific programs at the CSRS were to be integrated into the "système de programmation", or at least approved by the ministry; furthermore, the ministry reserved the right to authorize the import and export of scientific materials and to appoint a number of Ivorian scientists as research associates at the CSRS. On the other hand, the Ivorian government provided the land on which the CSRS was built free of charge and offered generous tax exemptions for the import of scientific devices and infrastructure.[88] During the negotiations, the Ivorian delegates once again made it clear that they would expect Swiss participation in the newly established IIRSDA.[89] From a scientific perspective, such collaboration would certainly be valuable: some of the key areas of CSRS expertise, such as taxonomy, parasitology or soil science, did not feature on the IIRSDA's research agenda. The main problem was that, as a nongovernmental body, the SNG could only participate in the Donors Committee, but not as a full member of the Board. However, the society's attempts to persuade the Swiss government to pursue membership of the IIRSDA were unsuccessful. While Federal Councillor Flavio Cotti remained uncommitted vis-à-vis official invitations from the Ivorian government, the SDC's position was quite clear: Côte d'Ivoire was not one of the SDC's priority countries; its economic situation had deteriorated to such an extent that it was not a good choice for further activities; and as far as agriculture and health were concerned, the SDC preferred to channel funds to the Consultative Group on International Agricultural Research (CGIAR) and the WHO's tropical

---

88   SCNAT, GA SANW 829, Auguste Kouassi, Beat Sitter, André Aeschlimann, Protocole d'accord entre le Gouvernement de la République de Côte d'Ivoire et la Société Helvétique de Sciences Naturelles (Académie Suisse des Sciences Naturelles) concernant le Centre Suisse de Recherches Scientifiques en Côte d'Ivoire, 29 March 1988.

89   ASTI, CSRS, Adresses, Commission, Principes, Sitter, Aeschlimann, Bericht, p. 7.

disease programs.[90] Accordingly, the above-mentioned SDC credit covering a three-year period was merely an interim solution.

In fact, the idea of an effective international research institute proved difficult to realize. As it turned out, neither France, Canada nor Côte d'Ivoire truly supported the IIRSDA – that is, their support was more based on political considerations than inspired by a wish for international scientific cooperation. The Ivorian government had originally intended to establish a forestry institute modeled on the existing Savanna Institute (IDESSA), but as France was not prepared to hand over the Adiopodoumé site, it decided to internationalize ORSTOM. Canada's commitment was based on a quid pro quo: the country already had a research institute in Côte d'Ivoire and made it clear that France could only expect Canadian commitment to the IIRSDA if the French provided financial backing for Canadian scientific projects in return. Critical voices could also be heard from within the French Ministry of Technical Cooperation, which, according to some observers, increasingly started to question whether the effort was worthwhile.[91] Between 1989 and 1991, scientific activities in Adiopodoumé almost came to a standstill. The Ivorian government decided that 75% of the French scientific personnel should be withdrawn from the site, and a number of laboratories closed down in quick succession. New statutes and a new Canadian director general were unable to reverse this trend. In 1991, the IIRSDA had four scientists on the site, and only one researcher was left by the end of that year.[92] In 1995, both the IIRSDA and the former Dutch research center were closed down.[93] Of the former colonial research institutions operating in Adiopodoumé, only the CSRS remained.

90   Ibid., Alassane Salif N'Diaye to Flavio Cotti, Invitation du Gouvernement de la Confédération Helvétique à adhérer à l'Institut International de Recherche Scientifique pour le Développement d'Adiopodoumé (IIRSDA), 26 April 1989; Flavio Cotti to Alassane Salif N'Diaye, Institut International de Recherche Scientifique pour le Développement Adiopodoumé (IIRSDA), 29 June 1989; Fritz Staehelin (SDC) to B. Hahnloser (EDI), Institut d'Adiopodoumé (Côte d'Ivoire), 23 August 1989, pp. 1–2.
91   Archive Centre Suisse de Recherches Scientifiques (ACSRS), Entwicklung IIRSDA – Stand Oktober 1989, pp. 1–3, here: pp. 1–2.
92   ASTI, CSRS, Kommissionssitzungen 1990–1997, Rapports Annuels 1990–1996, Liliane Ortega, Rapport Annuel 1993, CSRS, Centre Suisse de Recherche Scientifique en Côte d'Ivoire, 1 February 1994, pp. 1–10, here: p. 10.
93   Ibid., R. Leuthold, Protokoll der Sitzung der Kommission für das Centre Suisse de Recherches Scientifiques, Côte d'Ivoire, 8 March 1995, pp. 1–5, here: p. 4.

While Swiss science outlived the French and Dutch presence at the site, it did so with different purposes. With the departure of the French from Adiopodoumé and the signing of the framework agreement, the idea that the CSRS could be a vehicle for Swiss scientists to pursue their research interests was abandoned. Instead, all activities were to come under specific core areas reflecting the country's research priorities. In the 1990s, the areas of nature/ecology, nutrition/rural development and parasitology (medicine)/rural development were defined.[94] Later, the topic of urbanization and its health effects was added. This new area in particular called for close collaboration between the natural and social sciences.[95]

From Ivorization to Research Partnerships

The draft agreement of 1988 between the CSRS and the Ivorian government was crucial in transforming the negative discourse of Ivorization into the positive ideal of research partnerships, which has come to dominate current thinking.[96] Under the agreement, the Research Ministry[97] was entitled to assign Ivorian scientists to CSRS research programs. In the 1990s, thanks in particular to the efforts of CSRS director Peter Lehmann and his successor Liliane Ortega (a botanist and the center's first female director), a first group of Ivorian scientists participated in various new research programs. From the outset, however, Switzerland acted as a gatekeeper, with partnerships being subject to certain constraints. The first was financial: the Swiss Academy of Sciences (as the SNG is now called) insisted that, apart from modest social security contributions, the Ivorian ministry

94 Jean-François Graf, *Kommission für das Centre Suisse de Recherches Scientifiques en Côte d'Ivoire (CSRS)*, in: Jahrbuch der Schweizerischen Akademie der Naturwissenschaften, Bern 1990, pp. 24–27, here: p. 24; ASTI, CSRS, Kommissionssitzungen 1990–1997, Rodolphe Spichiger, Protocole de la séance de la Commission ad hoc du CSRS du 16.05.1990, pp. 1–4, here: p. 2; ASTI, CSRS, Adresses, Commission, Principes, Forschungsschwerpunkte am CSRS, Planungsperiode 1992–1995, p. 1.

95 Marcel Tanner, *Commission pour le Centre Suisse de Recherche Scientifique en Côte-d'Ivoire,* in: Jahrbuch der Schweizerischen Akademie der Naturwissenschaften, Bern 2000, pp. 95–97, here: p. 95.

96 Kent Buse, Andrew Harmer, *Power to the Partners? The Politics of Public-Private Health Partnerships,* in: Development, Vol. 47, No. 2, 2004, pp. 49–56, here: pp. 51–52.

97 In 1986, the Ministère de l'Education Nationale et de la Recherche Scientifique was reorganized to form a Ministère de l'Education Nationale under Balla Keita and a Ministère de la Recherche Scientifique under Alassane Salif N'Diaye.

should cover the African researchers' salaries and infrastructure. The second was the fear of a loss of research quality. Without a say in the selection of candidates, the CSRS was worried about "key functions" within its research structures being blocked by "incompetent local researchers".[98] This question was discussed at a meeting between a Swiss Academy of Sciences delegation and Ivorian officials in 1991, where the Research Minister promised that he would only send "highly qualified young researchers", who would complete their third-cycle education at the CSRS.[99] Some years later, the arrangements were changed, and it was agreed that the CSRS could now select future researchers from a group of the most promising candidates.[100] The fact that, from an institutional viewpoint, development took the form of nurturing the Ivorian elite was echoed in Liliane Ortega's statement that "le vrai développement, c'est, quand on le peut, d'aider les meilleurs dans le pays."[101]

One of the main features of research partnerships in the initial years was that the research priorities were defined by Switzerland.[102] Ivorian researchers could not pursue their own research interests but were given a specific topic within the predefined areas. Most of them worked together with Swiss PhD students who already had elaborate research plans and financial support. While this arrangement did not necessarily lead to interpersonal tensions between African and Swiss researchers, it was impervious to Ivorian inputs, thus undermining the whole idea of partnership. Recalling his first years at the CSRS, one of the African researchers said:

> In the past, it was like the Swiss researcher came with a research topic and with money, and it was here where he looked for support. He asked somebody to help him – another researcher or a student to support his work. So everything was prepared there [in Switzerland]. He probably had time to think about his topic for six

---

98 ASTI, CSRS, Adresses, Commission, Principes, Paul Walter, Besuch einer Delegation der SANW beim Centre Suisse de Recherches Scientifiques en Côte d'Ivoire (CSRS) in Abidjan vom 9.-24. März 1991, Inoffizieller Bericht, 6 April 1991, pp. 1–12, here: pp. 5–6.

99 Ibid., p. 10.

100 ASTI, CSRS, Kommissionssitzungen 1990–1997, Jakob Zinsstag, Maria Zinsstag, Centre Suisse de Recherches Scientifiques en Côte d'Ivoire, Rapport Annuel 1995, 8 February 1995, pp. 1–28, here: p. 17.

101 Catherine Morand, *Notre institut sous les tropiques africains*, in: Journal de Genève et Gazette de Lausanne, 14/15 December 1991.

102 ASTI, Adresses, Commission, Principes, Séry Bailly, Jakob Zinsstag, Compte rendu du séminaire sur le partenariat ivoiro-suisse entre l'Université d'Abidjan et le Centre Suisse de Recherches Scientifiques, jeudi, 23 mars 1994, pp. 1–3, here: p. 2.

months or even a year, and when he arrived here he had to start, he would not wait for three months to get the project started. He had to start immediately, and he then looked for a student. Sometimes, this student had no time [for preparation]. Matters were already difficult from the beginning ... [103]

For many of the first African researchers – disregarding their weak position in framing research proposals – partnership provided access to a competitive research environment and to a research infrastructure that could allow them to pursue their academic careers. However, individual career paths were not always favored by predefined research areas. One researcher, for instance, who was writing his thesis on mammals was at a disadvantage when CSRS research policies were readjusted, downgrading traditional zoological topics.[104] Similarly, some research fields at the CSRS proved to be more open to African researchers than others. In particular, the internationally renowned primatology group working in the Tai Forest under Christophe Boesch was criticized for its reluctance to collaborate with Ivorian scientists.

Towards a New World Order

This chapter sought to relate macroeconomic processes – the liberalization of African economies and the new transnational modalities between private and government actors in science and health care – to institutional changes occurring within the STIFL and the CSRS. It highlighted a series of contradictory processes within biomedical research and development practices conducted in the context of widespread poverty. The first is the fact that the economic downturn experienced by Tanzania and Côte d'Ivoire since the 1970s very much contributed to Switzerland's increasing power in Africa. The African continent's declining economic performance not only ushered in new forms of governmentality – with NGOs increasingly assuming roles that were once part of the core activities of governments – but also put an end to some long-established ties. As shown by the example of Côte d'Ivoire, the period saw the disruption of ties be-

103 Anonymized, Interview held in Adiopodoumé, 2009.
104 Anonymized, Interview held in Adiopodoumé, 2009.

tween Paris and its former colony. Despite the Janus-faced character[105] of French policies towards its former colonial possession still prevailing today, most historians and observers of international relations interpreted the end of the 1980s as a watershed in official French-African relations. The policy reorientation was rooted in economic and political considerations: with the end of the Cold War, Africa lost much of its former geostrategic importance, and France's attention turned towards more "profitable" and industrialized areas in Eastern Europe and Asia.[106] Additionally, France's adoption of the "Abidjan doctrine" in 1993 (making aid subject to compliance with IMF requirements), the disastrous role played in the Rwandan genocide a year later, and general doubts about the efficiency of development aid in Africa were all signs that the presence of the "grande nation" on the continent had become economically and politically unrewarding.[107] France's shifting relations to what was formerly one of its closest allies in francophone West Africa – Côte d'Ivoire – are a revealing example of the process described by James Ferguson as "global disconnect" within a world order for which connection is of the essence.[108]

These reconnects and disconnects on a global scale were reflected in the micropolitics of the two institutions. Largely shaped by the state of French science in Côte d'Ivoire, the activities of the CSRS were more strongly focused on the African country, both from the point of view of tackling local priorities and including African scientists in research programs. Ivorization was a process initially feared and later largely controlled by the members of the CSRS. Insofar as the CSRS could choose the most suitable candidates for participation in its research programs, scien-

---

105 Jean-François Bayart speaks of the "schizophrenic" nature of France's African policy during the 1990s, characterized by subjection to the requirements of the Bretton Woods institutions on the one hand, and continuing efforts to promote political stabilization – including military interventions – on the other; see: Jean-François Bayart, *Réflexions sur la politique africaine de la France*, in: Politique Africaine, Vol. 58, 1995, pp. 41–50.

106 Jean-François Bayart, *France-Afrique. La fin du pacte colonial*, in: Politique Africaine, Vol. 39, 1990, pp. 47–53, p. 50.

107 Philippe Marchesin, *La politique africaine de la France en transition*, in: Politique Africaine, Vol. 71, 1998, pp. 91–106.

108 James Ferguson, *Global Disconnect. Abjection and the Aftermath of Modernism*, in: Peter Geschiere, Birgit Meyer and Peter Pels (eds.), Readings in Modernity in Africa, Bloomington, Indiana 2008, pp. 1–8. For a similar argument, see: James Ferguson, *Transnational Topographies of Power. Beyond "the State" and "Civil Society" in the Study of African Politics*, in: Ferguson, Global Shadows. Africa in the Neoliberal World Order, Durham, London 2006, pp. 89–112.

tific abilities and skills became the key to upward social mobility. Decolonization was by and large a sociotechnical project, with older categories of race being transformed into "the possibility of boundless upward mobility through the acquisition of technological knowledge".[109]

In Tanzania, the integration of the STIFL also went hand in hand with both administrative reforms and a redistribution of responsibilities between the SDC and the STI/IC. Dissatisfied with what had been achieved in the Tanzanian health sector – especially in the area of PHC – the SDC and the STI tried to introduce new mechanisms so as to make medical research more demand-driven (the research user fund); to channel the flow of SDC funds more directly to the NIMR rather than the IC; to reinvent district collaboration with SolidarMed; and to expand the role of the Steering Committee as a private-public partnership now responsible for all innovations. However, the changes initiated were short-lived. The idea of the research user fund never really took off. According to former NIMR director Wenceslaus Kilama, the main problem (apart from resistance from the Tanzanian MOH) was finding research clients who would come up with research proposals. The mindset still prevalent was that policy implementers and other clients did not allow themselves to guide the work of scientists: "They said, you are the researchers, you know better, and we don't want to interfere with you doing a good job."[110]

More effective, however, were the SDC's efforts to separate health service provision from scientific research – the combination of which had been one of the major achievements of the KIHERE project. Bringing SolidarMed into the development equation, the SDC largely put an end to the health service activities. The IC, consequently, sought new donors and became a highly attractive center of excellence, especially in the areas of malaria research and vaccine development, which got off the ground with the Kilombero Malaria Project (KMP) in 1988 and gained unprecedented global attention from the 1990s. How malaria research took shape in Kilombero District and how it was interpreted by the local population are the topics of the next chapter.

109 Gabrielle Hecht, *Rupture-Talk in the Nuclear Age*, p. 719.
110 Interview with Wenceslaus Kilama, 9 February 2011.

Chapter 7
The Governance of Malaria Research in Tanzania

The previous chapter described the transition from a situation where medical research was negotiated locally and discussed under the headings of development and primary health care (PHC) to one where research practices on the ground in Tanzania were shaped by the diversification of the global health network.[1] One reason for this shift into a postdevelopment era was the redistribution of responsibilities between the SDC and the Ifakara Center (IC), as well as the widening gap between health research and the provision of health services in Kilombero District. In addition, research at the IC began to focus increasingly on malaria – the main health issue in the region. Apart from the testing of chloroquine by Swiss scientists at St. Francis Hospital, the topic of malaria had long been monopolized by Tanzanian research groups. Towards the end of the 1980s, however, the National Institute of Medical Research (NIMR) relaxed its monopoly on investigations of the disease. In 1988, in an attempt to diversify its resources, the STIFL embarked on the Kilombero Malaria Project (KMP), which aimed both to develop possible malaria vaccine candidates and to evaluate insecticide-treated nets (ITNs) for widespread use among the population.[2] This new research agenda called for new modes of collaboration, as the quest for a malaria vaccine, in particular, was a highly competitive endeavor involving research groups around the globe.[3] The renewed focus on malaria research during the 1990s can be explained by the assumption that the burden of the disease could be significantly reduced – not by an all-encompassing

---

1 I am deeply indebted to Jensen Charles and Ronald Munga for their assistance during fieldwork in Idete, Mingoyo, Mnolela and Nyengedi.

2 Archive Swiss Tropical and Public Health Institute, Basel (ASTI), Kilombero Malaria Project, Summary of the Kilombero Malaria Project, pp. 1–2, here: p. 1. The KMP was a joint undertaking involving the Swiss Tropical Institute (STI), the Swiss Tropical Institute Field Laboratory (STIFL), the Universities of Wageningen and Nijmegen, the WHO Immunology Research and Training Center (WHO-IRTC), Imperial College London, the Tanzanian National Institute of Medical Research (NIMR) and the District Health Office. The funds for the initial three-year period came from the SDC, the Dutch government and the WHO-IRTC.

3 ASTI, KIHERE Letters, 1985–1988, Antoine Degrémont to Don DeSavigny and Christoph Hatz, 18 July 1986, pp. 1–9.

"magic bullet", but through a number of more or less technical and integrated approaches which, collectively, would help to mitigate the devastating effects of the disease. Hence, as had been the case before African independence, health was again perceived as the "product of technical interventions divorced from economic, social and political contexts".[4] From the beginning of the 1990s, however, in striking contrast to earlier decades, the number of actors involved in malaria research rose exponentially. Malaria was (and still is) first and foremost a disease of the poor in Third World countries. But in the privileged North/Western hemisphere, malaria has become a powerful icon for raising funds and rallying politicians, global charities, scientific institutions, pharmaceutical companies and national governments behind a new humanitarian movement, which perhaps more than ever considers the fight against the disease as a moral imperative.

This chapter therefore examines certain aspects of the history of malaria research in Tanzania in order to address a major research question: under what conditions can science move beyond the stage of experimentation and have an impact at the level of national health policy? My attempt to answer this question involves two case studies, which form the core of the chapter. Both deal with the organization of malaria interventions (in twentieth- and twenty-first-century Tanzania) and their effects on power relations, but they do so from different vantage points. The first case study concerns the history of the vaccine candidate SPf66 (serum *Plasmodium falciparum*, version 66). SPf66 was produced by the Colombian scientist Manuel Patarroyo and tested in a Phase III trial in Idete, a small village within the catchment area of the KMP. The second case study deals with the intermittent preventive treatment in infants (IPTi) project, conducted in the southeastern Mtwara and Lindi Regions between 2004 and 2009.[5] IPTi involves the administration of a full dose of an antimalarial drug at specific times during the first year of life, regardless of the presence or absence of malaria parasites. At first sight, the two projects appear to be quite different. The SPf66 project involved attempts to transform African villages into veritable trial sites, where all external factors could be controlled. In contrast, the aim of the IPTi project was to introduce this method into the na-

---

4   Anne-Emanuelle Birn, *Gates's Grandest Challenge. Transcending Technology as Public Health Ideology*, in: Lancet, Vol. 366, No. 9484, 2005, pp. 514–519.

5   The most detailed history of these regions is: Felicitas Becker, *A Social History of Southeast Tanzania 1890–1950*, PhD Study Cambridge University, Cambridge 2002. For a political history of the colonial period, see: J. Gus Liebenow, *Colonial Rule and Political Development in Tanzania. The Case of the Makonde*, Evanston 1971.

tional health system. Examined from a distance, however, there are certain similarities: two overarching issues account for their failure. The first was the problem of "stabilization" of scientific facts. As we will see, not only was there a failure to control all the external factors at the trial site, but concurrent trials of SPf66 in other parts of the world, using different protocols, made it impossible to standardize the results. Secondly, there is the issue of health governance – a leitmotif of medical research in the new millennium. The term "governance" is used here not in a normative sense, but more neutrally to denote a "process of collective action between both state and non-state actors to resolve complex societal problems".[6] That the resolution of such problems in a collaborative manner is far from easy is one lesson to be drawn from the history of IPTi. It is argued here that this new partnership structure is marked by power inequalities among the different actors, and that the entanglement of science and policy is likely to produce unsatisfactory outcomes in health policymaking in Africa.

It may be said that the case studies chosen here paint a rather negative picture. It must be acknowledged that, in some cases, efforts to translate science into public health action have indeed been successful. The Tanzanian government is currently scaling up a national bed-net program which emerged from research conducted by the IC and the STI. This research, together with past interventions, had a measurable impact on the epidemiology of malaria around Ifakara.[7] It is nonetheless important to recall the history of SPf66 and IPTi because it raises the possibility that the problems in translating scientific results into public health policy may have to be sought within the scientific system itself. While SPf66 has now indeed become history, discussions about the implementation of IPTi in public

---

6   Till Förster, Lucy Koechlin, *The Politics of Governance. Power and Agency in the Formation of Political Order in Africa*, in: Basel Papers on Political Transformations, No. 1, 2011, pp. 1–24, here: p. 8.

7   David Schellenberg et al., *The Changing Epidemiology of Malaria in Ifakara Town, Southern Tanzania*, in: Tropical Medicine and International Health, Vol. 9, No. 1, 2004, pp. 68–76; Christian Lengeler, Don DeSavigny, Jacqueline Cattani, *From Research to Implementation*, in: Lengeler, DeSavigny and Cattani (eds.), Net Gain. A New Method for Preventing Malaria Deaths, Geneva 1996, pp. 1–15; Joanna Schellenberg, *KINET. A Social Marketing Programme of Treated Nets and Net Treatment for Malaria Control in Tanzania, with Evaluation of Child Health and Long-Term Survival*, in: Transactions of the Royal Society of Tropical Medicine and Hygiene, Vol. 93, No. 3, 1999, pp. 225–231; Happiness Minja, *Introducing Insecticide Treated Mosquito Nets in the Kilombero Valley (Tanzania). Social and Cultural Dimensions*, PhD Study University of Basel, Basel 2001.

health policy are ongoing. The history of IPTi lacks the historical "event" or "fact" which some think history is made of; it can be no more than a history of the "not yet" – history in the making.

SPf66 – A Vaccine Candidate from the South

In 1986, the eyes of the world's scientific community turned to Colombia, where Manuel Elkin Patarroyo, working at the Instituto Nacional de Inmunología in Bogotá, announced a new development that would have a strong impact on one of the world's most serious tropical diseases – SPf66, the first vaccine to be synthesized chemically rather than made from attenuated or dead pathogens (viruses or bacteria).[8] Patarroyo's vaccine also differed from earlier efforts in that it was designed, not to prevent blood-stage infection, but to reduce the number of parasites in the blood – preventing life-threatening malaria while allowing natural immunity to develop. Thus, the vaccine's major advantage was that it was not tailored to the needs of tourists or business travelers, but to those of people living in malaria-endemic areas.

Political Peptides

When, in the late 1980s, Manual Patarroyo proved SPf66 to be safe and immunogenic in *Aotus* monkeys and subsequently also in humans, hardly anybody in the scientific community would have questioned the need for what was seen as a scientific breakthrough. Soon after the publication of his results in *Nature*, however, several malariologists expressed skepticism as to the reproducibility of the results. Though criticisms were also voiced by Colombian scientists, by far the loudest objections came from the West, where such a success from the Third World "represents a blow to the scientific establishment that believes itself to be the trustee of malaria vaccine research".[9] Nevertheless, an ad hoc committee of the World Health Organization (WHO) and the Pan American Health Organization visiting Bogotá in

---

8   David Spurgeon, *Southern Lights. Celebrating the Scientific Achievements of the Developing World*, Ottawa 1995, p. 41.

9   Kirsten MacLeod, *Creation of First Malaria Vaccine Raises Troubling Questions about "Intellectual Racism"*, in: Canadian Medical Association Journal, Vol. 153, No. 9, 1995, pp. 1319–1321, here: p. 1321.

1990 concluded that "SPf66 merited further study" and recommended that "randomized, placebo-controlled trials should be carried out urgently among children living in areas of high transmission, particularly in Africa."[10] Setting up such trials was, however, highly contentious. The UK Medical Research Council (MRC), which operated large laboratories in the Gambia, twice refused to test the product on the grounds that the required technical information about the formulation of the vaccine was still lacking. On the basis of such limited information, the argument went, it would never allow a trial to be conducted in Britain and therefore it refused to do so in Africa.[11] The MRC's hesitation opened up possibilities for other research groups: Pedro Alonso – a Spanish malariologist collaborating with both Patarroyo in Colombia and Brian Greenwood, the principal investigator engaged for the Gambia trials – approached Marcel Tanner to explore whether the IC was willing and able to provide the infrastructure required for vaccine trials.[12]

When asked why the STI stepped into the breach and agreed to test the vaccine in rural Tanzania, Marcel Tanner replied that, from his point of view, there had – at that time – been no reason to hesitate. The primary objective of the first Phase III trial with SPf66 outside Latin America was to determine the efficacy of the vaccine in preventing malaria episodes in a hyperendemic area, highly representative of large parts of Africa.[13] To him and his collaborators, it was important to test the product independently of Manuel Patarroyo's group once all the ethical clearances were at hand.[14] Alonso's proposal also matched the overall aims of the KMP, which prioritized research on possible vaccine candidates.[15] Naturally enough, with the IC taking the lead in the SPf66 trial, the political tensions surrounding the vaccine did not vanish altogether. As it turned out, there was strains in the relationship between the principal co-investigators of the Tanzania

10 Pedro Alonso, Thomas Teuscher, Marcel Tanner, SPf66: Research for Development or Development of Research?, in: Vaccine, 1994, Vol. 12, No. 2, pp. 99–101, here: p. 99.
11 Phyllida Brown, *Colombia's Malaria Vaccine Approved for Trials*, in: New Scientist, 26 September 1992.
12 ASTI, KIVAC, Correspondence Pedro Alonso, Pedro Alonso to Marcel Tanner, 11 December 1991, pp. 1–2.
13 Secondary objectives were (a) to measure any immediate or delayed side effects associated with the administration of SPf66 in a semi-immune population and (b) to assess the immunogenicity of each dose of SPf66; see: ASTI, Pedro Alonso et al., A Trial of SPf66, A Candidate Synthetic Malaria Vaccine in Tanzania, Draft for Publication, p. 9.
14 Personal communication with Marcel Tanner, 10 May 2010.
15 ASTI, Kilombero Malaria Project, Summary of the Kilombero Malaria Project, pp. 1–2, here: p. 1.

trial – Marcel Tanner (STI), Pedro Alonso (Hospital Clinic i Provincial) and Thomas Teuscher (IC) – and the chair of the WHO TDR/IMMAL (Tropical Diseases Research/Immunology of Malaria) Steering Committee, Howard Engers. Although funds were released by the WHO, the investigators suspected the organization of giving priority to another SPf66 trial, led by Jerald Sadoff and the Walter Reed Army Institute of Research in Washington. The US Army researchers, collaborating closely with Patarroyo, used a vaccine developed in California (rather than Bogotá) in accordance with good clinical practice, so as to satisfy the requirements of the Food and Drug Administration (FDA).[16] The principal co-investigators' suspicions regarding the role played by the WHO stemmed from the fact that Patarroyo rejected a USD 70 million offer from the pharmaceutical industry for the SPf66 patent rights, assigning them instead to the WHO free of charge. In so doing, the Colombian scientist placed the WHO in a rather delicate position – being forced to choose between endorsing a product of as yet unproven efficacy for the Third World, or adopting the pharmaceutical industry's tactic of delaying the use of Patarroyo's product and supporting US efforts to develop a formulation that would gain the FDA's approval.[17] The impression that the WHO was eager to downplay the Tanzanian trial was also reflected in the media. In an article in the *New Scientist*, for example, Phyllida Brown gave a detailed account of the development of a new malaria vaccine without even mentioning the Tanzanian trial.[18] In a letter to Odile Puijalon, chair of the IMMAL/TDR subcommittee, Pedro Alonso expressed his concerns as follows:

> I would like to draw your attention to a recent news report which appeared in Science. This plus other circulating comments seem to be creating the distinct impression that the IMMAL supported Tanzanian trial is not the adequate trial. This is, to say the least, scientifically debatable. However, IMMAL may be seen as contributing to create this impression by recommending the urgent execution of another trial, which as we all know, intends to use the SPf66 molecule synthesized in the US. I am worried that IMMAL might be seen as promoting the use of a US synthesized product rather than one, at least equally good, coming from a developing country and which is already being used in a WHO supported trial.[19]

16 Phyllida Brown, *Colombia's Malaria Vaccine Approved.*
17 John Maurice, *Impfstoff, Zündstoff*, in: Die Zeit, No. 51, Dezember 1994, p. 37.
18 Phyllida Brown, *Colombia's Malaria Vaccine Approved*; see also: Phyllida Brown, *Malaria Vaccine Trials Stalled a Second Time*, in: New Scientist, 21/28 December 1991.
19 ASTI, KIVAC, Correspondence Pedro Alonso, Pedro Alonso to Odile Puijalon, 22 October 1992, pp. 1–3, here: p. 2.

Against this political backdrop, it was clear to Marcel Tanner and his collaborators that their trial should at least not be "criticized on design and operational grounds", and that their aim should be "to generate an efficacy figure that will be accepted by the scientific establishment".[20]

Standards and Standardization

The trial was a joint venture involving the IC, the Tanzanian National Institute for Medical Research (NIMR), the Swiss Tropical Institute (STI), the London School of Hygiene and Tropical Medicine (LSHTM), the Instituto de Parasitología (Spain) and the Foundation for Biomedical Research (Hospital Clinic i Provincial de Barcelona, Spain); it received funds from Spain and the UNDP/World Bank/WHO Special Program for Research and Training in Tropical Diseases (TDR).[21] This program was launched in the 1970s in an attempt to raise the profile of parasitological research and to focus on six diseases particularly prevalent in Africa – malaria, filariasis, schistosomiasis, trypanosomiasis, leishmaniasis and leprosy.[22] Like the (canceled) trial in the Gambia, the Tanzanian project was a placebo-controlled, double-blind vaccine trial. Important for the later history of SPf66 in Idete was the definition of malaria and the methods to be used for recording cases of the disease. It was clear that, in order to assess the impact of the vaccine on clinical malaria, a suitable definition had to be found for this endpoint. In areas where malaria is not highly endemic, case definition is relatively unproblematic: diagnosis is usually based on symptoms of fever and detection of malaria parasites in the blood. However, in most parts of sub-Saharan Africa, where malaria is endemic or hyperendemic, this case definition would be inadequate. There, "to assume that a child who presents with fever and who has parasitaemia is ill from malaria is not valid, and will result in over-diagnosis."[23] The researchers therefore defined clinical malaria as a combination of fever (37.5°C or higher) and high parasite density – the latter being uncommon in asymptomatic cases of malaria. The organization of the vaccine trial thus entailed adaptation to the new setting.

20 ASTI, KIVAC, Correspondence 1994, Marcel Tanner to Giuseppe del Guidice, 7 March 1994, pp. 1–2, here: p. 1.
21 Pedro Alonso et al., *A Trial of the Synthetic Malaria Vaccine SPf66 in Tanzania. Rationale and Design*, in: Vaccine, Vol. 12, No. 2, pp. 181–186, here: p. 182.
22 Max Charlesworth et al., *Life Among the Scientists*, p. 230.
23 Pedro Alonso et al., *A Trial of the Synthetic Malaria Vaccine*, p. 184.

The work of the anthropologist Adriana Petryna investigates the pharmaceutical industry's growing demand for "treatment-naïve" human subjects and the offshoring of clinical trials to mid- and low-income countries. In the logic of global research, this is legitimized by the fact that the trials constitute a social good in themselves, providing extensive health care for the people involved. Moreover, these experimental terrains are depicted in the language of "humanitarian crises", creating spaces of emergency where research easily transgresses what might be ethically justifiable.[24] The context of the SPf66 trial in Tanzania was different. On the one hand, the logistics of clinical trials and field trials are not readily comparable. On the other, the scientific product in question was developed in a laboratory in Colombia and was therefore seen as a successful example of "South-South collaboration", with Western assistance.[25] Petryna's argument is, however, compelling with regard to the different standards concerning risk-benefit ratios applied to medical research in Europe and Africa. The transfer of the vaccine from Latin America to rural Africa involved not merely the movement of a scientific object produced in Bogotá and formulated and bottled in Spain for injection into the right upper arm of 580 children aged 1 to 5 in rural Tanzania. It also involved the acceptance of certain risks associated with the administration of a substance tested on adults in countries of low malaria transmission to semi-immune children in an area of much higher disease prevalence.[26] While scientific objects and arrangements can be transferred from one place to another, health insurance schemes to

24   Adriana Petryna, *Globalizing Human Subjects Research*, in: Petryna, Andrew Lakoff and Arthur Kleinman (eds.), Global Pharmaceuticals. Ethics, Markets, Practices, Durham, London 2006, pp. 33–60, see especially p. 51; Adriana Petryna, *Clinical Trials Offshored. On Private Sector Science and Public Health*, in: BioSocieties, Vol. 2, 2007, pp. 21–40; Adriana Petryna, *When Experiments Travel. Clinical Trials and the Global Search for Human Subjects*, Princeton 2009.

25   ASTI, KIVAC, Correspondence Pedro Alonso, Marcel Tanner, Thomas Teuscher and Pedro Alonso, 3 September 1993.

26   Carlos Alonso noted: "The parameters of toxicity, safety and immunogenicity may vary from population to population due to the different genetic background of those populations and to the pressure of the disease. For that reason it is of the utmost importance to carefully determine those parameters before the main trial starts in order to avoid potential unwanted risks. Thus, it is recommended that the main trial should not be carried out until these parameters are clearly defined for the present situation." See: ASTI, KIVAC, Correspondence Pedro Alonso, Carlos Alonso, Chairman of the Committee, Centro de Biología Molecular, Ethical Evaluation of the Study Protocol on the "Trial of a Potential Synthetic Malaria Vaccine SPf66 in Tanzania", pp. 1–3, here: p. 1.

cover the adverse effects of a vaccine seem to be more bound to specific locations. In this regard, it is worth noting the response given by a Swiss legal firm when it was asked whether the villagers involved in the trial could be included in a comprehensive health insurance scheme:

> From a legal point of view, the insurance coverage of the vaccination test program has to be in conformity with the requirements in the country in which the program is executed. I assume that legislation and relevant guidelines in Tanzania reflect the absence of general health insurance in that country and do therefore not require health insurance in connection with a vaccination test program. Guidelines existing in Switzerland are designed to protect Swiss population along [sic] the standards of the Swiss social security and health care system and cannot be transferred to a developing country and applied to its inhabitants.[27]

In medical research, Africa thus evokes a double discourse and double standards. In the official discourse, the continent is an ideal site for testing new medications because diseases are widespread and the new products should reach those places where sufferers are living. At the same time, Africa constitutes a good testing ground because of the availability of more treatment-naïve subjects than in European countries and because the urgency of health interventions overshadows the lack of a legal framework that would protect individuals from adverse effects of the interventions in question. In stark contrast to the considerations about where research is to be carried out, how diseases are to be defined, and how trials are to be organized, are the collective anxieties and individual decisions concerning participation in this form of research at the local level.[28] It is to these aspects that we now turn.

Idete

Idete was established as a ujamaa village in 1974, as part of the socialist villagization program, and buoyed by its location on both the road and the TAZARA railway line to Zambia. Most of the village's older dwellers had

27 ASTI, KIVAC, Correspondence 1992/1993, Christian Brückner (Christ, Löw, Brückner, von Planta & Staehelin), Malaria Vaccination Program in Tanzania, 6 July 1992, pp. 1–2, here: p. 2.
28 James Fairhead, *Public Engagement with Science? Local Understandings of a Vaccine Trial in the Gambia*, in: Journal of Biosocial Science, Vol. 38, 2006, pp. 103–116.

been forcibly relocated and given a plot where they could grow maize and naturally irrigated rice. There were no health facilities in the 1970s, and a single bicycle was the only means of transportation in an emergency.[29] My own research conducted during 2010 revealed contradictory perceptions of malaria. The differences were due not just to varying individual statements but also to the different sources consulted. Not surprisingly, in an area of high malaria transmission, the record book kept at the village dispensary registered 600–800 cases of malaria each month in the early 1990s.[30] Almost 20 years later, many villagers reported that malaria was no longer much of a problem because of the widespread use of mosquito nets. Others, again, reported that the disease still takes a steady toll among the village community. There is no doubt, however, that Idete has been visited frequently over the years by researchers working for the Tanzanian government and for the IC (renamed the Ifakara Health Institute/IHI in 2008). The village was included as a research site in the KMP, and today fieldworkers from the IHI still meticulously record the health situation, patterns of migration, evidence of prosperity and destitution, and birth and death rates for all households and at regular intervals.[31] The IHI and Idete's dispensary staff were also the main disseminators of biomedical messages to villagers in Idete. They explained the connection between mosquitoes and malaria, advocated appropriate prevention measures and urged sufferers to seek medical advice as soon as the first symptoms appeared. In her study of community understanding of malaria, the anthropologist Susanna Hausmann Muela showed that the population living in and around Ifakara understood the biomedical message very well, but that this information coexisted and sometimes merged with pre-existing ideas about the disease – a phenomenon she termed "medical syncretism".[32]

Vaccines for the prevention of childhood diseases were a familiar biomedical tool, and the Expanded Program on Immunization (EPI) – launched

29   Interview with LR in Idete, 3 April 2010.
30   ASTI, KIVAC, Correspondence 1992/1993, Winnie Mpanju, Malcolm Molyneux, SPf66 (Candidate Malaria Vaccine) Trial Ifakara Centre, Tanzania. Report of Trial Monitors' visit 29.07–05.08.1992, pp. 1–12, here: p. 2.
31   Joanna Schellenberg et al., *Ifakara DSS, Tanzania*, in: International Development Research Centre (ed.), Population and Health in Developing Countries. Population, Health and Survival at INDEPTH Sites, Vol. 1, 2002, pp. 159–164.
32   Susanne Hausmann Muela, *Community Understanding of Malaria, and Treatment-Seeking Behavior in a Holoendemic Area of Southeastern Tanzania*, PhD Study University of Basel, Basel 2000.

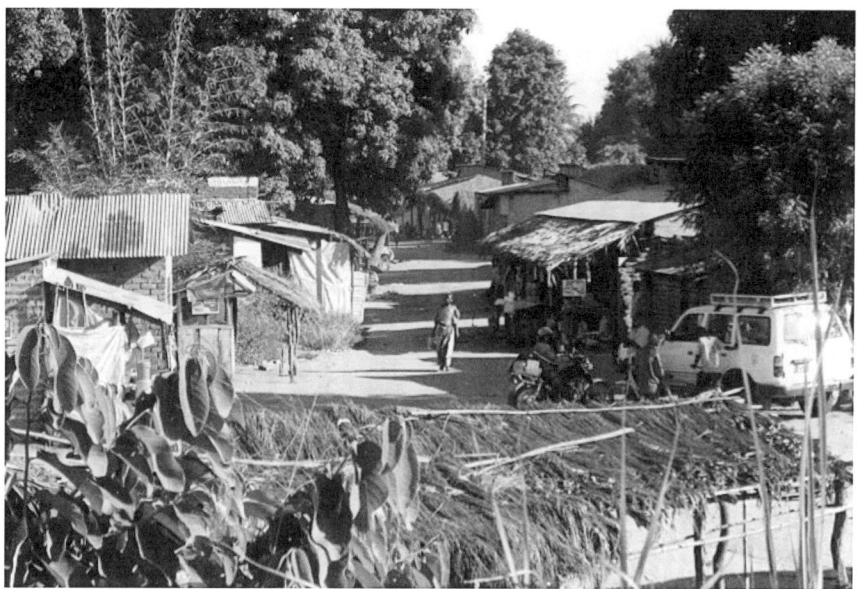

Idete, Kilombero District, picture: Lukas Meier, 2012

by the WHO and UNICEF in the mid-1970s to improve vaccine coverage among children – is still considered highly effective by the villagers. Nevertheless, the initial reaction to the announcement of the SPf66 trial included both relief and widespread unease.

Here, it is important to mention the methodological difficulties and constraints that I faced during my discussions with the trial population. Jensen Charles – the son of Charles Leutel, who was in charge of Idete's dispensary at the time of the SPf66 trial – still knew many of the parents who had allowed their children to be included in the vaccine trial and could easily arrange meetings with them. His close relationship with the participants could well explain a certain bias in their answers. More methodologically challenging, however, was the fact that our purposive sample included only those who had ultimately decided to participate in the trial and who were therefore assumed to have had a positive attitude towards the vaccination project. To counter methodological bias, I took an indirect approach, asking participants about the arguments of those who had refused to participate in the trial. I thus learned that the village had been very much divided on this issue: participants had been accused of rashly making their children available for a biomedical trial, the intention of which was to decimate the population – "quite similar to the family planning initiatives", as one of the interviewees remarked.[33] People had also been accused of agreeing to participate purely because of the material benefits involved, and it had been claimed that malaria was too severe a disease to be successfully controlled by a vaccine.[34] One mother recalled:

> First, we were very much afraid ... and why were we afraid? It was because people said that they take blood and the blood is for business, so they take a lot of blood from the bodies of the children, so they are going to die. Secondly, other mothers around us, they said, ah, why are you taking your children to the vaccination station, because of the soap? You don't have money to buy soap, so you bring your children because of the soap ... But I have taken the child to the hospital because there is malaria in the household. Because of Skola [her daughter], she was always suffering from malaria ... I said, ah, I don't try to hear these words around, so I will take my child – if she dies, OK, if she's not dying, OK. If I don't take my child to the vaccination station, she is going to die anyway. She is always suffering in the house. It is better to bring her to the hospital. If she dies, no problem. But around, some mothers insisted that I am going to take the child to the vaccination for the soap, and they asked: Why? Don't you have money to buy soap? Only 100 shillings for one piece of soap? But my child was still suffering from malaria, so I decided to take her – but there were some discussions around. [35]

The stories circulating within the village after the announcement of the vaccine trial stoked villagers' anxieties about having their children injected with an unknown substance.[36] The villagers' answers to the question of why they had participated in the trial fell into two broad categories. In the first of these, the severity of the disease was weighed against the risks of the vaccine – for example: "We did not know what the vaccine was about, but we are very aware what malaria is all about, and that is why we

---

33   Interview with JM, 3 April 2010.
34   Interview with AL, 17 April 2010.
35   Interview with GN, 22 March 2010; see also: Uli Beisel, René Gerrets, *The Public of Public Health. In Search of "Civil Society" within Contemporary Malaria Control in Africa* [unpublished draft] pp. 1–30, here: p. 16.
36   Melissa Leach, James Fairhead, *Vaccine Anxieties. Global Science, Child Health and Society*, London 2007; Wenzel Geissler, *"He is Now Like a Brother, I Can Even Give Him Some Blood" – Relational Ethics and Material Exchanges in a Malaria Vaccine "Trial Community" in the Gambia*, in: Social Science and Medicine, Vol. 67, 2006, pp. 696–707; James Fairhead, *Where Techno-Science Meets Poverty. Medical Research and the Economy of Blood in the Gambia*, in: Social Science and Medicine, Vol. 63, 2000, pp. 1109–1120.

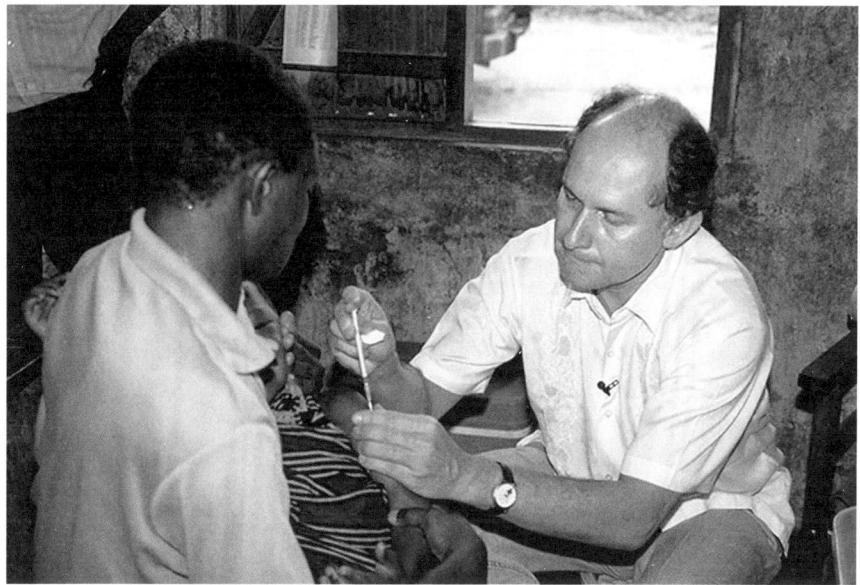

Manuel Elkin Patarroyo vaccinates a child against malaria, 1995, Archive STI

were happy to take our children to the vaccination station."[37] The second set of answers invoked social aspects and the vital role played by the village leadership in the villagers' decision-making: "The government would never be able to sacrifice their people."[38] Others again decided to participate because others were doing so, or were persuaded by villagers working at the dispensary.[39]

As it was not possible for villagers to assess the likely effects of SPf66 on the basis of their past experiences with vaccinations, their decisions on whether or not to participate in the trial were determined by perceptions of the threat of malaria, considerations about risks and potential benefits, and social and economic concerns. It is important to note that the uncertainties, concerns and mutual accusations arising at the local level were echoed among biomedical experts around the world: as we will see below, the scientific community was also deeply divided about the effects of SPf66.

37 Interview with MK, 22 March 2010.
38 Interview with AD, 3 April 2010.
39 Ibid.

The Interpretation of Truth

On October 29, 1994, the principal investigators and their collaborators published the data from the Idete trial in the *Lancet*. While they reported that the SPf66 vaccine "reduces the risk of malaria among children highly exposed to natural infection", the estimated efficacy of 31% (95% confidence interval 0–52%) warranted only cautious optimism.[40] The authors concluded: "The estimated efficacy of SPf66 is lower than that of most vaccines in use for other infections. However, since the burden of malaria morbidity and mortality is vast, measures with a moderate efficacy merit development."[41] But not everyone within the scientific community agreed that the efficacy figure justified consideration of the use of SPf66 as a public health measure. Worse still, critical voices were raised concerning the reliability of the data presented. After publication of the *Lancet* article, Pierre Druilhe of the Institut Pasteur in Paris complained: "We have no clear evidence about the efficacy or the inefficacy of SPf66." Echoing concerns expressed by Jean-François Trapé (ORSTOM) and Christophe Rogier (Institut Pasteur, Dakar), he claimed that "the ways … the data were collected on the spot were deficient" and that "the number of fever cases measured in nonvaccinated children was inexplicably low".[42]

For the purposes of my argument, several aspects of the ensuing scientific debate are of interest, as they indicate the instability of experimental terrains and the gap between scientific assumptions and local realities. In a draft reply to the criticisms from Dakar and Paris, the scientists involved in the Idete trial considered possible reasons why the number of episodes of clinical malaria was lower than would have been expected in an area of high malaria transmission.[43] It would appear that their idea of establishing standardized trial conditions, where all external factors could be brought under control, had been too optimistic. The first factor that could have explained the low number of cases reported was the free medical services provided at the dispensary during the trial – a finding of major public

---

40   Pedro Alonso et al., *Randomized Trial of Efficacy of SPf66 Vaccine Against* Plasmodium falciparum *Malaria in Children in Southern Tanzania*, in: The Lancet, Vol. 344, 1994, pp. 1175–1181, here: p. 1180.

41   Ibid., p. 1181.

42   ASTI, KIVAC, Correspondence 1995, Interrogations sur le vaccin colombien contre le paludisme. De l'envoyée spéciale de l'AFP, 14 April 1995, p. 1.

43   ASTI, KIVAC, Correspondence 1994, Draft Reply to Lancet Letters.

health relevance.[44] Secondly, the incidence was higher among children living closer to the dispensary, suggesting that reporting rates were lower for more remote parts of the village. Thirdly, the main data analysis depended on passive case detection (PCD), which meant that it included all cases of clinical malaria recorded at the dispensary. This approach was likely to exclude all cases of asymptomatic parasitemia. Fourthly, the frequency of clinical malaria was negatively correlated with age, meaning that the risk of clinical malaria decreased as trial subjects got older.[45] Thus, not only were the results dependent on an appropriate definition of malaria in a hyperendemic area, but the findings were influenced by the nature of the intervention itself (improved health service delivery, aging of the trial population). But if, as the scientists argued, the social fabric of the population is fundamentally changed by the performance of a trial, then the very notion of the medical trial is called into question.

Mechanisms of critical self-reflection are inherent in all scientific activities. The application of scientific results requires a certain level of approval and acceptance among the wider scientific community. The less one's results are accepted by outside experts, the more critical one tends to be of one's own products. The Idete scientists, at least, were preoccupied by the question whether or not the reactions to the *Lancet* study were justified. In a letter to a collaborator at the LSHTM headed "What are we trying to do?", an STI investigator reflected on how science progresses:

> I thought that I was trying to find out from the data as much as possible about what SPf66 is likely to be doing in these children. This involves making hypotheses, and testing them against the alternatives using not just the evidence from the trial but also what we already know from other sources. Since the primary effect (published in the Lancet) that we saw is so small, and subject to considerable uncertainty, nothing relating to clinical episodes can be expected to be free of reasonable doubt, and so we must hedge all conclusions with words like "likely", "suggest", "appear to indicate". You would not want to send anyone to prison on the strength of evidence as weak as this. However, this evidence is the best that we have. If someone comes along next week and shows that we are wrong, I would not be surprised. This is how science progresses.[46]

---

44   See also: Pedro Alonso et al., *Randomized Trial*, p. 1180.
45   Ibid.
46   ASTI, KIVAC, Correspondence, anonymized, What Are We Trying To Do?, pp. 1–6, here: p. 1.

The collaborator at the LSHTM, however, was less inclined to accept this Popperian view of science's progress and argued that SPf66 should not yet be abandoned: research should now focus on large-scale application and on the question of whether SPf66 would have any effect on severe disease and death.[47] In this, she shared the views of most public health experts pursuing effective means of protecting people from malaria. However, the future of SPf66 would depend on the outcomes achieved in other endemic settings. Two trials – in the Gambia and Thailand – sealed the fate of SPf66, ultimately making it just one more episode on the rocky road to a malaria vaccine.[48]

The Global Blow

The Gambian trial, conducted in collaboration with Patarroyo's group, included the vaccine produced in Colombia as well as the US formulation. But the results obtained with SPf66 were far from encouraging. In a letter to Patarroyo, Brian Greenwood wrote:

> I am afraid that we have some rather worrying data from the Gambian SPf66 trial … At the beginning of May, the MRC Trial Monitoring Committee, chaired by Malcolm Molyneux met to review the side effects and serological data that we had obtained after administration of the third dose of American or Colombian SPf66 to the children in our pilot trial. There were no major differences in the incidence of local or systemic side effects among children who had received SPf66 or IVP [polio vaccine]. However, the committee noted that more children in the malaria vaccine group had had a positive blood film with or without accompanying fever than had children given polio. The tendency was present with both the American and Colombian vaccines and was most prominent in the group that had received the high dose Colombian vaccine.[49]

The efficacy figure reported for the Gambian trial was a mere 3%, and the SPf66 and placebo groups did not differ significantly in parasite rates or in

---

47   ASTI, KIVAC, Documents IV, anonymized, 8 June 1995, pp. 1–3, here: p. 1.

48   Robert E. Desowitz, *The Malaria Capers. More Tales of Parasites and People, Research and Reality*, New York 1991.

49   ASTI, KIVAC Documents III, Brian Greenwood to Manuel Patarroyo, 26 May 1994, pp. 1–2, here: p. 1.

any other index of malaria.[50] However, Marcel Tanner believed that the results from this parallel study should not affect the decision to assess the efficacy of SPf66 in infants under one year of age: "Given the results from the Tanzanian trial for an area of high and perennial transmission, trials with immunization of infants and with severe malaria as endpoint represent a logical evolution." Pointing to major differences between the two trials in terms of the protocol and population, he argued that it would be premature to abandon SPf66 without having assessed its efficacy in infants living in the Kilombero valley.[51]

The argument based on differences in the local characteristics of study sites became more compelling after the publication of sobering news from Thailand. Here, the efficacy of SPf66 was assessed in a double-blind placebo-controlled trial involving Karen children at a military-controlled refugee camp. Principal investigator François Nosten (Mahidol University) and his co-workers concluded that "there is no evidence that SPf66 is effective against falciparum malaria" and that "there appears to be little justification for further trials with this vaccine".[52] As mentioned above, this trial had long been a thorn in the side of the Swiss-Spanish-British-Tanzanian team because it used a version of SPf66 manufactured in the US rather than in Colombia. While these results probably dealt the final blow to the vaccine, questions about the comparability of populations, sites and products remained. While Marcel Tanner and Pedro Alonso accepted the conclusions drawn by Nosten's group, they raised a number of questions:

> Firstly, we have no evidence as to the possible role that the genetic make-up of the population of parasites or volunteers may play in modulating efficacy. Secondly, there are a number of differences between the Thai trial and all other trials, including the type of placebo used, the very intense active daily case detection, and perhaps the specificity of the case definition used. Finally, and probably most important, the authors acknowledge that there is strong evidence that the US manufactured product is not identical to the Colombian manufactured SPf66. Not only are

50 ASTI, KIVAC, Correspondence 1995, The Lancet: Press Release. Malaria Vaccine not so Efficacious, 19 August 1995.
51 Ibid., Marcel Tanner to Howard Engers, Summary Document of Meeting to Discuss SPf66 Development 20th–21st March 1995, 17 April 1995, pp. 1–2.
52 François Nosten et al., *Randomized Double-Blind Placebo-Controlled Trial of SPf66 Malaria Vaccine in Children in Northwestern Thailand*, in: The Lancet, Vol. 348, No. 9029, 1996 pp. 701–707, here: p. 707; see also: Michael Day, *Malaria Vaccine Fails to Deliver*, in: New Scientist, 21 September 1996.

there differences in the proportion of monomer to polymer between the two products, but these differences have been shown to imply significant differences in immunogenicity both in mice and in humans, with the US manufactured version having been shown to be consistently less immunogenic than the Colombian SPf66.[53]

Besides the ethical question of why the persons in charge of the Thai trial had chosen a vaccine shown in previous studies to be less immunogenic than Colombian-manufactured SPf66, what the whole matter revealed was:

> once again the difficulty and importance of standardizing products for field trials ... as well as the need of standardizing protocols and procedures in order to allow for adequate comparison of results. The Thai trial has also highlighted the need to choose the trial sites and subsequently interpret the results in relation to the relevance to the different populations of the malaria endemic areas. In other words, how relevant are the results obtained in northern Thailand among refugees living in a camp under daily medical surveillance and the protection of the Thai army, to the malaria endemic populations of sub-Saharan Africa?[54]

Looking back, the history of malaria vaccine development has much to say about the difficulties encountered in translating medical research into sustained public health action. In the case of SPf66, two points should be mentioned in particular. Firstly, it suffered from a birth defect – rather than being "merely" a chemical substance, its life story was shaped by political and economic interests. The fact that SPf66 was produced in Colombia, and that the patent rights were not sold to the pharmaceutical industry but assigned to the WHO, was more than enough to provoke serious doubts about its efficacy and safety. Secondly, there is the difficulty of standardizing scientific products, trial sites and trial protocols. The SPf66 compound manufactured in the US laboratories was not identical to that produced in Colombia, and the differences between the results of the Gambian and Tanzanian trials were partly attributable to the different study protocols. However, quite apart from methodological differences, the attempt to establish laboratory conditions in African villages was impeded by "reality effects": the presence of Western experts in the village, the desires aroused by the objects (nets, sodas, soaps, etc.) they introduced, the renovation of the dispensary and provision of essential drugs, the aging of the trial population – all

---

53   ASTI, KIVAC Documents IV, Pedro Alonso, Marcel Tanner to J. Rodes (The Lancet), 15 October 1996, pp. 1–2, here: p. 1.
54   Ibid., p. 2.

these elements were not only beyond the scientists' control but influenced the results of the study. In contrast, IPTi – the subject of our second case study – did not involve attempts to turn African villages into laboratories. Here, the health system as a whole became the laboratory, but without the active intervention of scientists. Nevertheless, the problems of scaling up health interventions were similar, as discussed in the next section.

Intermittent Preventive Treatment of Malaria in Infants – History in the Making

At the beginning of the new millennium, the development mindset started to rule out other legitimate approaches to the remodeling of African societies. Now a mainstream concept, development cuts across different academic fields and policymaking areas. Today, it is scarcely possible to speak of agriculture, health, infrastructure, education or economics in sub-Saharan Africa without referring to development. The fact that development is ubiquitous does not, however, mean that development practices have not changed considerably over time. Development in 2010 is no longer necessarily a bilateral arrangement between industrialized and "underdeveloped" nations, but a matter for multilateral consortia and philanthropic institutions. Development in the new millennium is also an occasion for grand gestures. In 2003, multibillionaire Bill Gates announced that the Bill & Melinda Gates Foundation (BMGF) would donate USD 168 million to help alleviate the appalling health situation in sub-Saharan Africa. The BMGF funds were designed to address one of Africa's most tenacious scourges – malaria. Initially, the Foundation selected three areas of intervention: (a) using existing malaria drugs to prevent infants from becoming infected, (b) developing new drugs to combat drug-resistant malaria and (c) finding a malaria vaccine.[55] With the emergence of highly resistant malaria parasites in Africa and a renewed belief among Western scientists in the potential of an integrated approach to malaria control, the issue once again commanded the attention of the international donor community.

The new movement – attracting scientists, policymakers and philanthropists – saw a change in malaria research compared to previous de-

---

55   Bill Gates, *The World Must Do More to Conquer Malaria*, in: Financial Times, 22 September 2003.

cades. The emphasis was now to be placed on partnership between the various actors, and the governance structure for the new research practices comprised global charities, international organizations, pharmaceutical companies and scientific communities, as well as national governments.

The first part of the second case study is concerned with IPTi trials in West and East Africa – in particular, the organization and structure of the IPTi Consortium, the main coordinating body for IPTi research efforts on the continent. The second part examines the implementation of a specific IPTi trial in Tanzania, and the associated policy discussions. As in our review of the history of SPf66, local, national and global arenas will be considered in an attempt to elucidate the many factors that can inhibit the translation of research into health policy action.

Organization of Science

In a study of intermittent sulfadoxine-pyrimethamine (SP) treatment conducted in Ifakara between 1999 and 2001, the protective efficacy of IPTi against clinical malaria was 59%.[56] Like insecticide-treated nets, IPTi was hailed as an effective new tool in the fight against the disease. At the beginning of the new millennium, scientific meetings were held at short intervals to set up a comprehensive research program investigating the efficacy and safety of the intervention in various epidemiological settings across Africa. To support these efforts, the BMGF awarded USD 28 million to the multinational consortium established to coordinate trials in East and West Africa.[57] The Consortium's collaborative funding proposal covered a series of trials, all of which – with the exception of the Kenyan trial – were to use SP produced by the Basel-based company Hoffmann-La Roche.[58]

---

56 David Schellenberg et al., *Intermittent Treatment for Malaria and Anaemia Control at Time of Routine Vaccinations in Tanzanian Infants. A Randomized, Placebo-Controlled Trial*, in: The Lancet, Vol. 357, 2001, pp. 1471–1477.
57 Documents Marcel Tanner (DMT), IPTi, Bill and Melinda Gates Foundation (BMGF), New Grants to Accelerate Malaria Research and Development, pp. 1–2, here: p. 1.
58 Ibid., David Schellenberg, Jane Crawley, Intermittent Preventive Treatment with Antimalarial Drugs Delivered Through the Expanded Programme of Immunisation. A New Potential Public Health Strategy to Reduce the Burden of Malaria in Young African Children. A Proposal to the Bill and Melinda Gates Foundation from the IPTi Consortium, 18 April 2003.

In the previous section on SPf66, we saw the perils of competition between different research groups. In contrast, the IPTi trials were designed to proceed in an atmosphere of mutual trust and open communication. Responsibility for governance rested with the IPTi Consortium – a highly complex structure. From the bottom up, it comprised individual projects under the responsibility of collaborative research groups, to whom funds were directly channeled. Each project had a Data Safety Management Board (DSMB), responsible for reporting adverse effects occurring during trials and represented on the Consortium Safety Panel (CSP). The Investigators Committee provided a forum where the key investigators could discuss scientific issues emerging from the various trial sites. The Core Administration, based in Barcelona, ensured coordination and the smooth exchange of information between the different groups. The Consortium Executive Committee – with Brian Greenwood and Marcel Tanner as standing members and an otherwise rotating membership – was to oversee the whole consortium and provide guidance to the coordinators in Barcelona.[59] Finally, a WHO-based Policy and Programme Implementation Platform would liaise between the Consortium and the WHO/UNICEF, facilitate the translation of scientific evidence into policy recommendations, and "create in malaria endemic countries in Africa an environment that is conducive to the adoption of IPTi as national policy".[60] One of the Consortium's IPTi trials was held in southern Tanzania, in an area which would soon be referred to as the "forgotten southern zone".[61]

The Forgotten Southern Zone: Implementation Research in Mtwara and Lindi Regions 2004–2009

On April 22, 2004, at a workshop in Mtwara on Integrated Management of Childhood Illness, members of the Ifakara Health Research and Development Center (IHRDC) presented their IPTi research plans to key medical

---

59 DMT, IPTi, Meeting Minutes, 18–20 January 2004, pp. 1–10, here: p. 6.
60 Ibid., Jane Crawley, Planning for Success. A WHO-UNICEF Policy and Programme Implementation Platform of Intermittent Preventive Treatment in Infants. A Proposal to the Bill and Melinda Gates Foundation, 10 January 2004, pp. 1–9, here: p. 3.
61 Archiv Ifakara Health Institute Mtwara Branch (AIHI-MB), IPTi Project Reports, Dr. Budeba (RMO Mtwara) cited in: Introducing IPTi in the Southern Zone, Saturday, 24th April 2004, pp. 1–7, here: p. 5.

personnel from the southern districts. Highlighting the depressing statistics on malaria infection and childhood mortality, they explained the suitability of this area (given the lack of research undertaken to date) and the potential benefits of the project – also in terms of "employment opportunities in the southern regions".[62] The next day, the IHRDC team explored the country-side, visiting the Mahurunga Health Center and the Madimba dispensary of Mtwara Rural District, and enjoying breathtaking views of the tree-covered hillside of northern Mozambique just a few miles away. They were troubled to learn, however, that the NIMR was running a malaria trial in this area, and not in Mtwara Urban District, as previously assumed: "The team spent many hours on Friday evening poring over maps and discussing various pros and cons of alternative districts to Mtwara Rural."[63] They finally selected five districts in Lindi and Mtwara Regions (Lindi Rural, Nachingwea, Ruangwa, Newala and Tandahimba) for their intervention, ruling out Mtwara Rural District so as to avoid interference with the NIMR's plans. While regretting this decision, the Mtwara Regional Medical Officer (RMO) nevertheless welcomed the arrival of the experienced researchers, as it offered an opportunity for scientific and economic progress.

During these busy days spent gathering around maps and demarcating intervention and control areas, the RMOs and District Medical Officers (DMOs) learned, no doubt, that the IPTi study was based on an effectiveness protocol. In contrast to the controlled laboratory conditions of the SPf66 trial in Idete, the aim here was to see how an intervention worked under real-life conditions within the existing health system and without undue interference by the research team.[64] Among the research priorities

---

62 Ibid., p. 3.
63 Ibid., p. 1.
64 There was, however, one striking similarity to the Idete trial – several of the well-established research collaborators appeared on the funding application for the IPTi trial in southern Tanzania: the Hospital Clinic in Barcelona, the IHRDC, the LSHTM, the STI and the NMCP. See: Ibid., Official Documents (IPTi in Southern Tanzania), David Schellenberg, Community Effectiveness of Intermittent Preventive Treatment Delivered through the Expanded Program of Immunisation for Malaria and Anaemia Control in Tanzanian Infants. A Collaborative Funding Proposal, 19 April 2003, pp. 1–59. The Principal Investigator was David Schellenberg (LSHTM); the Co-Principal Investigators were, in Tanzania, Hassan Mshinda (IHRDC) and Joanna Armstrong Schellenberg (IHRDC/LSHTM) and, in Europe, Pedro Alsono (Hospital Clinic, Barcelona) and Marcel Tanner (STI); the co-investigators were Salim Abdulla (NMCP), Guy Hutton (STI), Clara Menendez (Hospital Clinic, Barcelona), Robert Pool (LSHTM) and Cally Roper (LSHTM). Almost CHF 7 million was awarded to the STI (the grant holder). All project expenditures in Tanzania were "posted at the headquarters of

were the development of a strategy for delivery of IPTi to rural communities, assessment of the safety profile of SP, and generation of information about acceptability, cost-effectiveness and drug resistance, as well as the impact of the intervention on mortality and morbidity.[65]

IPTi came to Mtwara and Lindi Regions in waves: in the first year, intense efforts were made to assess the shortcomings of the health system at the facility level, visits were paid to the Council Health Medical Teams (CHMTs) in all selected districts and stakeholders at all levels were informed about the project. At two stakeholder meetings, representatives of the Tanzanian health system and international organizations had an opportunity to discuss pressing issues, thus paving the way for the smooth translation of research into sustained public health action.[66] Since the term "IPTi" was not particularly catchy, the preintervention phase also involved efforts to find an appropriate "brand name" for the project. Various names and logos were field-tested, and the Swahili term "mkinge" (protect) emerged as the most suitable. In the second phase, staff at the regional, district and facility levels were trained to administer and meticulously record individual SP doses (a space for the three mkinge doses was included on an amended standard clinic card). Also preceding the implementation process were extensive household surveys, studies of health-seeking behavior and assessments of child health in the area.

The Expanded Program of Immunization and the Health Sector Reform of 1993

One of the main objectives of the project was to couple IPTi with the Expanded Program of Immunization (EPI). The three antimalarial doses were to be administered together with childhood vaccines and thus form part of the population's routine contacts with the health system. UNICEF introduced EPI to Tanzania in the early 1970s, and the childhood vaccination rate

---

IHRDC in Dar es Salaam, consolidated, locally audited and forwarded to STI"; see: ASTI, IPTi, U. Wasser, RE: Fragekatalog zum Tanzania Projekt, pp. 1–8, here: p. 5.

65 AIHI-MB, Schellenberg, Community Effectiveness, p. 12.

66 AIHI-MB, IPTi Project Report, David Schellenberg, Community Effectiveness, p. 14; for a description of the implementation stages, see also: Fatuma Manzi et al., *Intermittent Preventive Treatment for Malaria and Anaemia Control in Tanzanian Infants. The Development and Implementation of a Public Health Strategy*, in: Transactions of the Royal Society of Tropical Medicine and Hygiene, Vol. 103, No. 1, 2009, pp. 79–86.

was reported to have risen from 15% to almost 80% in the 1990s.[67] EPI was organized vertically and partly funded by foreign donors. The Ministry of Health (MOH) was responsible for planning, procurement, storage and delivery of EPI to the regions. Under the health sector reforms which followed the publication of the 1993 World Development Report (WDR93), Tanzania began to shift managerial and financial responsibility from the national to the district level. Former vertical programs such as EPI were not excluded from these efforts and were more closely integrated into a decentralized health system. Integration of EPI services started in 1996 and involved the transfer of responsibility for procurement, storage and distribution to the semi-autonomous Medical Stores Department (MDS), placed under the direction of the MOH. At the district level, decentralization included the establishment of District Councils as the main political entity responsible for health care delivery. While responsibility for EPI prior to the reform had rested with the DMOs, District Cold Chain Officers and District Executive Directors, EPI functions were now transferred to the CHMTs and District Councils. In fact, the latter were the major beneficiaries of the reform, taking on key functions in the running of EPI, such as planning, resource allocation and human resources.[68] The increased concentration of power in the hands of the District Councils worked to the detriment of the CHMTs, whose activities were restricted to unpopular tasks such as supervision tours or management of EPI delivery. As a consequence, morale declined considerably, and this in turn had an effect on national EPI coverage, which fell from a prereform level of 80% to a mere 50% in the postreform era.[69]

Whether the implementation of the IPTi project was also affected by the health sector reform remains an open question, given that District Council and CHMT personnel often overlapped.[70] However, concerns about the performance of the CHMTs were frequently expressed by the research team. One research team member recalled that CHMTs failed to supervise facilities regularly because of "competing activities" in the district or – more mundanely – a lack of appropriate transport. Consequently, dispensaries were often without either vaccines or drugs. On the rare occasions when CHMT members actually toured the area for EPI supervisions,

---

67   Innocent Semali, *Understanding Stakeholders' Roles in Health Sector Reform Process in Tanzania. The Case of Decentralizing the Immunization Program*, PhD University of Basel, Basel 2003, pp. 100–101.

68   Ibid., p. 128.

69   Ibid., p. 133.

70   Yuna Hamisi, personal communication, 28 February 2011.

they were sometimes well-supplied with vaccines but did not deliver SP tablets for mkinge, or they forgot to ask staff about mkinge interventions altogether.[71] At the dispensary level, the impact of mkinge was stronger, depending on personal interactions between patients and nurses.

Site of Negotiation: The Microlevel

The main implementer of the project was Yuna Hamisi (known to the nurses as "Dr. Yuna"), who toured the districts in order to check that the drugs were being correctly administered and the doses recorded. These issues needed careful attention because the administration of mkinge was demanding: during their training sessions, the nurses learned that SP tablets had to be halved or quartered, placed on a spoon and allowed to disintegrate in water before being administered to children. This procedure required the provision of safe water and a degree of cleanliness. Furthermore, each consultation had to be recorded in the mkinge section of the clinic cards and documented in the health management information system, and the drugs had to be ordered from the district drug stores in good time. One of the nurses admitted that mkinge added considerably to her already substantial workload, and mothers sometimes complained about overlong waiting periods in (seriously understaffed) dispensaries.[72] As the procedure became more routine, however, these problems disappeared. The nurses had a powerful role in the mkinge project. In fact, mkinge had its greatest impact at the microlevel of daily interactions and unequal power relations between dispensary personnel and patients' mothers. The nurses were crucial in educating mothers about the intervention. This was especially important given the fears and rumors about possible adverse effects of SP, and the fact that the Tanzanian government replaced SP with artemether-lumefantrine (produced by Novartis) as a first-line treatment in 2006. On the first day of the project at Mingoyo dispensary:

> [The nurse] then led a 10–15 minute health education session, sitting between two groups of around 10 mothers with their young children. She first asked whether any of the children were sick and needed to see the doctor quickly. She then reminded the mothers of IPT in pregnancy, and asked what drug they had taken. One said "Fansidar" but the answer she was looking for was "SP", which was volun-

71   Interview with Yuna Hamisi in Dar es Salaam, 28 February 2011.
72   Interview with dispensary staff in Mingoyo, 18 February 2011.

teered by another mother. She introduced Mkinge as being "sawa na dawa ya ndani – chanjo", i.e. similar to vaccines and explained that it is given after "sindano za begani" (i.e. BCG, at birth), "na sindano za pajani ya kwanza" (i.e. DPT-HB1), at the time of giving "sindano za pajani" at 2m and 3m (i.e. DPT-HB2 and 3) and "sindano za surua" (i.e. measles vaccine) at 9m. She mentioned that the dose was a quarter or half tablet, and that this was "dozi ndogo tu" (very small). She reassured them that there was nothing to be worried about, and that the drug would be given as directly-observed treatment at the clinic. One or two mothers replied that they had been listening and that they understood. [The nurse] went on to say that Mkinge had been used already in Ifakara and they now had "hamna kabisa malaria" (i.e. no malaria). She explained that the first children to get Mkinge in Lindi and Mtwara would be here, today, at this clinic, and pointed out the two posters, saying how they were real people and not hand-drawn pictures and the children looked very healthy.[73]

The equation of vaccines and medication not only featured in such educational efforts but was practiced on the ground. Since the two interventions were coupled, there was no vaccine without mkinge and vice versa. Whether nurses actually refused general treatment until the child had received its mkinge doses – as one mother claimed – remains unclear.[74] The power of dispensary staff to ensure the administration of all three doses was also reflected in a nurse's statement that they occasionally toured villages to detect negligent mothers.[75]

In general, interviews conducted with mothers revealed that mkinge was an acceptable intervention.[76] The acceptability of EPI vaccinations was high, and mkinge was regarded as an additional benefit.[77] In addition,

73   AIHI-MB, Mkinge, Mkinge, Start of Piloting of IPTi in Lindi and Mtwara Regions, 14th-17th Feb. 2005, Note for the Record, Preparations for Training of Facility Staff, p. 4.
74   Interview in Mingoyo, 18 February 2011. This perception was also reported in Robert Pool et al., *The Acceptability of Intermittent Preventive Treatment of Malaria in Infants (IPTi) Delivered Through the Expanded Programme of Immunization in Southern Tanzania*, in: Malaria Journal, Vol. 7, No. 213, 2008, pp. 1–11, here: p. 10.
75   Interview with staff in Mingoyo, 18 February 2011.
76   Interviews in Mingoyo, Mnolela and Nyengedi, 18, 21 and 22 February 2011.
77   Robert Pool et al., *The Acceptability of Intermittent Preventive Treatment of Malaria in Infants (IPTi) Delivered Through the Expanded Programme of Immunization in Southern Tanzania*, in: Malaria Journal, Vol. 7, No. 213, 2007, pp. 1-11, here: p. 10; for an in-depth analysis of the acceptability of IPTi, see: Adiel Mushi, *Reaching the Poorest Children in Rural Southern Tanzania. Socio-Cultural Perspectives for Delivery and Uptake of Preventive Child Health Interventions*, PhD Study London School of Hygiene & Tropical Medicine, London 2009; for opposing views concerning perceptions of SP, see: Vinay Kamat, *Cultural Interpretations of the Efficacy and Side-Effects of Antimalarials in Tanzania*, in: Anthropology of Medicine, Vol. 16, No. 3, 2009, pp. 293–305.

many mothers had received SP doses during pregnancy (IPTp), and it seemed to be a small step from IPTp to IPTi. Positive attitudes to this new intervention were maintained even when children again sickened with malaria during or after the mkinge interventions; in this case, the mothers reported that malaria returned in milder forms.[78]

The population's perceptions of this intervention in Mtwara and Lindi contrasted sharply with the vaccine trial in Idete. What made IPTi readily acceptable to the local population was that the project presented itself, not so much as research, but as an addition to daily routine. Thus, IPTi did not create divisions between villagers who abstained and others offering their offspring for a small reward. Science in this instance did not create laboratory conditions in a futile effort to keep every factor under control but remained in the background, observing how an existing health system performs when a new element is added. The researchers concluded that IPTi-SP was safe and highly cost-effective, with "a reduction in the prevalence of *P. falciparum* infection and of anemia, suggesting that existing levels of drug resistance were not preventing a beneficial effect of IPTi".[79]

Moreover, IPTi could be managed by weak health systems, with coverage levels being achieved similar to those of EPI vaccines.[80] The trial was designed so that the efforts of district health personnel would continue even after the withdrawal of the research team. So it was difficult for the nurse at Mingoyo dispensary to say how mkinge as currently practiced had changed. The main change for her was that activities were no longer monitored by "Dr. Yuna", and compliance had declined as a result.[81]

The effectiveness trial in Southern Tanzania contributed one small piece of evidence to the overall picture of the Consortium's trials. Towards the end of the first decade of the new millennium, the results of the various IPTi studies were published in the scientific journals. They revealed a heterogeneous picture as regards the pressing questions of safety, efficacy, resistance and a possible rebound effect. While this had been expected by the scientific community, the variety of answers to what was considered to be one problem gave policymakers nothing that could be readily translated into health policy.

---

78 Interviews with mothers in Mingoyo, Mnolela and Nyengedi.
79 Joanna Schellenberg et al., *Community Effectiveness of Intermittent Preventive Treatment of Infants (IPTi) in Rural Southern Tanzania*, in: American Journal of Tropical Medicine and Hygiene, Vol. 82, No. 5, 2010, pp. 772–781, here: p. 780.
80 Ibid., p. 779.
81 Interview in Mingoyo, 18 February 2011.

Stumbling Block of Governance: The Global Level

The Consortium scientists were aware that different IPTi trials conducted in different settings and with different endpoints were likely to generate different results as far as efficacy and safety were concerned:

> It is likely that the ongoing and planned research studies will demonstrate considerable variation in the efficacy of IPTi in different settings, and that some unexpected safety concerns may arise. The purpose of a WHO policy recommendation will, therefore, be to provide malaria-endemic countries with a comprehensive and balanced appraisal of the benefits and limitations of IPTi in a range of epidemiological settings.[82]

It was precisely the "considerable variation in efficacy" and "unexpected safety concerns" associated with SP that hampered the smooth translation of science into policy. After reviewing the essential information on the trials conducted by the IPTi Consortium, the WHO was reluctant to offer a clear policy recommendation for IPTi. Doubtless, history played a part here: all too often in the course of efforts to eradicate or contain malaria in Africa, the WHO had overhastily endorsed ineffective strategies (the most notorious example being DDT). With regard to the novel strategy of IPTi, the WHO identified various risks relating to SP and expressed concerns about the efficacy of IPTi. SP was associated with a risk of severe skin reactions, including Stevens-Johnson syndrome.[83] Furthermore, efficacy against clinical malaria varied widely in the trials under consideration. To reiterate, while the Ifakara trial showed a protective efficacy of 59%, the figures for other trial sites ranged between 20% and 33%, yielding overall efficacy of 30%.[84] Perhaps even more pressing was the question whether the effects are sustainable in the long term or whether a rebound effect occurs.[85] Three of the trials showed an increased incidence of anemia during

---

82 DMT, IPTi, Jane Crawley, Planning for Success, pp. 3–4.
83 Ibid., WHO's Position on the IPTi Strategy. Implications for Policy, June 2007, pp. 1–8, here: p. 3.
84 Ibid., The Facts, November 2007, pp. 1–3, here: p. 1.
85 "A rebound is normally said to have occurred when the incidence of clinical malaria in intervention-recipients is significantly higher than the contemporaneous incidence in the control arm"; see: DMT, IPTi, David Schellenberg, Response to Gates Foundation, 30 September 2009, pp. 1–4, here: p. 3.

the 8 months after the last dose of IPTi-SP.[86] As we have seen, several mothers interviewed at the dispensaries of Mingoyo, Mnolela and Nyengedi confirmed that their children were still suffering from malaria but suggested that the attacks were less severe than in the past. The pooled analysis of all the trials, however, showed that "there were no significant rebound episodes of clinical malaria, anemia or hospital admissions … [during] the 5 month period after the IPTi schedule was finished".[87] But the WHO remained unconvinced. In 2007, despite all the Consortium's efforts to bridge any gaps between science and policy, the WHO's Technical Expert Group (TEG) concluded:

> There remain significant safety concerns, particularly regarding the risk of severe skin reactions. Taking into account these safety concerns when IPTi would be administered to otherwise healthy children, the duration of protection against malaria, the uncertainty over the magnitude of the protective effect against anaemia and severe malaria, the uncertainty concerning the efficacy against highly SP resistant parasites and the optimal dose and timing of administration, the committee cannot recommend general deployment of SP-IPTi.[88]

The WHO's position met with incomprehension among the scientists. The whole research process was geared towards rapid propagation of IPTi as an effective new tool against malaria, and it was clear that national malaria control programs in Africa would never adopt the strategy without WHO policy support. The Consortium, and especially the BMGF, needed visible results because the logic of humanitarianism required high-profile interventions rather than abstract science. In the eyes of the scientists, the WHO's reaction demonstrated that "international health policy making is not necessarily an evidence-based process".[89] The rejection of a public health strategy which – according to the scientists – was effective, safe, cheap and relatively easy to deliver through the existing EPI system could

---

86 This was the case for the Navrongo, the Kumasi and the Tamale trial; see: DMT, IPTi, The Facts, p. 2.

87 Ibid.

88 WHO, Report of the Technical Expert Group (TEG) Meeting on Intermittent Preventive Therapy in Infancy (IPTi), Geneva, 8–10 October 2007, pp. 1–12, here: p. 7, www.who.int/malaria/publications/atoz/tegconsultiptioct2007report.pdf (accessed 7 March 2011).

89 DMT, IPTi, David Schellenberg, Marcel Tanner, Annual Progress Report. Community Effectiveness of Intermittent Preventive Treatment delivered through the Expanded Programme of Immunisation for Malaria and Anaemia Control in Tanzanian Infants, 01/2006 – 12/2006, pp. 1–22, here: p. 13.

barely pass uncontested. The response submitted to the WHO Global Malaria Program (GMP) was therefore blunt: the WHO had not only misinterpreted the scientific facts but also failed in its role of providing ministries of health in Africa with guidance on setting sound national health policies.[90] The response stated:

> In the past, WHO has been criticized, unfairly perhaps, for making policy decisions without a sound science base – often in difficult circumstances where no substantial data were available. With IPTi, WHO has been presented with an unprecedented science base for considering this tool for policy adoption. It remains unclear why the policy process at WHO around IPTi appears to have been abandoned, ignoring a substantial and well documented body of data.[91]

Two years later, in the light of new scientific evidence assembled on IPTi, the TEG reconsidered its position. The new evidence leading to a change of heart included (a) an analysis, conducted by the Consortium, of the severe skin reactions associated with SP-IPTi reported previously; (b) two additional randomized placebo-controlled trials on the safety and efficacy of IPTi; and (c) the experience of implementation studies conducted by UNICEF and another by the Consortium.[92] The TEG concluded that the skin reactions reported in two earlier trials were not to be classified as severe adverse reactions; that there was no evidence of an adverse effect of SP-IPTi on infants' serological response to EPI vaccines; and that a rebound effect was not evident in the pooled analysis. In 2010, the WHO therefore recommended the use of IPTi for *P. falciparum* malaria control in sub-Saharan Africa in areas "with moderate-to-high malaria transmission … and where parasite resistance to SP is not high".[93]

90   Ibid., The Policy Review Process at the World Health Organization's Global Malaria Program – has it gone off the tracks?, p. 1.
91   Ibid., Response to WHO-GMP Statement on IPTi policy process, 28 June 2007, pp. 1–2, here: p. 2.
92   WHO, Report of the Technical Consultation on Intermittent Preventive Treatment in Infants (IPTi),Technical Expert Group on Preventive Chemotherapy, 23rd–24th April 2009, WHO/HQ, Geneva, Switzerland, Room D46025, 2009, pp. 1–11, here: p. 2, www.who.int/malaria/publications/atoz/tegconsultiptiapr2009report.pdf   (accessed 7 March 2011).
93   WHO, Policy Recommendation on Intermittent Preventive Treatment during infancy with sulphadoxine-pyrimethamine (SP-IPTi) for *Plasmodium falciparum* malaria control in Africa, 2010, pp. 1–3, here: p. 2, www.who.int/malaria/news/WHO_policy_recommendation_IPTi_032010.pdf (accessed 7 March 2011).

The new millennium's global partnership in malaria research is not immune to vested interests and is apt to delay health policymaking. One of the consequences of the sheer amount of money distributed by the new global charities is that malaria research is now driven not just by the need for quick scientific results but by the urgency of translating science into policy. African policymakers are included in the scientific process, informed about research projects in their respective countries and invited to share their views at stakeholder meetings. But what is their role in the policy process itself? In the eyes of members of the Tanzanian National Malaria Control Program (NMCP), how do science and research contribute to the design and implementation of sound malaria control strategies deployed on a national scale?

Off the Desks: The National Level

Together with the NIMR, the IHI has privileged access to the highest levels of health policymaking in Tanzania. This is mainly due to the IHI's international contacts – especially with the STI – and the close network of personal relationships established over the years. For example, Hadji Mponda, the current Health Minister, worked on the KINET project (promotion of insecticide-treated nets via social marketing) in Kilombero and Ulanga Districts between 1996 and 2000, and Hassan Mshinda, the Director General of the Tanzanian Commission for Science and Technology (COSTECH), also studied under Marcel Tanner and succeeded Andrew Kitua as Director of the IC. There are, of course, both positive and problematic aspects to the close connections existing between the STI and scientists at the highest levels of the Tanzanian health system. On the one hand, these Tanzanian scientists embody the success of the STI's investments in manpower and training schemes over the years, enabling African scientists to write a PhD in London or Basel and to pursue their academic careers. On the other hand, there is a risk that these elements of partnership – following an interpersonal rather than an "official" logic – may be short-lived.

The NMCP has a very positive attitude towards participatory approaches. According to one of its members, the novel feature of the Roll Back Malaria initiative is that "we are now working as partners" to fight the deadly disease.[94] Asked whether the Tanzanian government is not in

94   Interview at the NMCP in Dar es Salaam, 8 February 2011.

danger of being submerged by the masses of foreign money, international donors, advocates and advisers, a respondent at the NMCP replies, with practiced ease: "The Tanzanian government is contributing a lot to these efforts." The government pays the salaries of NMCP staff and provides fuel and electricity for daily operations.[95]

IPTi-SP has not yet found its way into the minds of NMCP staff. This is due not so much to the WHO's reluctance to recommend IPTi as a national policy in African countries, but to the ambivalent governance structure described above. At the time of the IHRDC trial in Southern Tanzania, another Consortium-sponsored IPTi trial was conducted by the NIMR (Tanga Center). Comparing different regimens for IPTi, the NIMR team could not find any protective effect of SP against clinical malaria in infants.[96] For the NMCP, which draws up policies for the whole country, different findings from different epidemiological settings pose challenges:

> Yes, they also have IPTi results, but these results are not the same … They are giving us different information, so as a policymaker, what would you do? It is the task of them to settle, to go back and harmonize, and to see how best they can inform the government. Who has done the right job? What went wrong during the fieldwork? What is it that is different in the other part of the country? From Mtwara or from wherever? So we need to be guided. You cannot receive different information.[97]

Health policies are necessarily general, glossing over different local situations. In other words, science has to be detached from local characteristics before being translated into health policies. Bruno Latour famously described the creation of scientific "facts" as a process of "stabilization". According to him, scientific objects are affected by different statements and conversational exchanges: "more and more reality is attributed to the object and less and less to the statement *about* the object. Consequently, an inversion take [sic] place: the object becomes the reason why the statement was formulated in the first place."[98] By analogy, one can say that the process of stabilization has not yet divorced IPTi from the different statements

---

95   Ibid.
96   R. D. Gosling et al., *Protective Efficacy and Safety of Three Antimalarial Regimens for Intermittent Preventive Treatment for Malaria in Infants. A Randomised, Double-Blind, Placebo-Controlled Trial*, in: Lancet, Vol. 374, 2009, pp. 1521–1532.
97   Interview at the NMCP in Dar es Salaam, 8 February 2011.
98   Bruno Latour, Steve Woolgar, *Laboratory Life. The Construction of Scientific Facts*, Princeton 1986, p. 177.

it is exposed to. It has not yet become a scientific fact, living a life outside interpretation. The NMCP policymakers still attributed the different results about IPTi to a "mistake" in the system of scientific production. The scientists have to go back to find out what "went wrong" during fieldwork and to haggle over "who has done the right job" in order to be of any use to the NMCP. According to another long-serving member of the NMCP:

> We cannot say, "Now let us go to the southern zone, we do this, and in the northern zone, we do that!" No, we take it that once it [an intervention] is effective, it will also be effective in every zone, you see? So, since the researchers know how to go about doing research which will be representative of the country, we normally don't want to question the credibility of the research and the methodology and the like. We say, "We have this problem, can you please do this for us?" They come up with the budget, we give them the money, and they do it. And fortunately, we never had experienced problems that the research on this thing did not materialize in the southern part but did work in the northern [part], we never experienced that kind of problem, you get it? And if you see the interventions, malaria control is not defined that this is for the southern and this is for the northern – it will cut across all the regions, all the zones, all the areas in the same package, you see?[99]

The exclusion of IPTi from the desks and minds of NMCP staff is attributable not only to contradictory scientific information but also to increasing parasite resistance to SP. This phenomenon has attracted considerable attention, and even when the drug was introduced as a first-line treatment of malaria, it was clear that it would not last for ever.[100] The replacement of SP as a first-line treatment did not, however, affect its use in intermittent preventive treatment during pregnancy (IPTp), which has already been adopted as a national policy. But the NMCP was reluctant to see IPTp as a precedent for IPTi:

> We don't know even if it [SP] is working well, even for IPTp. Probably it does, but we are not monitoring because we don't have that capacity. We don't have a lot of information on IPTp, and on SP for IPTp. How do we monitor this drug because we cannot do it at national level. It has to be done with the research institutions … Well, SP worked, it works for parasitemia in pregnancy but then does it still work even today, we don't know. That is the challenge I think.[101]

99 Interview at the NMCP in Dar es Salaam, 10 February 2011.
100 Joanna Schellenberg, personal communication.
101 Interview at the NMCP in Dar es Salaam, 8 February 2011.

The same institution that introduced IPT-SP as a national policy for pregnant mothers is more than cautious in extending the intervention to infants. This reluctance should not be dismissed as "irrational" behavior. What it reveals, however, are the contradictions involved and the inability of the NMCP to control malaria through single technical approaches.

Beyond the Laboratory

The aim of this chapter was to shift the analysis from the microlevel of scientific practices – which dominated previous chapters – to the wider question of how scientific results can be translated into national health policy. One of the major difficulties illustrated by the example of the failed malaria vaccine candidate SPf66 was the problem of standardization. Even though standardization of trial protocols and populations was seen as the basis for successful execution of the SPf66 trial, the results from various sites around the world were far too heterogeneous for SPf66 to represent an effective solution. In the particular case of SPf66, there is good reason to suspect that the efforts were undermined by the WHO and the pharmaceutical industry, but the suggestion here is that, even if all partners had worked together, the complexities of local malaria situations would not have allowed for a one-size-fits-all approach.

Perhaps even more than the SPf66 case study, the discussion of IPTi showed that health research and policymaking in the new millennium is enmeshed in a governance structure comprising global charities, scientists, pharmaceutical companies and international organizations. These new features of what is euphemistically known as "health governance" invite more general reflection on the relationship between science and policymaking in the era of a new humanitarianism. Above all, health governance stands for dissolving boundaries between science and policy. As shown by the example of IPTi in Mtwara and Lindi Regions, scientists very much intrude into the policy realm, introducing new elements into the health system (e.g., the amended clinic card) and seeking to make lasting changes to health performance. The example of implementation research demonstrates, however, that the scientific and policy level are separated once again when the implementation of IPTi results on a national scale is at stake. The partnership concept is destabilized by different results obtained in different parts of the world, and by the interplay of local, national and global actors striving for national health solutions.

Epilogue
Science and Decolonization Revisited

Colonial Science

Côte d'Ivoire and Tanganyika played different roles within the larger framework of the French and British Empires. While the former, rich in natural resources, was of vital political and economic importance for metropolitan France, the unprofitable trust territory of Tanganyika was not a source of imperial pride for London. But despite their different rankings on the imperial scale, the two African territories had similar experiences. For example, both were drawn into a process that has been described as a "second colonial occupation" after World War II, when the resources of France and Britain had been depleted and supplies from overseas were again desperately needed for metropolitan consumption. Science and technology played an important part in the valorization of the colonies. In the 1940s, for the first time, Paris and London provided substantial funds for colonial research and development. There can be few places in sub-Saharan Africa that embody the value attached to science and technology more than Adiopodoumé near Abidjan. In 1945, Adiopodoumé became a center within the periphery. The Office de la Recherche Scientifique et Technique Outre-Mer (ORSTOM) transformed the village into a major scientific site. It attracted substantial funds from Paris, and high-ranking scientists wove a politico-scientific web between Paris and the political elite in Abidjan. Adiopodoumé came to symbolize a change in France's imperial policy of seeking to curb political resistance within Côte d'Ivoire, offering instead an image of what could be expected from Franco-African ties. Science and development played an important part in Tanganyika, too. However, the similarities between the two territories are somewhat reduced if different regions within the colonies are taken into consideration. The rural Ulanga (Mahenge) District of Tanganyika never caught the imagination of imperial social reformers in Britain to the extent that Adiopodoumé did in Paris. In this vast district, many days' journey from the country's main urban centers, the art of governing was left to district commissioners, ruling indirectly through local chiefs. Their impact on the district's political and economic history depended on their individual efforts to implement policies drafted in distant colonial offices. Still, the remoteness of the sites, the money invested or the importance attached to particular scientific projects says little about how Western science and technology was experienced locally. While ORSTOM, as a specific project of domination, was too exclusive and too much of a foreign body to have had any impact on the local population, the attempt to contain the spread of sleeping sickness in Ulanga did indeed disrupt the lives of people in the area. Historian Michael Worboys once noted that, in their efforts to control the spread of the disease, the British focused on the tsetse fly, the Belgians on the movement of humans and the Germans on the trypanosome.[1] However, as we have seen, District Commissioner Arthur Theodore Culwick very much promoted a spatial approach to the disease, attempting to concentrate people in sleeping sickness settlements, thereby controlling human movement and reducing man-fly contacts. Whether these interventions actually had an effect on the spread of the disease was not Culwick's primary concern; he was more interested in the economic and social benefits of people living closer together. Thus, health policy in Ulanga had become the model for social policy – a concept that would linger on in postcolonial times. It would be wrong, however, to see colonial health policy as a homogeneous set of principles and actions implemented along the dichotomy between government agents and rural populations. Not only was there a gap between technocrats and social reformers within the colonial health department, but the resettlement of large parts of Ulanga's population called for the cooperation of local chiefs, without whom the district authorities would have been unable to conduct such large-scale social engineering projects.

The different geographical constituencies, historical legacies and social networks operating in Adiopodoumé and Ifakara very much determined the character of Swiss science at the two sites. Largely unaffected by the ravages of war and devoid of colonial possessions, Switzerland became a prominent player on the imperial stage in the decade after 1945. Swiss scientists were able to forge new connections with the major imperial powers in Africa, ultimately leading to the creation of two Swiss research laboratories in Adiopodoumé and Ifakara. Regarding the first years of their operation, three main points are worth repeating. Firstly, scientific practices at these two sites were too diverse for the notion of "colonial science" to be tenable. Beyond the fact that Thierry Freyvogel and Fritz Haerdi both

---

1   Michael Worboys, *The Comparative History of Sleeping Sickness*.

worked at the same location in Tanganyika, their activities – studying malaria parasites in monkeys, or the vernacular names of local plants – had little in common. Diversity was also the main characteristic of Swiss science as practiced in Côte d'Ivoire. Science at the CSRS did not necessarily follow a strict agenda, nor did it aim at continuity. Rather, for more than 40 years, each of the CSRS directors arriving at the Ebrié Lagoon had his own research agenda, depending on his particular educational background or scientific interests. Yet, especially during the 1950s, Switzerland's scientific efforts were marked by the wish to assemble substantial collections, to describe unknown species and to inventorize the tropics. Secondly, Switzerland's penchant for collections did not accord with French conceptions of science after World War II. In the eyes of ORSTOM, Switzerland's fervor for collecting specimens and sending them back home for scientific scrutiny, or to enrich museum displays, was anachronistic: it belonged to a bygone age in the history of colonial science or was at least incompatible with the more technology-driven late-colonial approach which should also offer benefits for local populations. Thirdly, Swiss colonial science does not necessarily correspond to the image of a "tool of empire", which was assumed to help sustain the overall colonial project. It may be argued that collecting scientific specimens and rendering the unknown tropical world meaningful according to a Western epistemology are indeed forms of cultural domination that sustained the colonial project.[2] On the other hand, it must be acknowledged that, during the late 1950s, not only were Swiss scientific activities doomed to fail, but their impact on the local African population remained limited. The weakness of Swiss science is also apparent when one considers the relations between the French and Swiss scientists in Côte d'Ivoire. It was not only that the Swiss required approval from their French neighbors for their scientific activities. Switzerland's subordinate position was also evident in every aspect of social life – from budgetary constraints to the inability to meet social obligations in the colony (a source of deep resentment). The fact that notions of "smallness" and "weakness" had a firm place in the historical repertoire of Swiss self-representation (and could be deployed strategically when needed) should not obscure the fact that colonial societies did not operate along the colonizer/colonized divide but displayed various shades of gray within the dominant white society. This insight is also important for meth-

---

2   Nicholas B. Dirks, *Introduction. Colonialism and Culture*, in: Dirks (ed.), Colonialism and Culture, Michigan 1992, pp. 1–25, here: p. 3.

odological reasons since it implies that, in order to understand Switzerland's history in a wider imperial context, it is important to consider transfers not only between metropoles and peripheries and vice versa, but also within empires, individual colonies and small social networks within the colonies.

Development

Science and health became important reference points within the political and symbolic borders of the new African nations after independence. Investment in these fields, in particular, was considered a break with the colonial past, and African leaders such as Julius Nyerere or Félix Houphouët-Boigny were eager to exploit the symbolic value of these topics, sending strong signals to their electorate that the winds of political change would soon bring better education, health care and scientific infrastructure. Within the decolonization process, Switzerland had a special role to play. In the years after African independence, the formal ending of the British and French Empires transformed the country's weak position into one of relative strength. On account of Switzerland's political neutrality and untainted (colonial) past, Swiss development experts were highly esteemed guests at the round tables where Africa's future role was discussed. The problem was, however, that the Empire could not simply be "switched off", like blowing out the candles of an antiquated candelabra. As we have seen from the example of Côte d'Ivoire, the forces of colonialism and the paternalistic system of personal relations imposed by France were still very much alive after Ivorian independence and beyond. The perception of Côte d'Ivoire as remaining under French tutelage very much restricted Switzerland's room to maneuver. Members of the DftZ – the official Swiss development aid body that emerged in 1961 – were reluctant to embark on substantial development projects in the West African country for fear of possible French political reactions. Swiss science experienced and resented both France's influence and Switzerland's caution. While the colonial period was marked by a "Gleichzeitigkeit des Ungleichzeitigen" (synchronicity of the nonsynchronous) in scientific practices, the two centers' scientific styles increasingly converged after independence, so that the boundaries between Swiss and French science disappeared.

The example of Tanganyika involved not only a different trajectory of decolonization but also a variety of possibilities for Swiss foreign policy.

From 1964 onwards, Julius Nyerere actively forged new political relations with various Asian and European donor countries, which gradually came to replace British domination. In Tanzania, Switzerland found one of its most rewarding locations for development assistance. In the early 1960s, development activities were the business of private actors. Members of the STI and the pharmaceutical industry were able to offer the DftZ prepackaged development plans, especially in the area of health care, where Switzerland's official development agencies lacked expertise. Perhaps the most important lesson to be drawn from the empirical evidence presented in the previous chapter is that development was not just the application of Western technology in Third World countries, nor merely colonialism by other means, as is often argued in the works of development thinkers such as Wolfgang Sachs or Arturo Escobar.[3] As the rise of social medicine in Tanzania demonstrated, Tanzanian actors were able to shape the outlook of Swiss development projects on the ground, in turn triggering changes in development concepts back in Switzerland. More importantly, development aid was not an instrument to prevent the spread of communist ideology in Africa. Swiss development actors not only embraced African socialism as formulated by Nyerere but also became what Michael Jennings has called "surrogates of the state", spreading the socialist ideology in remote areas beyond the reach of the Tanzanian state.[4] It is therefore necessary to deconstruct Cold War ideology and embrace the more historically informed view that the Cold War was not the overarching ideological principle structuring East-West or North-South relations. Rather, historical actors could choose whether or not to exploit the metanarrative of a bipolar world order, depending on their particular interests.

Medical Research and Development

In the period between 1970 and the mid-1990s, medical research and development ideologies converged. True, development has always involved questions of knowledge: the field was (and still is) populated by many consultants whose expertise derives from their ability to reduce complex economic relationships to neat statistics, or to elaborate economic models

---

3   Wolfgang Sachs, *The Development Dictionary*; Arturo Escobar, *Encountering Development*.
4   Michael Jennings, *Surrogates of the State*.

providing guidance for future action. The point here is that, during this period, Swiss basic medical research in Africa was regarded as compliant with overall development aims. This was evident in the case of the STIFL, which at the beginning of the 1980s – guided by a broader understanding of disease causation – started to work more closely together with and within African societies. The step from the laboratory to the field, taken in the name of development and primary health care (PHC), entailed new forms of experimentation. These contrasted with the long tradition of the laboratory being a more or less confined space where scientific facts were produced for subsequent application within society. Operational research in Africa differed in that it introduced new elements into African society, while studying the effects at the same time. Africans were not just passive objects of Western science. The impact of Swiss science in rural Ulanga District increased exponentially as African researchers were attached to Swiss research teams and new collaborations were sought with Tanzanian institutes and the population. The events of the 1980s show that the concepts of experimentation and development have very strong affinities. Both are oriented towards an as yet unknown future state; both trigger transformative processes and both strive for a "systematic production of novelty".[5] However, medical research could also involve what might be called the "systematic production of differences". The history of the Nestlé Foundation in Côte d'Ivoire reminds us that powerful transnational corporations and their humanitarian offshoots were not bound by the same restrictions as political actors. Switzerland's ability to embark on development projects did not depend on the postcolonial political constituencies of African countries, but on the bargaining power of individual actors. The food company's close relations with the Ivorian government made it relatively easy for it to launch long-term research projects in the country. For Nestlé, notions of "science" and "development" served to camouflage more mundane economic interests. Nestlé researchers on the ground sought to establish protein deficiency as a major health concern in rural areas, which – as a scientifically proven fact – would in turn provide a strong argument for the sale of protein-rich nutrients. It is not that Côte d'Ivoire did not have a malnutrition problem at all, but it was a problem of poverty encountered in the outskirts of Abidjan and not in rural areas. The historical account of the Nestlé Foundation's activities is not intended as an indictment of the company, but rather to indicate the divergent voices and internal struggles be-

5   John Pickstone, *Ways of Knowing*, p. 13.

tween Nestlé, the Nestlé Foundation and individual researchers working in the field. Moreover, the history of nutritional research highlights the more general problems of research ethics, which have only been touched on superficially throughout the study – a shortcoming which cannot be remedied here. Suffice it to say that medical research in the 1970s and 1980s was strongly biased towards innovation and implementation, without paying sufficient attention to the validation of research results.

Switzerland's Late Decolonization

Though different in many respects, the history of the two African countries – especially in the 1970s and 1980s – showed certain similarities. This is especially true of the long shadow cast on Côte d'Ivoire and Tanzania by the economic and political crisis. Along with historian Frederick Cooper, we may well ask whether the year of the oil crisis and global recession did not leave a stronger imprint on the fate of African societies than the much-trumpeted independence a decade earlier.[6] The period of structural adjustment, market liberalization and heavy dependence on moneylenders such as the IMF and the World Bank marked the beginning of what James Ferguson called "transnational governmentality". Rather than portraying African states as "failed", "weak", or otherwise "hollowed out", transnational governmentality referred to a new mode of political action involving new forms of collaboration between private and public actors across national borders and the outsourcing of former state functions to innumerable NGOs operating in the field of African politics.[7] The history of the two Swiss scientific institutions in the 1980s and 1990s provides strong empirical support for this view. Contrary to the "lost development decade" discourse at home, the STIFL was by then more closely integrated into the Tanzanian health system, as well as the global health network, and scientific activities on the ground became more intense. Being part of a transnational political apparatus does not necessarily mean losing sight of national priorities. However, as shown by the examples of recent malaria research in Tanzania, the process of translating scientific results into public health action can be seriously impeded by diverging interests on the part of the various actors involved. In other words, future research will require atten-

6   Frederick Cooper, *Africa since 1940*, p. 87.
7   James Ferguson, Akhil Gupta, *Spatializing States*, p. 990.

tion not only to new forms of transnational governmentality but also to the functioning of policy networks and the power inequalities within them.

The effects of global political changes were also evident in the case of the CSRS. With the forced retreat of ORSTOM from Côte d'Ivoire and France turning its back on its former colony, the CSRS emerged as the sole actor on the scientific stage in Adiopodoumé. However, the end of the colonial pact between France and Côte d'Ivoire placed the CSRS in a difficult position, for the institution was obliged to jettison the view of science as mainly serving Swiss purposes, to open up the CSRS to African scientists and to seek new collaborations with both African and international institutions.[8] From the perspective of African researchers, the process of Africanization did not necessarily mean taking over a European institutional or cultural legacy, but being engaged in the new participatory models known as "research partnerships". Though initially little more than a euphemism for continuing power imbalances between Swiss and African researchers, the partnership concept became more balanced during the latter half of the 1990s. It was at this time that the STI became more involved in the overall policies of the CSRS. Drawing on experiences in Tanzania, the STI had a strong interest in collaborating with the CSRS, especially in the fields of public health and veterinary sciences. In 1997, STI Director Marcel Tanner became a member – and a year later President – of the Commission for the CSRS. He had a strong wish to transform the CSRS into a center of excellence, on the model of the IHI in Tanzania. This ambitious enterprise was facilitated by a series of legal measures. In 1998, the Swiss Undersecretary of State Charles Kleiber and the Ivorian Research and Education Minister Francis Wodié signed a framework agreement on scientific cooperation which brought an end to the legal uncertainty which the CSRS had endured since the end of the ORSTOM era. Under the agreement, the Swiss party was to train Ivorian scientists in the context of scientific projects and to provide scientific infrastructure; in return, major advantages were secured in the form of tax exemptions. The host country agreement signed two years later was even more significant in that it fostered the partnership idea and granted the CSRS quasi-diplomatic status.[9]

---

8   In 1992, a new agricultural and health research site supported by Nestlé and Syngenta was inaugurated in Bringakro (central Côte d'Ivoire) in the context of the research axis led by Niklaus Weiss of the STI.

9   The normative concept of a research partnership has served as the basis for a series of new regulations and funding mechanisms within a broader institutional setting in Switzerland. In 1998, the Commission for Research Partnerships with Developing Coun-

In 2004, Guéladio Cissé, a researcher originating from Mauritania, was named Director of the CSRS. His election proved to be crucial during the years of crisis, when questions of Ivorian identity became the subject of violent ethnic conflicts. Since 2000, more than 20 MSc and 25 PhD students from African and European universities have graduated from the CSRS.[10] At the same time, the CSRS was organized as an international trust – on the model of the IHI governance structure – with African partners holding a majority of seats on the Board of Governors.

Thus, it would appear that both the IHI and the CSRS have a strong impact on the societies in which they operate. Both institutes attract the most committed African and European researchers, seeking to improve the health situation or to offer scientific solutions for pressing societal problems.

Writing a Swiss History of Science in Africa

This book has sought to trace the development of formerly Swiss scientific institutions, not from within the narrow confines of the nation, but in the field, where science has been practiced and reshaped and from where new ideas have traveled back home. Adopting this perspective not only requires a history of the sciences which can be connected to social, economic and cultural histories, but also an acknowledgement that Switzerland was what Latour called a "center of calculation" within the French and British Empires. The approach chosen here was to compare scientific practices in Adiopodoumé and Ifakara, including the various transfers of people, technology and concepts between these sites and across continents. However,

tries (KFPE) published its "11 Principles for Research in Partnership", which provided guidelines and focused more strongly on the research process itself, from the setting of priorities to the dissemination of results. In the Federal Council's Dispatch on the Promotion of Education, Research and Technology for 2000–2003, the Swiss government proposed the establishment of so-called National Centers of Competence in Research (NCCR). After a selection process, the NCCR "North-South – Research Partnerships for Mitigating Syndromes of Global Change" was launched in 2001, with support provided by the SDC as well as the Swiss National Science Foundation (SNSF). More recently, the KFPE's 11 principles have been revised, and a new funding mechanism has been established by the SDC and the SNSF to tackle global themes through participatory approaches.

10 Bassirou Bonfoh et al., *Research in a War Zone*, in: Nature, Vol. 474, 2011, pp. 569–571, here: p. 570.

"multi-sited history" – as this endeavor could be termed in analogy to George Marcus's multi-sited ethnography – does not only mean paying attention to the various geographical factors that shaped the course of scientific developments. It also involves switching back and forth between the local, national and international arenas where science was produced, experienced, accepted, rejected and interpreted. While such an approach is more common among British and French historians, Swiss historiography has not yet come to terms with the empire. Looking at Swiss history from different geographical angles helps to destabilize the foundational categories underlying Switzerland's self-conceptions. Science and technology are no longer regarded as homogeneous entities shifted from the center to the periphery. Rather, these terms disclose their local rootedness, their different and changing meanings over time, and their resistance to any attempts at standardization. Moreover, this perspective focuses attention on the movement of concepts between sites, as was relevant in those parts of the study dealing with Swiss development aid. The emphasis on connectivity and mutual entanglements should not be read as an invitation to neglect processes of exclusion and suppression or the disconnects which also characterize the history of Swiss-African encounters. It is, however, assumed that the adoption of a relational approach to Swiss history will promote greater modesty and a more nuanced understanding of the extent to which the notions of "self" and "other" are mutually constitutive.

References
Archives, Sources, Publications

Archives and unpublished Sources

Switzerland

Staatsarchiv Basel-Stadt (StABS)

Universitätsarchiv I 71.1, (Schweizerisches Tropeninstitut), 1942–1944
Universitätsarchiv X 3.5 158, Adolphe Sicé, 1946–1957
ED-REG 42a, 2-2-6 (10), Rudolf Geigy, 1960–1972
ED-REG 1a, 1, 1266, Sicé, Prof. Dr. Adolphe, –1964
ED-REG 1c 190-2-5 (1), Schweizerische Tropenschule, 1943–1964
ED-REG 1c, 190-2-6 (1), Protokolle (Kuratorium, Geschäftsausschuss), 1944–1968
ED-REG 1c, 190-2-8 (1), Ifakara, Schulungszentrum, 1959–1968
ED-REG 1c, 190-4 (1), Schweizerische Forschungsstation Elfenbeinküste (Adiopodoumé),
    1951–1968
FD-REG 1d, 37.2, (Schweizerisches Tropeninstitut), 1943–1959
PA 212a, T2, Sarasinisches Familienarchiv, XLIV 92
PA 212a, T2, 28–28a, Rudolf Geigy, 1936
PA 1095, (A), Rudolf Geigy, Biographisches, –1995
PD-REG 1a, 1969–471, (Schweizerisches Tropeninstitut), 1945–1958

Archiv Museum der Kulturen Basel (AMKB)

Museumskommission, Protokolle, 1960–1964

Archive Musée d'Histoire Naturelle de Genève (AMHN)

360.B.4.4, Mission scientifique en Côte d'Ivoire, 1953–1957

Schweizerisches Wirtschaftsarchiv Basel (SWA)

Institute 196

Archiv Schweizerische Akademie der Naturwissenschaften, Depot Burgerbibliothek Bern (SCNAT)

GA SANW 350, Zentralvorstand Lausanne, Korrespondenz, 1953–1958
GA SANW 448, Senat, 1977–1984
GA SANW 457, CSRS, 1974–1984
GA SANW 458, CSRS

GA SANW 825, Sitzungen der Kommission CSRS, 1951–1990
GA SANW 826, Kommissionen CSRS, Varia I, 1951–1970
GA SANW 826, ORSTOM Korrespondenz, 1951–1976
GA SANW 829, Kommissionen CSRS, Akten Generalsekretariat, 1984–1990
GA SANW 830, Centre Suisse, Varia, Korrespondenz, Geschichte der Station, 1981–1987

Schweizerisches Bundesarchiv Bern (BAR)

Direktion Internationale Organisationen

E 2003-03 (-), 1976/44, (Schweizerisches Tropeninstitut Basel), 1960–1963
E 2003-03 (-), 1976/44, 46, Basler Stiftung zur Förderung von Entwicklungsländern Basel, 1961–1964
E 2003-03 (-), 1976/44, 205, Lumemo-River, Bewässerungsprojekt, 1961–1963

Direktion für Entwicklungszusammenarbeit und Humanitäre Hilfe (DEH)

E 2005 (A), 1978/137, 80, t.311-Elfenbeinküste, Projekte und Aktionen, 1964–1966
E 2005 (A), 1978/137, 83, Ecole de médicine Conakry, Bd. 1, 1963–1966
E 2005 (A), 1978/137, 155, t. 311, Tanzania – Projekte und Aktionen, 1964–1966
E 2005 (A), 1980/82, 243, t. 311-Tanzania – Medical School Dar es Salaam, 1967
E2005 (A), 1983/18, 361, Rural Medical Aid Centre Ifakara,1970–1972
E2005 (A), 1983/18, 364, Flying Doctor Service in Tanzania, 1967–1972
E 2005 (A), 1985/101, 11, Arbeitsgruppe Bevölkerungsprobleme und medizinische Entwicklungszusammenarbeit, 1975
E 2005 (A), 1985/101, 688, Medicus Mundi Basel, 1973–1975
E 2005 (A), 1991/16, 400, Tansania Allgemeines, 1976–1978

Direktion für Entwicklung und Zusammenarbeit (DEZA)

E 2025 (A), 1991/168, 812, Schweizerisches Tropeninstitut, Bde I-II, 1979–1981
E 2025 (A), 1993/130, 456, t.311-Tansania.45, Recherches médicales au Swiss Tropical Institute Field Lab à Ifakara, Vols. I–II, 1981–1984
E 2025 (A), 1997/200, 642, t.311-Tansania.45, Recherches médicales au Swiss Tropical Institute Field Lab à Ifakara, Vols. 1–2, 1985–1987
E 2025 (A), 2000/138, 752, t.311-Tansania.45, Recherches médicales au Swiss Tropical Institute Field Lab à Ifakara, Vols. 1–2, 1988–1989
E 2025 (A), 2000/138, 753, t.311-Tansania.45, Recherches médicales au Swiss Tropical Institute Field Lab à Ifakara, Vols. 1–2, 1989–1990
E 2025 (A), 2000/253, 9, t.311-Tansania.69, Abk. CH/Tansania betr. "The Kilombero District Health Support" – Phase I, 1994–1997
E 2025 (A), 2002/145, 802, t.311-Tansania.45, Recherches médicales au Swiss Tropical Institute Field Lab à Ifakara, Vols. 5-7, 1992–1993
E 2025 (A), 2002/145, 803, t.311-Tansania.45, Recherches médicales au Swiss Tropical Institute Field Lab à Ifakara, Vol. 8, 1993
E 2026 (A), 2005/9, 861, t.311-Tansania.69, Kilombero District Health Support (KDHS), Vol. 1, 1993–1994
E 2026 (A), 2005/9, 861, t.311-Tansania.69, Kilombero District Health Support (KDHS), Vol. 2, 1994

Eidgenössisches Politisches Departement (EPD), Postenberichte Abidjan

E 2200.5 (-), 1969/217, 2, Correspondances officielles, 1952

E 2200.5 (-), 1969/217, 4, Agence Consulaire de Suisse à Abidjan

E 2200.5 (-), 1979/93, 8, Faculté de médecine en Côte d'Ivoire

E 2200.5 (-), 1979/93, 10, Centre technique Suisse de Recherche Scientifique en Côte d'Ivoire, 1961–1965

E 2200.5 (-), 1979/94, 6, Centre Suisse de Recherches Scientifiques en Côte d'Ivoire, 1966–1968

E 2200.5 (-), 1998/4, 13, Associations et institutions scientifiques, 1985–1988

E 2400, 1000/717, 1, Abidjan, Jahresberichte, 1953–1959

Eidgenössisches Politisches Departement (EPD), Postenberichte Dar es Salaam

E 2200.83 (A), 1983/26, 3, Dienst für technische Zusammenarbeit, Agricultural Development (Lumemo), 1962–1963

E 2200.83 (A), 1983/26, B 8, Dienst für technische Zusammenarbeit, 1961–1965

E 2200.83 (A), 1983/26, 3, B. 8.15.1, Experten, Spezialisten, Schweizerärzte, 1962–1963

E 2200.83 (A), 1983/26, 4, Rural Aid Centre Ifakara, 1960–1965

E 2200.83 (B), 1990/26, 10, 771.22.8, Pathologisches Institut Dar es Salaam

E 2200.83 (B), 1999/351, 10, Schweizerisches Tropeninstitut, 1982–1984

E 2200.83 (B), 2000/281, 8, Technische Zusammenarbeit Schweiz-Tansania, Allgemeines

Generalsekretarat Eidgenössisches Departement des Innern (EDI)

E 3001 (B), 1978/30, 62, Fondation pour un Centre Suisse de Recherches Scientifiques en Côte d'Ivoire, 1951–1954

Eidgenössische Finanzverwaltung

E 6100 (C), 1998/106, 1, Antrag auf Einsetzung einer nichtständigen Expertenkommission zur Erarbeitung von Grundlagen für ein BG über Krankheitsvorbeugung, 1979–1984

Diplomatische Dokumente der Schweiz [Dodis], www.dodis.ch

Firmenarchiv der Novartis AG, Basel

Bestand CIBA:

RE 15.04.1, Basler Stiftung zur Förderung von Entwicklungs- ländern, 1960–1975

RE 15.04.11, Basler Stiftung zur Förderung von Entwicklungsländern, Protokolle der Stiftungsratssitzungen, 1960–1982

Bestand J. R. Geigy AG:

SP 5, "Entwicklungshilfe", Entwicklungsländer

VW 8, Wirtschaftspolitisches Komitee

Archive Historique Nestlé, Vevey (AHN)

9564-1, Administration, 1972–1979

9564-4, Séances du Conseil, 1973–1975

9564-22, Communication interne, 1967–1970

Rapport Annuels, 1971, 1974, 1977

Private Holdings

Archive Swiss Tropical and Public Health Institute, Basel (ASTI)

Entwicklungshilfe

DEH/DDA, Arbeitsgruppe Gesundheit
DEH/DDA, Arbeitsgruppe Gesundheit, Dokumente allgemein, II, 1979/80
DEH/DDA, Arbeitsgruppe Gesundheit, Dokumente allgemein, III
DEH/DDA, Arbeitsgruppe Gesundheit, Korrespondenz allgemein
Pathologie-Block, Dar es Salaam
Courses, 1966–1971
Ifakara I, BSFEL u.a.
Ifakara, 1980–1982 (vor DEH)

Swiss Tropical Institute Field Laboratory (STIFL)

STIFL, Correspondence, 1981–1987
STIFL, KIHERE, Administration, 1986
STIFL, NIIE/KIK
STIFL, Evolution/Integration, 1988–1994
STIFL, 1.2. General, Policy, Evaluation
STIFL, PHC, 3.2 (P.1)
STIFL, Correspondence, 1981–1987

Kilombero Health and Research Project (KIHERE)

KIHERE Letters, 1985–1988
KIHERE Letters, 1989–
KIHERE File, 1988, January–Juni
KIHERE File, 1990, January–June
KIHERE File, 1993, August–October, Phase V
KIHERE File, 1994, 15. Dezember–20. März, Phase V
KIHERE File, 1994, 21. März–30. Juni, Phase V
P. 40

Centre Suisse de Recherches Scientifiques (CSRS)

CSRS, Kommissionssitzungen, 1990–1997
CSRS, Adresses, Commission, Principes

Kilombero Malaria Project

KIVAC, Correspondence Pedro Alonso
KIVAC, Correspondence 1994
KIVAC, Documents IV
KIVAC, Documents III
KIVAC, Correspondence 1992/1993,
KIVAC, Correspondence 1995
IPTi

Personal Correspondence

Korrespondenz Thierry Freyvogel, 1972–1987
Documents Marcel Tanner (DMT)
Unterlagen Antoine Degrémont
Korrespondenz Appert, Eichenberger, Schuppler, Ifakara

Archiv Novartis Stiftung für Nachhaltige Entwicklung, Basel (ANSNE)

Protokolle, Korrespondenzen, 1971–1978

Archiv Novartis Stiftung für Nachhaltige Entwicklung, Basel (ANSNE)

Protokolle, Korrespondenzen, 1971–1978

Archive Nestlé Foundation, Lausanne

Rapport au Gouvernement, 1972

Archiv Medicus Mundi Schweiz (AMMS)

DEH, Documents base, 1967–1981

Archive Jardin Botanique de Genève (AJBG)

Correspondance Jaques Miège, –1976

Private Archive André Aeschlimann

Fonds André Aeschlimann (FAA), Correspondance Côte d'Ivoire 1959–1962

Private Archive Urs Rahm

Fonds Urs Rahm (FUR), Correspondance Côte d'Ivoire 1951–1953

Private Archive Thierry A. Freyvogel

Tagebuch, No. 1, Expédition de l'Institut Tropical Suisse de Bâle au Tanganyika, Ifakara Mai 1954–Juli 1954
Lettres d'Ifakara 1956, 1957, 1959–1985

Private Archive Fritz Haerdi

Afrika-Tagebuch II, 01.09.1958–05.02.1959
Afrika-Tagebuch III, 06.02.1959–05.08.1959
Afrika-Tagebuch IV, 06.08.1959–20.03.1960
Afrika-Tagebuch V, 21.03.1960–13.12.1960

Private Archive Rolf Wilhelm

Rolf Wilhelm (in collaboration with Marcel Tanner and Thierry Freyvogel), Das Projekt des
"Rural Aid Center" in Ifakara, Tanzania, [Typescript], 06.04.2004

France

Archives Nationales Fontainebleau, Paris (ANF)

Archives de l'ORSTOM, 19900236, Art. 1
Archives de l'ORSTOM, 19900236, Art. 2, Conseil supérieur de la recherche scientifique
Archives de l'ORSTOM, 19910536, Art. 8, Côte d'Ivoire, 1971–1978
Archives de l'ORSTOM, 19900236, Art. 53
Archives de l'ORSTOM, 19900236, Art. 57
Archives de l'ORSTOM, 19900236, Art. 58

Tanzania

Tanzania National Archive, Dar es Salaam (TNA)

450, 653, Ifakara Station, 1936–1948
61/104/G, Sleeping Sickness Mahenge
61/104/H, Sleeping Sickness Ulanga-District
450/66/Infectious Diseases, Spirillum Relapsing Fever, 1948–1957
450/87/20, Scientific (Tanganyika) Expedition by Profs. R. Geigy and H. Mooser and
    Dr. Freyvogel, 1954–1956
450/HE/1172, Medical Development Plan, 1963
450/HEH/30/7, Primary Health Care
461/16/2, Sleeping Sickness General, 1930–1940
No. 28446, Sleeping Sickness Concentrations Ulanga
No. 33041, Development and Reconstruction Ulanga District
Microfilm (MF), 21, Ulanga District

Ministry of Health (MOH) Library, Dar es Salaam

Annual Report on Health Services 1959
Budget Speeches, 1970/71, 1972/73, 1973/74

Tanzanian National Library (NBA Section), Dar es Salaam

Annual Reports Provincial Commissioners, Eastern Province, 1945, 1947, 1948

Diocesan Archives Kwiro (DAK)

Parish Ifakara 1956–1969, Correspondence Edgar Maranta 1958

Provincial Archive Dar es Salaam (PADSM)

Correspondence Pater Oswin 1954

Private Holdings

Archiv Ifakara Health Institute, Ifakara (AIHI)
Unbeschriftet

Archiv Ifakara Health Institute Mtwara Branch (AIHI-MB)
IPTi Project Reports
Official Documents IPTi in Southern Tanzania
Mkinge

Côte d'Ivoire

Archive Ministère de la Recherche Scientifique Côte d'Ivoire (AMRSCI)
Correspondances
Commission-Mixtes Franco-Ivoiriennes

Published Sources

Aellen Villy, *Animaux en Côte d'Ivoire,* in: Bulletin de la Société Neuchâteloise des Sciences Naturelles, Vol. 82, 1959, p. 329

Aellen Villy, *Chiroptères Nouveaux d'Afrique,* in: Archives des Sciences, Vol. 12, No. 2, 1959, pp. 217–235

Aellen Villy, *Description d'un nouvel Hipposideros (chiroptera) de la Côte d'Ivoire,* in: Revue Suisse de Zoologie, Vol. 61, No. 24, 1954, pp. 474–483

Aeschlimann André, *Développement embryonnaire d'Ornithodorus moubata (Murray) et transmission transovarienne de Borrelia duttoni,* Inauguraldissertation Universität Basel, Basel 1958

Anonymous, *In Memoriam Dr. h.c. René Wyniger,* 1921–2006, in: Mitteilungen der Entomologischen Gesellschaft Basel, Vol. 56, No. 4, 2006, pp. 178–188

Baer Jean-Georges, *"Charles Joyeux" (1881–1966),* in: Bulletin de la Société Neuchâteloise des Sciences Naturelles, Vol. 90, 1967, pp. 293-296

Baer Jean-Georges, *Ecology of Animal Parasites,* Urbana 1952

Bech Margunn M., *Changing Policies and their Influence on the Interaction between Health Workers and Patients. A Government Health Worker Perspective from Rural Mbulu District, Tanzania,* paper presented at the international conference "The History of Health Care in Africa. Actors, Experiences, and Perspectives in the 20th Century," Basel, 12th–14th September 2011

Beck A. D., *The Kilombero Valley of South-Central Tanganyika,* in: East African Geographical Review, Vol. 2, 1964, pp. 37–43

Berry Veronica (ed.), *The Culwick Papers,* 1934–1944. Population, Food and Health in Colonial Tanganyika (now Tanzania), London 1994

Biro Stephan, *Investigations on the Bionomics of Anopheline Vectors in the Ifakara Area (Kilombero District, Tanzania),* Inaugural-Dissertation zur Erlangung der Würde eines Doktors der Philosophie vorgelegt der Philosophisch-Naturwissenschaftlichen Fakultät der Universität Basel, Basel 1987

Bourlière, F., Bertrand M., Hunkeler C., L'écologie de la mone de Lowe (Cercopithecus campbelli lowei) en Côte d'Ivoire, in: Terre Vie, Vol. 23, 1969, pp. 135–163

Bourlière, F., Bertrand M., Hunkeler C., *Ecology and Behaviour of Lowe's guenon (Cercopithecus campbelli lowei) in the Ivory Coast,* in: J. R. Napier and P.H. Napier (eds.), Old World Monkeys. Evolution, Systematics, and Behavior, New York, London 1970, pp. 297–350

Brock J. F., Autret M., *Kwashiorkor in Africa,* Geneva 1952

Chevalier Auguste, *Un jeune africain prodige. Aké Assi, préparateur à l'Institut biologique d'Adiopodoumé (Côte d'Ivoire),* in: Revue Internationale de Botanique Appliquée et d'Agriculture Tropicale, 1948, p. 179

Commission on Health Research for Development (ed.), *Health Research. Essential Link to Equity in Development,* New York 1990

Cornaz Immita, *Santé et développement. Exposé à l'Association Suisse de Médecine Tropicale et de Parasitologie. 18.11.1988,* in: Bulletin Medicus Mundi Schweiz, Vol. 45, 1990, pp. 5–15

Culwick Arthur T., *New Beginning,* in: Tanganyika Notes and Records, Vol. 15, 1943, pp. 1–6

Culwick Arthur T., *The Laborer and his Hire,* in: Tanganyika Notes and Records, Vol. 17, 1944, pp. 26-33

Dasen Pierre et al., *Naissance de l'intelligence chez l'enfant Baoulé en Côte d'Ivoire,* Bern 1978

Dasen Pierre, *The Cross-Cultural Study of Intelligence. Piaget and the Baoulé,* in: International Journal of Psychology, Vol. 19, No. 4/5, 1984, pp. 407–434

Degrémont Antoine et al., *Longitudinal Study of the Health Status of Children in a Rural Tanzanian Community. Comparison of Community-Based Clinical Examinations, the Diseases seen at Village Health Posts and the Perception of Health Problems by the Population,* in: Acta Tropica, Vol. 44, 1987, pp. 175-190

Dobbing John (ed.), *Infant Feeding. Anatomy of a Controversy, 1973–1984,* London 1988

Douglas Steven, Schopfer Kurt, *Phagocyte Function in Protein-Calorie Malnutrition,* in: Clinical & Experimental Immunology, Vol. 17, No. 1, 1974, pp. 121–128

Dubois Georges, *Naturalistes Neuchâteloises du XXᵉ siècle (Cahiers de l'Institut Neuchâtelois),* Neuchâtel 1976

ETH Zürich (ed.), *Schweizer bauen und planen im Ausland – Les Suisses construisent à l'étranger. Ausstellung an der ETH-Hönggerberg Zürich – Exposition organisée par l'école polytechnique de Zurich,* Zürich 1978

Food and Agricultural Organization (ed.), *The Rufiji Basin Tanganyika. FAO Report to the Government of Tanganyika on the Preliminary Reconnaissance Survey of the Rufiji Basin,* Rome 1961

Favarger Claude, *Recherches taxonomiques sur les Mélastomacées d'Afrique Occidentale,* in: Lyeuria, Vol. 10, 1952, pp. 53–56

Favarger Claude, *Systématique et morphologie dans la botanique moderne. Leçon inaugurale prononcée le 30 avril 1947 à son installation comme Professeur ordinaire à la chaire de botanique,* in: Bulletin de la Société Neuchâteloise des Sciences Naturelles, Vol. 70, 1947, pp. 21–32

Freyvogel Thierry, *Eine Sammlung geflochtener Matten aus dem Ulanga-Distrikt Tanganyikas,* in: Acta Tropica, Vol. 16, No. 4, 1959, pp. 289–301

Freyvogel Thierry, *"Entwicklungshilfe" in Tanganyika. Separatdruck aus dem Schweizerischen Jahrbuch "Die Ernte",* 1963, pp. 55–66

Freyvogel Thierry, *Flussblindheit und ihre Bekämpfung in Westafrika,* in: Bulletin Medicus Mundi Schweiz, Vol. 49/50, 1992, pp. 37–45

Freyvogel Thierry, *The Work at the Rural Aid Center (RAC) Ifakara, Tanganyika,* in: Acta Tropica, Vol. 21, No. 1, 1964, pp. 91–95

Freyvogel Thierry, *Zur Frage der Wirkung des Höhenklimas auf den Verlauf akuter Malaria. Malaria in tiefer und mittlerer Höhenlage. Untersuchungen in endemischen Gebieten Tanganyikas,* PhD Study University of Basel, Basel 1955

Gaschen Hans, *Moustiques et paludisme dans le canton de Vaud à l'heure actuelle,* in: Bulletin de la Société Vaudoise des Sciences Naturelles, Vol. 62, No. 262, pp. 379–390

Geigy Rudolf, *Action de l'ultra-violet sur le pole germinal dans l'oeuf de Drosophila melanogaster (Castration et mutabilité). Thèse présentée à la faculté des sciences de l'université de Genève pour l'obtention du grade de docteur des sciences naturelles,* Genève 1931

Geigy Rudolf, *Zum Geleit,* in: Acta Tropica, Zeitschrift für Tropenwissenschaften und Tropenmedizin, Vol. 1, No. 1, 1944, pp. 1–3

Geigy Rudolf, Höltker Georg, *Mädchen-Initiationen im Ulanga-Distrikt von Tanganyika,* in: Acta Tropica, Vol. 8, No. 4, 1951, pp. 289–344

Geigy Rudolf, *Erforschung der Natur im Feld und Laboratorium,* in: Verhandlungen der Schweizerischen Naturforschenden Gesellschaft (wissenschaftlicher Teil), 150. Jahresversammlung in Basel, 1970, pp. 9–20

Geigy Rudolf, Herbig Adelheid, *"Erreger und Überträger tropischer Krankheiten",* Basel 1955

Geigy Rudolf, *Malaria in der Schweiz,* in: Acta Tropica, Vol. 2, No. 1, 1945, pp. 1–16

Geigy Rudolf, *L'expédition scientifique de l'Institut Tropical Suisse en Afrique Equatoriale,* in: La Revue Coloniale Belge, Vol. 6, 1946, pp. 10–12

Geigy Rudolf, *Elevage de Glossina palpalis,* in: Acta Tropica, Vol. 5, No. 1, 1948, pp. 201–218

Geigy Rudolf, Mooser Hermann, *Untersuchungen zur Epidemiologie des afrikanischen Rückfallfiebers in Tanganyika,* in: Acta Tropica, Vol. 12, No. 4, 1955, pp. 327–345

Geigy Rudolf, Freyvogel Thierry, *On the Influence of High Altitudes on the Course of Infection of Chicken Malaria (P. gallinaceum),* in: Acta Tropica, Vol. 11, No. 2, 1954, pp. 167–171

Geigy Rudolf, *Der Sprung in die Selbständigkeit. "Entwicklungshilfe" und Menschheitsproblem. Rektoratsrede gehalten an der Jahresfeier der Universität Basel am 23. November 1962,* Basel 1962

Geigy Rudolf, Siri, top secret, Basel 1977

Geigy Rudolf, *Training on the Spot. Swiss Development Aid in Tanzania 1960–1976,* in: Acta Tropica, Vol. 33, No. 4, 1976, pp. 290–306

Geigy Rudolf, *Neue Aufgaben des Tropeninstituts,* in: Mitteilungsblatt der Tropenschule des Schweizerischen Tropeninstituts in Basel, No. 9, Basel 1960, pp. 6–9

Geigy Rudolf, *Rural Medical Training at Ifakara. Swiss Help to Tanzania,* in: The Lancet, Vol. 285, No. 7400, 1965, pp. 1385–1387

Gigon Alfred, *Etwas über Medizin und Sozialpolitik,* in: Sonderabdruck aus der Schweizerischen Medizinischen Wochenschrift, Vol. 75, No. 18, 1945, pp. 394–501

Gigon Alfred, *Die Arbeiterkost nach Untersuchungen über die Ernährung Basler Arbeiter bei freigewählter Kost,* in: Institut für Gewerbehygiene in Frankfurt (ed.), Schriften aus dem Gesamtgebiet der Gewerbehygiene, Heft 3, Berlin 1914

Gontard Jean-Pierre, *Aperçu global de la coopération Suisse au développement dans le do-maine de la santé,* 1960–1993, in: Jahrbuch Schweiz-Dritte Welt, 1994, pp. 169–184

Graf Jean-François, *Kommission für das Centre Suisse de Recherches Scientifiques en Côte d'Ivoire (CSRS),* in: Jahrbuch der Schweizerischen Akademie der Naturwissenschaften, Bern 1990, pp. 24–27

Haerdi Fritz, *Die Eingeborenen-Heilpflanzen des Ulanga-Distriktes Tanganjikas (Ostafrika),* in: Acta Tropica (Supplementum 8), 1964

Heisch R. B., Grainger W. E., *On the Occurrence of Ornithodorus moubata Murray in Bur-rows,* in: Annals of Tropical Medicine and Parasitology, Vol. 44, 1950, pp. 153–155

Heisch R. B., *Ornithodorus moubata (Murray) in a Porcupine Burrow near Kitui,* in: East African Medical Journal, Vol. 31, 1954, p. 483

Herbig-Sandreuter Adelheid, *Untersuchungen über den Einfluss des Höhenklimas auf Hüh-nermalaria (Plasmodium gallinaceum Brumpt),* in: Acta Tropica, Vol. 10, No. 1, 1953, pp. 1–27

Hunkeler C., Bourlière F., Bertrand M., *Le comportement social de la Mone de Lowe (Cerco-pithecus campbelli lowei),* in: Folia primat, Vol. 17, 1972, pp. 218–236

International Bank for Reconstruction and Development (ed.), *The Economic Development of Tanganyika,* Baltimore 1961

Jelliffe Derrick, *Commerciogenic Malnutrition? Time for a Dialogue,* in: Food Tech, Vol. 25, No. 2, 1971, pp. 55–56

Jelliffe Eleanore F. P., *Maternal Nutrition and Lactation,* in: Ciba Foundation Symposium, No. 45, Breast Feeding and the Mother, Amsterdam, Oxford, New York 1976, pp. 119–143

Laraisse P., *La Colonie Suisse en Côte d'Ivoire,* in: Echo. Zeitschrift der Schweizer im Aus-land, Vol. 12, No. 33, 1953, pp. 28–29

Latham Michael C., *Protein-Calorie Malnutrition in Children and Its Relation to Psycho-logical Development and Behavior,* in: Physiological Reviews, Vol. 54, No. 3, 1974, pp. 541–565

Lauber Edgar, Reinhardt Michael, *Studies on the Quality of Breast Milk During 23 Months of Lactation in a Rural Community of the Ivory Coast,* in: The American Journal of Clin-ical Nutrition, Vol. 32, 1979, pp. 1159–1173

Lauterburg-Bonjour Mark, *"Gedanken über das Studium der Tropenmedizin in der Schweiz",* in: Schweizerische Ärztezeitung für Standesfragen, Vol. 28, No. 1, 1947, pp. 2–3

Lwihula George, *Human Behaviour and Social Factors Influencing S. Haematobium Trans-mission in Kikwawila (Kilombero District, Morogoro Region) Tanzania,* London 1985

Mémoires de l'Institut Français d'Afrique Noire (Centre du Caméroun), Série Science Na-turelles, No. 1, *Résultats de la mission zoologique Suisse au Cameroun,* Dakar 1951

Meyer Gustave, *Un demi-siècle en terre ivoirienne,* Paris 1975

Ministry of Health (ed.), *National Guidelines for the Implementation of the Primary Health Care Program in Tanzania,* Dar es Salaam 1983

Monckeberg Fernando B., *Effects of Nutrition on Brain Growth and Intellectual Develop-ment,* in: Frederick Richardson (ed.), Brain and Intelligence. The Ecology of Child Devel-opment, Hyatssville, Maryland 1973, pp. 207–228

Mooser Hermann, *Die Beziehungen des murinen Fleckfiebers zum klassischen Fleckfieber,* in: Acta Tropica (Supplementum 4), Basel 1945

Nyerere Julius, *Freedom and Socialism,* in: Nyerere, Nyerere on Socialism, Dar es Salaam 1969

Nyerere Julius, *Decentralization,* Dar es Salaam 1972

Parin Paul, Morgenthaler Fritz, Parin-Matthèy Goldy, *Die Weissen denken zuviel. Psycho-analytische Untersuchungen bei den Dogon in Westafrika,* Zürich 1963

Perret-Gentil André, *L'observation des réfugiés malariens dans la section clinique et le laboratoire de l'Institut Tropical Suisse,* in: Acta Tropica, Vol. 2, No. 1, 1945, pp. 97–121

Piaget Jean, *La naissance de l'intelligence chez l'enfant,* Neuchâtel 1959

Preiswerk Roy, *La coopération technique. Dimension nouvelle de la politique étrangère Suisse,* in: Annuaire Suisse de Science Politique, Vol. 6, 1966, pp. 75–97

Rahm Urs, *La Côte d'Ivoire. Centre de Recherches Tropicales. Possibilités pour la participation suisse à l'exploration de la Côte d'Ivoire,* in: Acta Tropica, Vol. 11, 1954, pp. 222–295

Rahm Urs, *Die innersekretorische Steuerung der postembryonalen Entwicklung von Sialis lutaria L. (Megaloptera). Inauguraldissertation Universität Basel,* Basel 1952

Rahm Urs, *Zur Ökologie des Zooplanktons der Lagune Ebrié (Elfenbeinküste),* in: Acta Tropica (Separatum), Vol. 21, No. 1, Basel 1964

Rahm Urs, *Beobachtungen an Atherurus africanus (Gray) an der Elfenbeinküste,* in: Acta Tropica, Vol. 13, No. 1, 1956, pp. 86–94

Rahm Urs, *Beobachtungen an den Schuppentieren Manis tricuspis und Manis longicaudata an der Elfenbeinküste,* in: Revue Suisse de Zoologie, Vol. 62, No. 2 /29, 1955, pp. 361–367

Rahm Urs, *Einige Schlangen des westafrikanischen Urwaldes,* in: Die Aquarien- und Terrarien-Zeitschrift (DATZ), Vol. 6, No. 11, 1953, pp. 292–294

Rahm Urs, *Einige Urwaldsäuger der Elfenbeinküste,* in: Leben und Umwelt, Vol. 9, 1952, pp. 1–5

Rahm Urs, *Einige Urwaldsäuger der Elfenbeinküste (II),* in: Leben und Umwelt, Vol. 9, 1953, pp. 114–118

Rahm Urs, *Quelques notes sur le Botto de Bosman. Extrait du Bulletin de L'Institut Français d'Afrique Noire (IFAN),* Vol. 22, No. A/1, 1960, pp. 331–342

Ravelli Gian Paolo, *Study of Malnutrition among Preschool-Age Children in a Village of the African Brush – Ivory Coast,* in: Frederick Richardson (ed.), Brain and Intelligence. The Ecology of Child Development, Hyatssville, Maryland 1973, pp. 257–265

Ravelli Gian Paolo, *Enquête nutritionnelle en milieu rural africain. Village d'Adahou, S/P de Toumodi, Côte d'Ivoire,* Thèse présentée à la Faculté de Médecine de l'Université de Berne, pour l'obtention du titre de Docteur en Médecine, Berne 1972

Regamey Gustave, *Etudes relatives à la malaria. La distribution des Anophèles dans le canton de Genève en relation avec les anciens foyers de malaria,* Thèse faculté des sciences, Lausanne 1927

Roux Wilhelm, *Die Entwicklungsmechanik der Organismen. Eine anatomische Wissenschaft der Zukunft,* Wien 1890

Schmalenbach Werner, *Grundsätzliches zur primitiven Kunst,* in: Acta Tropica, Vol. 15, No. 4, 1958, pp. 289–323

Schopfer Kurt, Douglas Steven, *Neutophil Function in Children with Kwashiorkor,* in: The Journal of Laboratory and Clinical Medicine, Vol. 88, No. 3, 1976, pp. 450–461

Schopfer Kurt, Douglas Steven, *Fine Structural Studies of Peripheral Blood Leucocytes from Children with Kwashiorkor. Morphological and Functional Properties,* in: British Journal of Haematology, Vol. 32, No. 4, 1976, pp. 573–577

Schweizerisches Tropeninstitut in Basel, *Jahresberichte 1944, 1947*

Shortt H. E., Garnham P. C. C., *Pre-erythrocytic Stage in Mammalian Malaria,* in: Nature, Vol. 161, 1948, p. 126

Spichiger Rodolphe, *"Jacques Miège" (1914–1993)*, in: Candollea, Vol. 49, No. 1, 1994, pp. 1–22

Suter Reto, *The Plant Molluscicide Swartzia Madagascariensis and its Application in Transmission Control Measures against Schistosoma Haematobium. Experience from Kikwawila (Kilombero District, Tanzania)*, Inaugural-Dissertation zur Erlangung der Würde eines Doktors der Philosophie vorgelegt der Philosophisch-Naturwissenschaftlichen Fakultät der Universität Basel, Basel 1986

Tanganyika African National Union (ed.), *The Arusha Declaration and TANU's Policy on Socialism and Self-Reliance*, Dar es Salaam 1967

Tanner Marcel, Kitua Andrew, Degrémont Antoine, *Developing Health Research Capability in Tanzania. From a Swiss Tropical Institute Field Laboratory to the Ifakara Centre of the Tanzanian National Institute of Medical Research*, in: Acta Tropica, Vol. 57, 1994, pp. 153–173

Tanner Marcel et al., *Longitudinal Study on the Health Status of Children in Kikwawila Village, Tanzania: Study Area and Design*, in: Acta Tropica, Vol. 44, 1987, pp. 119–136

Tanner Marcel, De Savigny Don, *Monitoring Community Health Status. Experience from a Case Study in Tanzania*, in: Acta Tropica, Vol. 44, 1987, pp. 260–270

Tanner Marcel, Lukmanji Zohra, *Food Consumption Patterns in a Rural Tanzanian Community (Kikwawila Village, Kilombero District, Morogoro Region) During Lean and Post-Harvest Season*, Tanzania Food and Nutrition Centre Report No. 940, 1985

Tanner Marcel et al., *Community Participation within a Primary Health Care Programme*, in: Tropical Medicine and Parasitology, Vol. 37, 1986, pp. 164–167

Tanner Marcel, *From the Bench to the Field. Control of Parasitic Infections within Primary Health Care*, in: Parasitology, Vol. 99, 1989, pp. 81-92

Tanner Marcel, *Monitoring of Community Health Status. Experience from a Case Study in Tanzania*, in: Acta Tropica, Vol. 44, 1987, pp. 260–270

Tanner Marcel, *Commission pour le Centre Suisse de Recherche Scientifique en Côte-d'Ivoire*, in: Jahrbuch der Schweizerischen Akademie der Naturwissenschaften, Bern 2000, pp. 95–97

Tappan Jennifer, *The True Fiasco. Efforts to Combat Protein Malnutrition in Uganda and the World 1950–1974, Background paper for the Mellon Biennial Zuckerman Conference*, April 2011

Titmuss Richard M., *The Health Services of Tanganyika. A Report to the Government*, London 1964

Walton G. A., *Ornithodorus moubata in Warthog and Porcupine Burrows in Tanganyika Territory*, in: Transactions of the Royal Society of Tropical Medicine and Hygiene, Vol. 47, 1953, pp. 410–411

Widmer Edgar, *Zur Geschichte der schweizerischen ärztlichen Mission in Afrika unter besonderer Berücksichtigung des medizinischen Zentrums von Ifakara, Tanganyika*, Basel 1963

Wiesmann Ernst, *Hermann Mooser 1891–1971*, in: Verhandlungen der Schweizerischen Naturforschenden Gesellschaft (wissenschaftlicher Teil), 152. Jahresversammlung in Luzern, 1972, pp. 322–324

Wilhelm Arthur, *Von den kulturellen Aufgaben Europas in Afrika*, in: Ciba-Blätter, Vol. 170, 1960, pp. 2–11

Wilhelm Rolf, *Auch die Gesundheit gehört zur Entwicklungsarbeit* in: Antenne, Vol. 2, 1976, pp. 1–2

Williams Cicely D., *Kwashiorkor. A Nutritional Disease of Children Associated with a Maize Diet*, in: The Lancet, Vol. 229, 1935, pp. 1151–1152

Wyniger René, *Dr. Dr. h.c. Robert Wiesmann,* in: Mitteilungen der Entomologischen Gesellschaft Basel, 22. Jahrgang 1972, pp. 69–70

Wyniger René, *Aus dem Tagebuch eines Entomologen,* in: Mitteilungsblatt der Tropenschule des Schweizerischen Tropeninstituts in Basel, No. 7, Basel 1959

Von Muralt Alexander, *Colloque pour le 25e anniversaire de la Fondation Ciba "L'Avenir des Fondations Philanthropiques",* Londres, 16-19 juin 1974, 18.07.1974, pp. 1–4

Von Muralt Alexander, *Preface,* in: Von Muralt, (ed.), Protein-Calorie Malnutrition. A Nestlé Foundation Symposium, Berlin 1969

Von Muralt Alexander, *Influence of Early Protein-Calorie Malnutrition on the Intellectual Development. The Point of View of a Physiologist,* in: M. A. B. Brazier (ed.), Growth and Development of the Brain. Nutritional, Genetic and Environmental Factors, New York 1974, pp. 307–314

Zanolli Noa, *Aus der Praxis lernen. Über die Aufgaben der Arbeitsgruppe Gesundheit,* in: Antenne, Vol. 2, 1976, pp. 5–6

Zanolli Noa, *Gesundheitliche Entwicklungszusammenarbeit des Bundes. Anfänge, Erfahrungen und die Projekte heute,* in: Sozial und Präventivmedizin, Vol. 24, 1979, pp. 192–194

Zehnder Andreas, *Agricultural Production in Kikwawila Village, Southeastern Tanzania,* in: Acta Tropica, Vol. 44, 1987, pp. 245–260

Zumstein Adrian, *A Study of Some Factors Influencing the Epidemiology of Urinary Schistosomiasis at Ifakara (Kilombero District, Morogoro Region, Tanzania),* in: Acta Tropica, Vol. 40, No. 3, 1983, pp. 187–204

Newspapers and Online Publications

Brown Phyllida, *Colombia's Malaria Vaccine Approved for Trials,* in: New Scientist, 26.09.1992

Brown Phyllida, *Malaria Vaccine Trials Stalled a Second Time,* in: New Scientist, 21./28.12.1991

Day Michael, *Malaria Vaccine Fails to Deliver,* in: New Scientist, 21.09.1996

Entwicklungshilfe in Tanganjika. Ein Vortrag von Prof. Rudolf Geigy, in: Neue Zürcher Zeitung (NZZ), 05.12.1963

Gates Bill, *The World Must Do More to Conquer Malaria,* in: Financial Times, 22.09.2003

Geigy Rudolf, *Lehrzentrum Ifakara in Südtansania. Völkerverbindende Entwicklungshilfe,* in: Basler Nachrichten, 31.01.1976

Kouassi Joseph, *La Fondation* Nestlé *quitte définitivement la région,* in: Fraternité Matin, Lundi, 21.09.1981

Maurice John, *Impfstoff, Zündstoff,* in: Die Zeit, No. 51, Dezember 1994

Morand Catherine, *Notre institut sous les tropiques africains, in:* Journal de Genève et Gazette de Lausanne, 14./15. décembre 1991

WHO, Report of the Technical Expert Group (TEG) Meeting on Intermittent Preventive Therapy in Infancy (IPTi), Geneva, 8–10 October 2007 Geneva, 8-10 October 2007, pp. 1-12, here: p. 7, http://www.who.int/malaria/publications/atoz/tegconsultiptioct2007report.pdf (accessed 07.03.2011)

WHO, Report of the Technical Consultation on Intermittent Preventive Treatment in Infants (IPTi), Technical Expert Group on Preventive Chemotherapy, 23rd-24th April 2009, WHO/HQ, Geneva, Switzerland, Room D46025, 2009, pp. 1–11, here: p. 2, http://www.who.int/malaria/publications/atoz/tegconsultiptiapr2009report.pdf (accessed 07.03.2011)

WHO, Policy Recommendation on Intermittent Preventive Treatment During Infancy with Sulphadoxine-Pyrimethamine (SP-IPTi) for Plasmodium Falciparum Malaria Control in Africa,
2010, pp. 1-3, here: p. 2, http://www.who.int/malaria/news/WHO_policy_recommendation_
IPTi_032010.pdf (accessed 07.03.2011)

Interviews

Abdulla Salim, Dar es Salaam, 12.02.2009
Aeschlimann André, Rochefort, 21.07.2010, 24.01.2011
Aeschlimann Lily, Rochefort, 21.07.2010
Betsche Peter, Zollikofen, 13.10.2006
Eichenberger Gerhard, Basel, 31.10.2008
Freyvogel Thierry, Arisdorf, 01.12.2008, 21.01.2010
Haerdi Fritz, Binningen, 12.11.2010
Hamisi, Yuna, Dar es Salaam, 28.02.2011
Hunkeler Pierre, Yverdon les Bains, 17.05.2010
Kilama Wenceslaus, Dar es Salaam, 09.02.2011
Kitua Andrew, Geneva, 22.01.2011
Likumi Twaibu, Kikwawila-Kilama, 04.04.2010
Limo Mzee, Kikwawila-Kikwawila, 08.02.2009
Logon Jean, Adiopodoumé, 06.08.2011
Mayombana Charles, Dar es Salaam, 09.02.2011
Mganda Ambros, Ifakara, 09.01.2009
Rahm Urs, Himmelried, 28.04.2009
Schopfer Kurt, Uettligen (BE), 12.04.2012
Tanner Marcel, Basel, 03.02.2012, 30.05.2009
Vogel Peter, Morges, 11.08.2010

Interview with Village Health Workers in Kikwawila, 2009/2010
Interviews with Villagers of Idete, 2010
Interview with Staff and "Users" of Dispensaries in Mingoyo, Mnolela and Nyengedi, 2011
Interview with Staff, National Malaria Control Program, Dar es Salaam, 2011

Publications

Agamben Giorgio, *Homo Sacer. Die Souveränität der Macht und das nackte Leben,* Frankfurt am Main 2003
Alonso Pedro et al., *A Trial of the Synthetic Malaria Vaccine SPf66 in Tanzania. Rationale
and Design,* in: Vaccine, Vol. 12, No. 2, pp. 181–186
Alonso Pedro et al., *Randomized Trial of Efficacy of SPf66 Vaccine Against Plasmodium
Falciparum Malaria in Children in Southern Tanzania,* in: The Lancet, Vol. 344, 1994,
pp. 1175–1181

Amrith Sunil S., *Decolonizing International Health. India and Southeast Asia,* 1930–1965, New York 2006

Anderson Benedict, *Imagined Communities. Reflections on the Origin and Spread of Nationalism,* London, New York 1991

Anderson Warwick, *Colonial Pathologies. American Tropical Medicine, Race, and Hygiene in the Philippines,* Durham, London 2006

Appadurai Arjun, *Modernity at Large. Cultural Dimensions of Globalization,* Minneapolis, London 1996

Arnold David, *Colonizing the Body. State Medicine and Epidemic Disease in Nineteenth-Century India,* Berkeley, Los Angeles 1993

Arnold David, *Medicine and Colonialism,* in: William F. Bynum and Roy Porter *(eds.), Companion Encyclopedia of the History of Medicine,* Vol. 2, London, New York 1993, pp. 1393–1416

Ash Mitchell G., *Wissenschaft und Politik als Ressourcen für einander,* in: Rüdiger vom Bruch and Brigitte Kaderas (eds.), Wissenschaften und Wissenschaftspolitik – Bestandaufnahmen zu Formationen, Brüchen und Kontinuitäten im Deutschland des 20. Jahrhunderts, Stuttgart 2002, pp. 32–51

Augé Marc, *Théorie des pouvoirs et idéologie. Etude de cas en Côte d'Ivoire,* Paris 1975

Banerji Debabar, *Primary Health Care. Selective or Comprehensive,* in: World Health Forum, Vol. 5, No. 4, 1984, pp. 312–315

Banerji Debabar, *Report of the Commission on Health Research for Development and the Countries of the South,* in: International Journal of Health Services, Vol. 22, No. 1, 1992, pp. 169–177

Basalla George, *The Spread of Western Science. A Three-Stage Model Describes the Introduction of Modern Science into any Non-European Nation,* in: Science, Vol. 156, No. 3775, 1967, pp. 611–622

Bates Margaret, *Tanganyika. The Development of a Trust Territory,* in: International Organization, Vol. 9, No. 1, 1955, pp. 32–51

Bayart Jean-François, *Réflexions sur la politique africaine de la France,* in: Politique Africaine, Vol. 58, 1995, pp. 41–50

Bayart Jean-François, *France-Afrique. La fin du pacte colonial,* in: Politique Africaine, Vol. 39, 1990, pp. 47–53

Becker Felicitas, *A Social History of Southeast Tanzania 1890–1950,* PhD Study Cambridge University, Cambridge 2002

Behrendt Richard, *Die Schweiz und der Imperialismus. Die Volkswirtschaft des hochkapitalistischen Kleinstaates im Zeitalter des politischen und ökonomischen Nationalismus,* Zürich 1932

Bell Heather, *Frontiers of Medicine in the Anglo-Egyptian Sudan,* 1899–1940, Oxford 1999

Bhabha Homi, *The Location of Culture,* London 1994

Birn Anne-Emanuelle, *Gates's Grandest Challenge. Transcending Technology as Public Health Ideology,* in: Lancet, Vol. 366, No. 9484, 2005, pp. 514–519

Bloch Marc, *L'étrange défaite. Témoignage écrit en 1940,* Paris 1946

Bonfoh Bassirou et al., *Research in a War Zone,* in: Nature, Vol. 474, 2011, pp. 569–571

Bonneuil Christophe, *Development as Experiment. Science and State Building in Late Colonial and Postcolonial Africa, 1930–1970,* in: Roy MacLeod (ed.), Nature and Empire. Science and the Colonial Enterprise, Chicago 2001, pp. 258–281

Bonneuil Christophe, Petitjean Patrick, *Les chemins de la création de l'ORSTOM. Du Front Populaire à la libération en passant par Vichy, 1936–1945,* in: Patrick Petitjean (ed.), Les sciences coloniales. Figures et institutions, Paris 1996 (Série sous la Direction de Roland Waast), pp. 113–161

Brown Theodore, Cueto Marcos, Fee Elizabeth, *The World Health Organization and the Transition from "International" to "Global" Public Health,* in: American Journal of Public Health, Vol. 96, No. 1, 2006, pp. 62–72

Brown Peter J., *Failure-As-Success. Multiple Meanings of Eradication in the Rockefeller Foundation Sardinia Project, 1946–1951,* in: Parassitologia, Vol. 40, No. 1-2, 1998, pp. 117–130

Brown Peter J., *Malaria, Miseria, and Underpopulation in Sardinia. The "Malaria Blocks Development" Cultural Model,* in: Medical Anthropology, Vol. 17, No. 3, 1997, pp. 239–254

Bruchhausen Walter, *Medizin zwischen den Welten. Geschichte und Gegenwart des medizinischen Pluralismus im südöstlichen Tansania,* Bonn 2006

Bryceson Deborah F., *Agrarian Fundamentalism or Foresight? Revisiting Nyerere's Vision for Rural Tanzania,* in: Kjell Havnevik and Aida C. Isinika (eds.), Tanzania in Transition. From Nyerere to Mkapa, Dar es Salaam 2010, pp. 71–98

Bucher Erwin, *Zwischen Bundesrat und General. Schweizer Politik und Armee im Zweiten Weltkrieg,* Zürich 1993

Bürgi Jürg, Imfeld Al, *Mehr geben, weniger nehmen. Geschichte der Schweizer Entwicklungspolitik und der Novartis Stiftung für Nachhaltige Entwicklung,* Zürich 2004

Büschel Hubertus, Speich Daniel, *Einleitung – Konjunkturen, Probleme und Perspektiven der Globalgeschichte von Entwicklungszusammenarbeit,* in: Büschel and Speich (eds.), Entwicklungswelten. Globalgeschichte der Entwicklungszusammenarbeit, Frankfurt am Main 2009, pp. 7–29

Buse Kent, Harmer Andrew, *Power to the Partners? The Politics of Public-Private Health Partnerships,* in: Development, Vol. 47, No. 2, 2004, pp. 49–56

Carpenter Kenneth J., *Protein and Energy. A Study of Changing Ideas in Nutrition,* Cambridge 1994

Cetina Karin Knorr, *Epistemic Cultures. How the Sciences Make Knowledge,* Cambridge, London 1999

Chabal Patrick, *Power in Africa. An Essay in Political Interpretation,* London 1992

Chafer Tony, *The End of Empire in French West Africa. France's Successful Decolonization?,* Oxford 2002

Chagula Wilbert, Tarimo Eleuther, *Meeting Basic Health Needs in Tanzania,* in: Kenneth W. Newell (ed.), Health By the People, Geneva 1975, pp. 145–168

Chambers David Wade, Gillespie Richard, *Locality in the History of Science. Colonial Science, Technoscience, and Indigenous Knowledge,* in: Osiris, Vol. 15, 2001, pp. 221–240

Charlesworth Max et al., *Life Among the Scientists. An Anthropological Study of an Australian Scientific Community,* Oxford 1989

Clarke Sabine, *A Technocratic Imperial State? The Colonial Office and Scientific Research,* 1940–1960, in: Twentieth Century British History, Vol. 18, No. 4, 2007, pp. 453–480

Conklin Alice L., *A Mission to Civilize. The Republican Idea of Empire in France and West Africa, 1895–1930,* Stanford 1997

Conrad Sebastian, Osterhammel Jürgen (eds.), *Das Kaiserreich transnational. Deutschland in der Welt, 1871–1914,* Göttingen 2004

Cooper Frederick, *Modernizing Bureaucrats, Backward Africans, and the Development Concept,* in: Cooper and Randall Packard (eds.), International Development and the Social Sciences. Essays on the History and Politics of Knowledge, Berkeley 1997, pp. 64–92

Cooper Frederick, *Africa since 1940. The Past of the Present,* Cambridge 2002

Cooper Frederick, *Decolonization and African Society. The Labor Question in French and British Africa,* Cambridge 2005

Cooper Frederick, *Writing the History of Development,* in: Journal of Modern European History, Vol. 8, No. 1, 2010, pp. 5–23

Cooper Frederick, Stoler Ann Laura, *Between Metropole and the Colony. Rethinking a Research Agenda,* in: Cooper and Stoler (eds.), Tensions of Empire. Colonial Cultures in a Bourgeois World, Berkeley, Los Angeles, London 1997, pp. 1–56

Coquery-Vidrovitch Catherine, *L'impact des intérêts coloniaux. SCOA et CFAO dans l'Ouest Africain, 1910–1965,* in: Journal of African History, Vol. 16, No. 4, pp. 595–621

Coulson Andrew, *Tanzania. A Political Economy,* Oxford 1982

Crook Richard C., *Politics, the Cocoa Crisis, and Administration in Côte d'Ivoire,* in: The Journal of Modern African Studies, Vol. 28, No. 4, 1990, pp. 649–669

Crouch Susan C., *Western Responses to Tanzanian Socialism, 1967–1983,* Aldershot 1987

Cueto Marcos, *The Origins of Primary Health Care and Selective Primary Health Care,* in: American Journal of Public Health, Vol. 94, No. 11, 2004, pp. 1864–1874

Curtin Philip D., *The Image of Africa. British Ideas and Action, 1780–1850,* Madison 1964

Daniel Ute, *Einleitung: Kulturgeschichte – und was sie nicht ist,* in: Daniel, Kompendium Kulturgeschichte. Theorien, Praxis, Schlüsselwörter, Frankfurt am Main 2001, pp. 7–25

David Thomas, Etemad Bouda, *Gibt es einen schweizerischen Imperialismus?,* in: Traverse. Schweiz-"Dritte Welt." Von der Expansion zur Dominanz, No. 2, 1998, pp. 17–27

David Thomas, Etemad Bouda, *L'expansion économique de la Suisse en Outre-mer (XIXe-XXe siècles). Un état de la question,* in: Schweizerische Zeitschrift für Geschichte, Vol. 46, No. 2, 1996, pp. 226–231

Deleuze Gilles, *Was ist ein Dispositiv?,* in: François Ewald and Bernhard Waldenfels (eds.), Spiele der Wahrheit. Michel Foucaults Denken, Frankfurt am Main 1991, pp. 153–162

Desowitz Robert E., *The Malaria Capers. More Tales of Parasites and People, Research and Reality,* New York 1991

Dieng Alioune, *La Suisse et l'Afrique au lendemain des indépendances. Le cas de la Côte d'Ivoire,* Mémoire de Master en Etudes Internationales (MEI), Histoire et Politique Internationale (HPI), Graduate Institute Geneva, 2010

Dirks Nicholas B., *Introduction. Colonialism and Culture,* in: Dirks (ed.), Colonialism and Culture, Michigan 1992, pp. 1–25

Dreier Marcel, *Healthcare, Welfare, and Development in Rural Africa. The Case of the Catholic Health Services in Ifakara/Tanzania in the 20th Century,* PhD University of Basel 2014 [forthcoming]

Driver Felix, Martins Luciana (eds.), *Tropical Visions in an Age of Empire,* Chicago 2005

Eckert Andreas, *Herrschen und Verwalten. Afrikanische Bürokraten, staatliche Ordnung und Politik in Tansania, 1920–1970,* München 2007

Eckert Andreas, *Kolonialismus,* Frankfurt am Main 2006

Eckert Andreas, *Regulating the Social. Social Security, Social Welfare, and the State in Late Colonial Tanzania,* in: Journal of African History, Vol. 45, 2004, pp. 467–489

Eckert Andreas, *"Tropics",* in: Akira Iriye and Pierre-Yves Saunier (eds.), Palgrave Dictionary of Transnational History, Basingstoke, London 2009, pp. 1059–1061

Ellis Stephen, *Writing Histories of Contemporary Africa,* in: Journal of African History, Vol. 43, 2002, pp. 1–26

Escobar Arturo, *Encountering Development. The Making and Unmaking of the Third World,* Princeton 1995

Espagne Michel, *Au-delà du comparatisme,* in: Espagne, Les transferts culturels franco-allemands, Paris 1999

Etemad Bouda, *Le commerce extérieur de la Suisse avec le tiers monde aux XIXe et XXe siècles. Une perspective comparative internationale,* in: Les Annuelles. La Suisse sur la ligne bleue de l'Outre-mer, Vol. 5, Lausanne 1994, pp. 19–41

Etemad Bouda, *Structure géographique du commerce entre la Suisse et le Tiers Monde au XXe siècle,* in: Paul Bairoch and Martin Körner (eds.), Die Schweiz in der Weltwirtschaft – La Suisse dans l'économie mondiale, Zürich 1990, pp. 165–183

Fairhead James, *Public Engagement with Science? Local Understandings of a Vaccine Trial in the Gambia,* in: Journal of Biosocial Science, Vol. 38, 2006, pp. 103–116

Fairhead James, *Where Techno-Science Meets Poverty. Medical Research and the Economy of Blood in the Gambia,* in: Social Science and Medicine, Vol. 63, 2000, pp. 1109–1120

Feierman Steven, *Struggles for Control. The Social Roots of Health and Healing in Modern Africa,* in: African Studies Review, Vol. 28, No. 2–3, 1985, pp. 73–147

Ferguson James, Gupta Akhil, *Spatializing States. Towards an Ethnography of Neoliberal Governmentality,* in: American Ethnologist, Vol. 29, No. 4, 2002, pp. 981–1002

Ferguson James, *Expectations of Modernity. Myths and Meanings of Urban Life on the Zambian Copperbelt,* Berkeley 1999

Ferguson James, *Global Disconnect. Abjection and the Aftermath of Modernism,* in: Peter Geschiere, Birgit Meyer and Peter Pels (eds.), Reading in Modernities in Africa, Bloomington, Indiana 2008, pp. 1–8

Ferguson James, *Transnational Topographies of Power. Beyond «the State» and «Civil Society» in the Study of African Politics,* in: Ferguson, Global Shadows. Africa in the Neoliberal World Order, Durham, London 2006, pp. 89–112

Fischer-Tiné Harald, *Low and Licentious Europeans. Race, Class and "White Subalternity" in Colonial India,* New Delhi 2009

Fisher Eleanor, Arce Alberto, *The Spectacle of Modernity. Blood, Microscopes, and Mirrors in Colonial Tanganyika,* in: Arce and Norman Long (eds.), Anthropology, Development and Modernities. Exploring Discourses, Counter-Tendencies and Violence, London, New York 2000, pp. 74–99

Fleury Antoine, Joye Frédéric, *Die Anfänge der Forschungspolitik in der Schweiz. Gründungsgeschichte des Schweizerischen Nationalfonds zur Förderung der wissenschaftlichen Forschung 1934–1952,* Baden 2002

Fleury Antoine, *La Suisse et la préparation à l'après-guerre,* in: Michel Dumoulin (ed.), Plans des temps de guerre pour l'Europe d'après-guerre, 1940–1947 – Wartime Plans for Postwar Europe 1940–1947, Bruxelles 1995, pp. 175–195

Fluri Branka, *Umbruch in Organisation und Konzeption. Die technische Zusammenarbeit beim Bund, 1958–1970,* in: Peter Hug and Beatrix Mesmer (eds.), Von der Entwicklungshilfe zur Entwicklungspolitik, Studien und Quellen, Vol. 19, Bern 1993, pp. 382–393

Ford John, *The Role of the Trypanosomiases in African Ecology. A Study of the TseTse Fly Problem,* Oxford 1971

Förster Till, Lucy Koechlin, *The Politics of Governance. Power and Agency in the Formation of Political Order in Africa,* in: Basel Papers on Political Transformations, No. 1, 2011, pp. 1–24

Franc Andrea, *Wie die Schweiz zur Schokolade kam. Der Kakaohandel der Basler Handelsgesellschaft mit der Kolonie Goldküste, 1893–1960,* Basel 2008

Garrett Laurie, *The Coming Plague. Newly Emerging Diseases in a World Out of Balance,* New York 1994

Geissler Wenzel, Molyneux Catherine (eds.), *Evidence, Ethos and Experiment. The Anthropology and History of Medical Research in Africa,* New York, Oxford 2011

Geissler Wenzel, *He is Like a Brother I can Even Give Him Some Blood. Relational Ethics and Material Exchanges in a Malaria Vaccine "Trial Community" in the Gambia,* in: Social Science and Medicine, Vol. 67, 2006, pp. 696–707

Gilomen Hans-Jörg, Müller Margrit, Tissot Laurent (eds.), *Dienstleistungen. Expansion und Transformation des "dritten Sektors" (15.–20. Jahrhundert) – Les services. Essor et transformation du "secteur tertiaire" (15ᵉ–20ᵉ siècles),* Zürich 2007, pp. 319–327

Gish Oscar, *Planning the Health Sector. The Tanzanian Experience,* London 1975

Gosling R. D. et al., *Protective Efficacy and Safety of Three Antimalarial Regimens for Intermittent Preventive Treatment for Malaria in Infants. A Randomized, Double-Blind, Placebo-Controlled Trial,* in: Lancet, Vol. 374, 2009, pp. 1521–1532

Graboyes Melissa, *Surveying the "Pathological Museum." A History of Medical Research Ethics in East Africa, 1940–1965,* PhD Boston University 2010

Graf Christoph, *Die Schweiz und die Dritte Welt. Die Anerkennungspraxis und Beziehungsaufnahme der Schweiz gegenüber dekolonisierten aussereuropäischen Staaten sowie die Anfänge der schweizerischen Entwicklungshilfe nach 1945,* in: Studien und Quellen, No. 12, Bern 1986, pp. 37–112

Green Maia, *Participatory Development and the Appropriation of Agency in Southern Tanzania,* in: Critique of Anthropology, Vol. 20, No. 1, 2000, pp. 67–89

Green Maia, *Priests, Witches and Power. Popular Christianity After Mission in Southern Tanzania,* Cambridge 2003

Green Maia, *Public Reform and the Privatisation of Poverty. Some Institutional Determinants of Health Seeking Behaviour in Southern Tanzania,* in: Culture, Medicine and Psychiatry, Vol. 24, 2000, pp. 403–430

Hall Budd L., *Mtu ni Afya – Man is Health. Tanzania's Health Campaign,* Washington 1978

Harries Patrick, *Butterflies and Barbarians. Swiss Missionaries and Systems of Knowledge in South-East Africa,* Oxford 2007

Harries Patrick, *Field Sciences in Scientific Fields. Entomology, Botany and the Early Ethnographic Monograph in the Work of H.-A. Junod,* in: Saul Dubow (ed.), Science and Society in Southern Africa, Manchester, New York 2000, pp. 11–41

Harries Patrick, Miescher Giorgio, *Immer etwas Neues aus Afrika. Einige Überlegungen zur Geschichte Afrikas in Basel,* in: Regio Basiliensis, Vol. 45, No. 2, 2004, pp. 87–97

Harrison Mark, *Disease and the Modern World. 1500 to the Present Day,* Cambridge 2004

Hausmann Muela Susanne, *Community Understanding of Malaria, and Treatment-Seeking Behavior in a Holoendemic Area of Southeastern Tanzania,* PhD Study University of Basel, Basel 2000

Havinden Michael, Meredith David, *Colonialism and Development. Britain and its Tropical Colonies, 1859–1960,* London, New York 1993

Hayden Cori, *Taking as Giving. Bioscience, Exchange, and the Politics of Benefit-Sharing,* in: Social Studies of Science, Vol. 37, No. 5, 2007, pp. 729–758

Headrick Daniel R., *The Tools of Empire. Technology and European Imperialism in the Nineteenth Century,* New York 1981

Hecht Gabrielle, *Introduction,* in: Hecht (ed.), Entangled Geographies. Empire and Technopolitics in the Global Cold War, Cambridge, Massachusetts, London 2011

Hecht Gabrielle, *Rupture-Talk in the Nuclear Age. Conjugating Colonial Power in Africa,* in: Social Studies of Science, Vol. 32, No. 5-6, 2002, pp. 691–727

Heesen Anke te, Spary E. C., *Sammeln als Wissen,* in: Anke te Heesen and E. C. Spary (eds.), Sammeln als Wissen. Das Sammeln und seine wissenschaftsgeschichtliche Bedeutung, Göttingen 2001, pp. 7–21

Hesse Philippe-Jean, Jean-Pierre Le Crom (eds.), *La protection sociale sous le régime de Vichy,* Rennes 2001

Hillier S. M., *Preventive Health Work in the People's Republic of China, 1949-82,* in: Hillier and J. A. Jewell (eds.), Health Care and Traditional Medicine in China, 1800–1982, London 1983, pp. 149–217

Hoag Heather J., *Transplanting the TVA? International Contributions to Postwar River Development in Tanzania,* in: Comparative Technology Transfer and Society, Vol. 4, No. 3, 2006, pp. 247–268

Hodge Joseph Morgan, *Triumph of the Expert. Agrarian Doctrines of Development and the Legacies of British Colonialism,* Athens 2007

Holdgate Martin, *The Green Web. A Union for World Conservation,* London 1999

Holenstein René, *Was kümmert uns die Dritte Welt. Zur Geschichte der internationalen Solidarität in der Schweiz,* Zürich 1998

Holenstein René, *Wer langsam geht kommt weit. Ein halbes Jahrhundert Schweizer Entwicklungshilfe,* Zürich 2010

Hug Peter, Mesmer Beatrix (eds.), *Von der Entwicklungshilfe zur Entwicklungspolitik,* Studien und Quellen, Vol. 19, Bern 1993

Humphreys Margaret, *Kicking a Dying Dog. DDT and the Demise of Malaria in the American South,* 1942–1950, in: Isis, Vol. 87, No. 1, 1996, pp. 1–17

Hunt Nancy Rose, *A Colonial Lexicon. Of Birth Ritual, Medicalization, and Mobility in the Congo,* Durham, London 1999

Hunt Nancy Rose, *"Le Bébé en Brousse". European Women, African Birth Spacing and Colonial Intervention in Breast Feeding in the Belgian Congo,* in: The International Journal of African Historical Studies, Vol. 21, No. 3, 1988, pp. 401–432

Iliffe John, *A Modern History of Tanganyika,* Cambridge 1979

Iliffe John, *East African Doctors. A History of the Modern Profession,* Cambridge 1998

Illies Joachim, *Das Geheimnis des Lebendigen. Leben und Werk des Biologen Adolf Portmann,* München 1976

Jacobs Nancy, *The Intimate Politics of Ornithology in Colonial Africa,* in: Comparative Studies in Society and History, Vol. 48, 2006, pp. 564–603

Jeffries Charles, *A Review of Colonial Research, 1940–1960,* London 1964

Jennings Michael, *"A Very Real War." Popular Participation in Development in Tanzania During the 1950s & 1960s,* in: The International Journal of African Historical Studies, Vol. 40, No. 1, 2007, pp. 71–95

Jennings Michael, *"Development is Very Political in Tanzania." Oxfam & the Chunya Integrated Development Programme, 1972–1976,* in: Ondine Barrow and Michael Jennings (eds.), The Charitable Impulse. NGOs and Development in East and North-East Africa, Oxford, Bloomfield CT 2001, pp. 109–132

Jennings Michael, *Surrogates of the State. Oxfam and Development in Tanzania, 1961–1979,* London 1998

Jennings Michael, *We Must Run While Others Walk. Popular Participation and Development Crisis in Tanzania, 1961-1969,* in: Journal of Modern African Studies, Vol. 41, No. 2, 2003, pp. 163–187

Joye-Cagnard Frédéric, *La construction de la politique de la science en Suisse. Enjeux scientifiques, stratégiques et politiques (1944–1974),* Neuchâtel 2010

Kaelble Hartmut, *Die Debatte über Vergleich und Transfer und was jetzt?*, in: H-Soz-u-Kult, 08.02.2005, http://hsozkult.geschichte.hu-berlin.de/forum/id=574&type=artikel (accessed, 15.03.2012)

Kägi Ulrich, *Die Schweizerische Entwicklungshilfe*, in: Entwicklungsländer (BRD), Vol. 5, 1960, pp. 150–152

Kalt Monica, *Tiersmondismus in der Schweiz der 1960er und 1970er Jahre. Von der Barmherzigkeit zur Solidarität*, Bern 2010

Kamat Vinay, *Cultural Interpretations of the Efficacy and Side-Effects of Antimalarials in Tanzania*, in: Anthropology of Medicine, Vol. 16, No. 3, 2009, pp. 293–305

Kamat Vinay, *"This Is Not Our Culture!" Discourses of Nostalgia and Narratives of Health Concerns in Post-Socialist Tanzania*, in: Africa, Vol. 78, No. 3, 2008, pp. 359–383

Katzenstein Peter J., *Corporatism and Change. Austria, Switzerland and the Politics of Industry*, New York 1984

Kaufmann Lyonel, *Guillaume Tell au Congo. L'expansion Suisse au Congo Belge, 1930–1960*, in: Bouda Etemad and Thomas David (eds.), Les Annuelles. La Suisse sur la ligne bleue de l'Outre-mer, Vol. 5, 1994, pp. 43–94

Keese Alexander, *First Lessons in Neo-Colonialism. The Personalisation of Relations between African Politicians and French Officials in Sub-Saharan Africa, 1956–1966*, in: The Journal of Imperial and Commonwealth History, Vol. 35, No. 4, 2007, pp. 593–613

Kilama W., Nhonoli A. M., Makene W. J., *Health Care Delivery in Tanzania*, in: Gabriel Ruhumbika (ed.), Towards Ujamaa. 20 Years of TANU Leadership. A Contribution of the University of Dar es Salaam to the 20th Anniversary of TANU, Kampala 1974, pp. 191–217

King Nicholas B., *Security, Disease, Commerce. Ideologies of Postcolonial Global Health*, in: Social Studies of Science, Vol. 32, No. 5-6, 2002, pp. 763–789

Kiondo Andrew, *Structural Adjustment and Non-Governmental Organizations in Tanzania. A Case Study*, in: Peter Gibbon (ed.), Social Change and Economic Reform in Africa, Uppsala 1993, pp. 161–183

Kipré Pierre, *Memorial de la Côte d'Ivoire. La Côte d'Ivoire Coloniale*, Abidjan 1988

Kirby Maurice W., *Operational Research in War and Peace. The British Experience from the 1930s to 1970*, London, Birmingham 2003

Kirchberger Ulrike, *German Scientists in the Indian Forest Service. A German Contribution to the Raj?*, in: Journal of Imperial and Commonwealth History, Vol. 29, 2001, pp. 1–26

Kiwara Angwara D., *Health and Health Care in Structurally Adjusting Tanzania*, in: Lucian Msambichaka, Humphrey P.B. Moshi and Fidelis P. Mtatifikolo (eds.), Development Challenges and Strategies for Tanzania. An Agenda for the 21st Century, Dar es Salaam 1994, pp. 296–290

Kjekshus Helge, *Ecological Control and Economic Development in East African History. The Case of Tanganyika 1850–1950*, London 1977

Kocka Jürgen, Haupt Heinz-Gerhard, *Comparison and Beyond. Traditions, Scope, and Perspectives of Comparative History*, in: Kocka and Haupt (eds.), Comparative and Transnational History. Central European Approaches and New Perspectives, New York 2009, pp. 1–32

Kohler Robert E., Kuklick Henrika, *Introduction*, in: Kohler and Kuklick (eds.), Science in the Field, Osiris, Vol. 11, 1996, pp. 1–14

Kuhn Konrad, *Entwicklungspolitische Solidarität. Die Dritte-Welt-Bewegung in der Schweiz zwischen Kritik und Politik, 1975–1992*, Zürich 2011

Lachenal Guillaume, *Biomédecine et décolonisation au Cameroun, 1944–1994. Technologies, figures et institutions médicales à l'épreuve.* Thèse de doctorat Université Paris 7 – Denis Diderot, Paris 2006

Lachenal Guillaume, *Franco-African Familiarities. A History of the Pasteur Institute of Cameroon, 1945–2000,* in: Mark Harrison, Margaret Jones, Helen Sweet (eds.), From Western Medicine to Global Medicine. The Hospital Beyond the West, New Delhi 2009, pp. 441–444

Lachenal Guillaume, *Le médecin qui voulut être roi. Médecine coloniale et utopie au Cameroun,* in: Annales HSS, Vol. 1, 2010, pp. 121–156

Lachenal Guillaume, *L'invention africaine de l'écologie française. Histoire de la station de Lamto (Côte d'Ivoire), 1942–1976,* in: La Revue pour l'histoire du CNRS, Vol. 13, 2005, pp. 1–15

Langwick Stacey, *Geographies of Medicine. Interrogating the Boundary between "Traditional" and "Modern" Medicine in Colonial Tanganyika,* in: Tracy J. Luedke and Harry G. West (eds.), Borders and Healers. Brokering Therapeutic Resources in Southwest Africa, Bloomington, Indianapolis 2006, pp. 143–165

Larson Lorne, *A History of the Mahenge (Ulanga) District, 1860–1957,* PhD Study University of Dar es Salaam, Dar es Salaam 1976

Latour Bruno, Woolgar Steve, *Laboratory Life. The Construction of Scientific Facts,* Princeton 1986

Leach Melissa, Fairhead James, *Vaccine Anxieties. Global Science, Child Health and Society,* London 2007

Lengeler Christian, DeSavigny Don, Cattani Jacqueline, *From Research to Implementation,* in: Lengeler, DeSavigny, Cattani (eds.), Net Gain. A New Method for Preventing Malaria Deaths, Geneva 1996, pp. 1–15

Lengwiler Martin, *Risikopolitik im Sozialstaat. Die schweizerische Unfallversicherung 1870–1970,* Köln 2006

Lenzin René, *Schweizer im kolonialen und postkolonialen Afrika. Statistische Übersicht und zwei Fallbeispiele,* in: Studien und Quellen, Vol. 28, Die Auslandschweizer im 20. Jahrhundert – Les Suisses de l'étranger au XXème siècle, Bern, Stuttgart, Wien 2002, pp. 299–326

Liebenow Gus J., *Colonial Rule and Political Development in Tanzania. The Case of the Makonde,* Evanston 1971

Lienhard Marina, *"Abenteurer sterben aus." Weisssein, Othering und Tropendiskurs in den Schriften und Korrespondenzen der Schweizerischen Tropenschule und ihrer ehemaligen Schüler (1943-1981),* MA thesis University of Zürich 2013

Lilienfeld Robert, *The Rise of Systems Theory. An Ideological Analysis,* New York, Chichester, Brisbane, Toronto 1978

Litsios Socrates, *The Long and Difficult Road to Alma-Ata. A Personal Reflection,* in: International Journal of Health Services, Vol. 32, 2002, pp. 709–732

Livingstone David, *Putting Science in Its Place. Geographies of Scientific Knowledge,* Chicago 2003

Lohrmann Ulrich, *Voices from Tanganyika. Great Britain, the United Nations and the Decolonization of a Trust Territory, 1946–1961,* Berlin 2007

Lorcin Patricia M. E., *Imperialism, Colonial Identity, and Race in Algeria, 1830–1870. The Role of the French Medical Corps,* in: Isis, Vol. 90, No. 4, 1999, pp. 653–679

Losch Bruno, *Libéralisation économique et crise politique en Côte d'Ivoire,* in: Critique Internationale, Vol. 19, No. 2, 2003, pp. 48–60

Losch Bruno, *Côte d'Ivoire, la tentation ethnonationaliste,* in: Politique Africaine, Vol. 78, 2000, pp. 5–25

Low Anthony, Lonsdale John, *Towards the New Order, 1945–1963,* in: Low and Alison Smith (eds.), History of East Africa, Vol. 3, 1976, pp. 12–16

Löwy Ilana, *Yellow Fever in Rio de Janeiro and the Pasteur Institute Mission (1901–1905). The Transfer of Science to the Periphery,* in: Medical History, Vol. 34, 1990, pp. 144–163

Luck Murray James, *Science in Switzerland,* New York, London 1967

Lyons Maryinez, *From "Death Camps" to Cordon Sanitaire. The Development of Sleeping Sickness Policy in the Uele District of the Belgian Congo, 1903–1914,* in: Journal of African History, Vol. 26, No. 1, 1985, pp. 69–91

Lyons Maryinez, *The Colonial Disease. A Social History of Sleeping Sickness in Northern Zaire, 1800–1940*, Cambridge 1992

MacLeod Roy, Milton Lewis, *Disease, Medicine and Empire,* London 1988

MacLeod Kirsten, *Creation of First Malaria Vaccine Raises Troubling Questions about "Intellectual Racism",* in: Canadian Medical Association Journal, Vol. 153, No. 9, 1995, pp. 1319–1321

Mandara M.P., *Health Services in Tanzania. A Historical Overview,* in: G. M. P. Mwaluko et al. (eds.), Health and Disease in Tanzania, London, New York 1991, pp. 1–7

Manzi Fatuma et al., *Intermittent Preventive Treatment for Malaria and Anaemia Control in Tanzanian Infants. The Development and Implementation of a Public Health Strategy,* in: Transactions of the Royal Society of Tropical Medicine and Hygiene, Vol. 103, No. 1, 2009, pp. 79–86

Marchesin Philippe, *La politique africaine de la France en transition, in:* Politique Africaine, Vol. 71, 1998, pp. 91–106

Marjanen Jani, *Undermining Methodological Nationalism. Histoire croisée of Concepts as Transnational History,* in: Mathias Albert et al. (eds.), Transnational Political Spaces. Agents – Structures – Encounters, Frankfurt, New York 2009, pp. 239–263

Marks Shula, *What is Colonial about Colonial Medicine? And What has Happened to Imperialism and Health?,* in: Social History and Medicine, Vol. 10, No. 2, 1997, pp. 205–219

Marsland Rebecca, *Community Participation the Tanzanian Way. Conceptual Contiguity or Power Struggle?,* in: Oxford Development Studies, Vol. 34, No. 1, 2006, pp. 65–79

Matzinger Albert, *Die Anfänge der schweizerischen "Entwicklungshilfe" 1948–1961,* Bern, Stuttgart 1991

Mayombo Rudolf Peter, *Economic Structural Changes and Population Migration in Kilombero Valley,* PhD Study University of Dar es Salaam, Dar es Salaam 1990

Mazrui Ali A., *Tanzaphilia,* in: Transition, Vol. 31, 1967, pp. 20–26

Mbembe Achille, *The Power of the Archive and its Limits,* in: Carolyn Hamilton et al. (eds.), Refiguring the Archive, Dordrecht, Boston, London 2002, pp. 19–26

Mbosa Mkeli, *Colonial Production and Underdevelopment in Ulanga District, 1894–1950,* Dar es Salaam 1988

McCulloch Jock, *Colonial Psychiatry and the African Mind,* Cambridge 1995

Meier Lukas, *The Other's Colony. Switzerland and the Discovery of Côte d'Ivoire,* in: Patricia Purtschert, Harald Fischer-Tiné (eds.), Colonial Encounters of the Swiss Kind. Imperial Entanglements and Postcolonial Assemblages, Cambridge 2014 (forthcoming)

Meier Lukas, *Die Macht des Empfängers. Gesundheit als Verhandlungsgegenstand zwischen der Schweiz und Tansania, 1970–1980,* in: Sara Elmer, Konrad Kuhn, Daniel Speich Chassé (eds.), Handlungsfeld Entwicklung. Schweizer Erwartungen und Erfahrung in der Geschichte der Entwicklungsarbeit, Itinera, Vol. 35, Basel 2014, pp. 125–144

Minder Patrick, *La Suisse coloniale? Les représentations de l'Afrique et des Africains en Suisse au temps des colonies, 1880–1939,* Bern 2011

Minja Happiness, *Introducing Insecticide Treated Mosquito Nets in the Kilombero Valley (Tanzania). Social and Cultural Dimensions,* PhD Study University of Basel, Basel 2001

Monson Jamie, *Africa's Freedom Railway. How a Chinese Development Project Changed Lives and Livelihoods in Tanzania,* Bloomington, Indiana 2009

Monson Jamie, *Rice and Cotton, Ritual and Resistance. Cash Cropping in Colonial Tanganyika, 1920–1940,* in: Allan Isaacman and Richard Roberts (eds.), Cotton, Colonialism and Social History in Sub-Saharan Africa, Portsmouth, London 1995, pp. 268–284

Monson Jamie, *The Tribal Past and the Politics of Nationalism in Mahenge District, 1940–1960,* in: Gregory H. Maddox and James Giblin (eds.), In Search of a Nation. Histories of Authority and Dissidence in Tanzania, Oxford, Dar es Salaam, Athens 2005, pp. 103–113

Munishi Gaspar K., *Intervening to Address Constraints through Health Sector Reforms in Tanzania. Some Gains and the Unfinished Business,* in: Journal of International Development, Vol. 15, No. 1, 2003, pp. 115–131

Murray Christopher, Lopez Alan (eds.), *The Global Burden of Disease. A Comprehensive Assessment of Mortality and Disability from Diseases, Injuries and Risk Factors in 1990 and Projected to 2020,* Cambridge 1996

Mushi Adiel, *Reaching the Poorest Children in Rural Southern Tanzania. Socio-Cultural Perspectives for Delivery and Uptake of Preventive Child Health Interventions,* PhD Study London School of Hygiene & Tropical Medicine, London 2009

Nader Laura, *Up the Anthropologist – Perspectives Gained from Studying Up,* in: Dell Hymes (ed.), Reinventing Anthropology, New York 1969, pp. 284–311

Niangoran-Bouah G., *Les Ebrié et leur organisation politique traditionnelle,* in: Annales de l'Université d'Abidjan (Ethnosociologie), Vol. 1, No. 1, 1969, pp. 51–91

Nosten François et al., *Randomized Double-Blind Placebo-Controlled Trial of SPf66 Malaria Vaccine in Children in Northwestern Thailand,* in: The Lancet, Vol. 348, No. 9029, 1996 pp. 701–707

Nugent Paul, *Africa Since Independence,* Basingstoke 2004

Osterhammel Jürgen, *Transkulturell vergleichende Geschichtswissenschaft,* in: Osterhammel, Geschichtswissenschaft jenseits des Nationalstaats. Studien zu Beziehungsgeschichte und Zivilisationsvergleich, Göttingen 2003, pp. 11–45

Osterhammel Jürgen, *Transnationale Gesellschaftsgeschichte. Erweiterung oder Alternative,* in: Geschichte und Gesellschaft, Vol. 27, No. 3, 2001, pp. 464–479

Packard Randall, *Malaria Dreams. Visions of Health and Development in the Third World,* in: Medical Anthropology, Vol. 17, 1997, pp. 279–296

Packard Randall, *The Making of a Tropical Disease. A Short History of Malaria,* Baltimore 2007

Packard Randall, *Visions of Postwar Health and Development and Their Impact on Public Health Interventions in the Developing World,* in: Cooper and Packard (eds.), International Development and the Social Sciences. Essays on the History and Politics of Knowledge, Berkeley 1997, pp. 93–115

Patel Kiran Klaus, *Nach der Nationalfixiertheit. Perspektiven einer transnationalen Geschichte.* Öffentliche Antrittsvorlesung an der Humboldt-Universität zu Berlin, Berlin 2004

Paulmann Johannes, *Internationaler Vergleich und interkultureller Transfer. Zwei Forschungsansätze zur europäischen Geschichte des 18. bis 20. Jahrhunderts,* in: Historische Zeitschrift, Vol. 267, 1998, pp. 649–685

Perrenoud Marc, *Guerres, indépendance, neutralité et opportunités. Quelques jalons historiques pour l'analyse des relations économiques de la Suisse avec l'Afrique (des années 1920 aux années 1960),* in: Suisse-Afrique (18e–20e siècles). De la traite des Noirs à la fin du régime de l'Apartheid, Münster 2005, pp. 85–104

Person Yves, *French West Africa and Decolonization,* in: Prosser Gifford and W. M. Roger Louis (eds.), The Transfer of Power in Africa. Decolonization 1940–1960, New Haven, London 1982, pp, 141–172

Petryna Adriana, *When Experiments Travel. Clinical Trials and the Global Search for Human Subjects,* Princeton 2009

Petryna Adriana, *Globalizing Human Subjects Research,* in: Petryna, Andrew Lakoff and Arthur Kleinman (eds.), Global Pharmaceuticals. Ethics, Markets, Practices, Durham, London 2006, pp. 33–60

Petryna Adriana, *Clinical Trials Offshored. On Private Sector Science and Public Health,* in: BioSocieties, Vol. 2, 2007, pp. 21–40

Pickstone John, *Ways of Knowing. A New History of Science, Technology and Medicine,* Manchester 2000

Pool Robert et al., *The Acceptability of Intermittent Preventive Treatment of Malaria in Infants (IPTi) Delivered Through the Expanded Programme of Immunization in Southern Tanzania,* in: Malaria Journal, Vol. 7, No. 213, 2008, pp. 1–11

Pratt Cranford, *The Critical Phase in Tanzania 1945–1968. Nyerere and the Emergence of a Socialist Strategy,* Cambridge 1976

Purtschert Patricia, Lüthi Barbara, Falk Francesca (eds.), *Postkoloniale Schweiz. Formen und Folgen eines Kolonialismus ohne Kolonien,* Bielefeld 2012

Redfield Peter, *Space in the Tropics. From Convicts to Rockets in French Guiana,* Berkeley, Los Angeles, London 2000

Redfield Peter, *The Half-Life of Empire in Outer Space,* in: Social Studies of Science, Vol. 32, No. 5-6, 2002, pp. 791–825

Renschler Regula, *Die Entwicklung der Entwicklungshilfe zur Entwicklungspolitik,* in: Richard Gerster (ed.), Die Entdeckung der Schweiz. 25 Jahre Helvetas. Jubiläumsschrift, Basel 1980, pp. 113–123

Reubi Serge, *Gentlemen, prolétaires et primitifs. Institutionalisation, pratiques de collection et choix muséographiques dans l'ethnographie Suisse, 1880–1950,* Thèse Université de Neuchâtel 2008

Reubi Serge, *L'ethnologue, prestataire de service pour l'industrie dans la Suisse des années 1930–1960,* in:

Rheinberger Hans-Jörg, *Gaston Bachelard und der Begriff der "Phänomenotechnik",* in: Marc Schalenberg and Peter Th. Walther (eds.), "... immer im Forschen bleiben." Rüdiger vom Bruch zum 60. Geburtstag, Stuttgart 2004, pp. 297–310

Rifkin Susan, Walt Gill, *Why Health Improves. Defining the Issues Concerning "Comprehensive Primary Health Care" and "Selective Primary Health Care,"* in: Social Science and Medicine, Vol. 23, 1986, pp. 559–566

Ritter Markus, *Die Biologie Adolf Portmanns im zeitgenössischen Kontext,* in: Basler Zeitung für Geschichte und Altertumskunde, Vol. 100, 2000, pp. 207–254

Roemer Milton I., *Internationalism in Medicine and Public Health,* in: William F. Bynum and Roy Porter (eds.), Companion Encyclopedia of the History of Medicine, Vol. 2, 1993, pp. 1417–1435

Rose Nikolas, Novas Carlos, *Biological Citizenship,* in: Aihwa Ong and Stephen J. Collier (eds.), Global Assemblages. Technology, Politics, and Ethics as Anthropological Problems, Malden 2008, pp. 439–463

Rottenburg Richard, *Social and Public Experiments and New Figurations of Science and Politics in Postcolonial Africa,* in: Postcolonial Studies, Vol. 12, No. 4, 2009, pp. 423–440

Ruxin Joshua N., *Hunger, Science, and Politics. WHO, and Unicef Nutrition Policies, 1945–1978,* PhD Study, University College London, London 1996

Sabrié Marie-Lise, *Histoire des principes de programmation scientifique à L'ORSTOM (1944–1994),* in: Patrick Petitjean (eds.), Les sciences coloniales. Figures et institutions, Paris 1996, pp. 223–233

Sachs Wolfgang (ed.), *The Development Dictionary. A Guide to Knowledge as Power,* London 1992

Sarasin Philipp, *Stadt der Bürger. Bürgerliche Macht und städtische Gesellschaft. Basel 1846–1914,* Göttingen 1992 (2nd edition)

Schär Bernhard, *Tropenliebe. Basler Naturforscher, holländische Imperialisten und die "Entdeckung" von Celebes um 1900,* Dissertation Universität Bern 2013 [forthcoming]

Schär Manuel, *Wie entwickeln wir die "Dritte Welt"? Kontinuitäten und Brüche im Entwicklungsverständnis um 1968 in der Schweiz,* in: Janick Marina Schaufelbuehl (ed.), 1968–1978. Ein bewegtes Jahrzehnt in der Schweiz. Unter Mitarbeit von Nuno Pereira und Renate Schär, Zürich 2009, pp. 99–111

Schellenberg David et al., *The Changing Epidemiology of Malaria in Ifakara Town, Southern Tanzania,* in: Tropical Medicine and International Health, Vol. 9, No. 1, 2004, pp. 68–76

Schellenberg David et al., *Intermittent Treatment for Malaria and Anaemia Control at Time of Routine Vaccinations in Tanzanian Infants. A Randomized, Placebo-Controlled Trial,* in: The Lancet, Vol. 357, 2001, pp. 1471–1477

Schellenberg Joanna, *KINET. A Social Marketing Programme of Treated Nets and Net Treatment for Malaria Control in Tanzania, with Evaluation of Child Health and Long-Term Survival,* in: Transactions of the Royal Society of Tropical Medicine and Hygiene, Vol. 93, No. 3, 1999, pp. 225–231

Schellenberg Joanna et al., *Ifakara DSS, Tanzania,* in: International Development Research Centre (ed.), Population and Health in Developing Countries. Population, Health and Survival at INDEPTH Sites, Vol. 1, 2002, pp. 159–164

Schellenberg Joanna et al., *Community Effectiveness of Intermittent Preventive Treatment of Infants (IPTi) in Rural Southern Tanzania,* in: American Journal of Tropical Medicine and Hygiene, Vol. 82, No. 5, 2010, pp. 772–781

Schmid Pascal, *Medecine, Faith, and Politics in Agogo. A History of Health Care Delivery in Rural Ghana, 1925-1980, PhD University of Basel, 2013*

Schmidt Elizabeth, *Anticolonial Nationalism in French West Africa. What Made Guinea Unique?,* in: African Studies Review, Vol. 52, No. 2, 2009, pp. 1–34

Schneider Leander, *Freedom and Unfreedom in Rural Development. Julius Nyerere, Ujamaa Vijijini, and Villagization,* in: Canadian Journal of African Studies, Vol. 38, No. 2, 2004, pp. 344–393

Schuknecht Rohland, *British Colonial Development Policy after the Second World War. The Case of Sukumaland, Tanganyika,* Berlin 2010

Schumaker Lyn, *Africanizing Anthropology. Fieldworks, Networks and the Making of Cultural Knowledge in Central Africa,* Durham, N.C., London 2001

Schumaker Lyn, *Malaria,* in: Roger Cooter and John Pickstone (eds.), Medicine in the Twentieth Century, Amsterdam 2000, pp. 703–717

Schuwey Jérome, *La Suisse et la Guinée de Sékou Touré. Les enjeux de la coopération technique au lendemain de l'indépendance (1958–1974),* Mémoire de licence en histoire contemporaine présenté à la Faculté des Lettres de l'Université de Fribourg, Fribourg 2005

Scott James, *Seeing Like a State. How Certain Schemes to Improve the Human Condition have Failed,* New Haven 1998

Semali Innocent, *Understanding Stakeholder's Roles in Health Sector Reform in Tanzania. The Case of Decentralizing the Immunization Program,* PhD Study University of Basel, Basel 2003

Semi-Bi Zan, *La politique coloniale des travaux publics en Côte d'Ivoire 1900–1940,* in: Annales de l'Université d'Abidjan, Vol. 1, No. 2, 1973–1974

Sidel Ruth, Sidel Victor W., *The Health of China. Current Conflicts in Medical and Human Services for One Billion People,* Boston 1982

Simon Christian, *DDT. Kulturgeschichte einer chemischen Verbindung,* Basel 1999

Simon Christian, *Natur-Geschichte. Das Naturhistorische Museum Basel im 19. und 20. Jahrhundert,* Basel 2009

Simon Christian, *Naturwissenschaft in Basel im 19. und 20. Jahrhundert. Die Philosophisch-Naturwissenschaftliche Fakultät der Universität,* published online 2010, www.unigeschichte.unibas.ch/cms/upload/FaecherUnd-Fakultaeten/Downloads/CSimon_Naturwissenschaften-Basel.pdf (accessed 16.02.2012)

Slater Leo B., *War and Disease. Biomedical Research on Malaria in the Twentieth Century,* New Brunswick, New Jersey, London 2009

Spalding N. J., *State-Society Relations in Africa. An Exploration of the Tanzanian Experience,* in: Polity, Vol. 29, 1996, pp. 65–96

Speich Daniel, *Helvetische Meliorationen. Die Neuordnung der gesellschaftlichen Naturverhältnisse an der Linth (1783–1823),* Zürich 2003

Spurgeon David, *Southern Lights. Celebrating the Scientific Achievements of the Developing World,* Ottawa 1995

Stepan Nancy, *The Idea of Race in Science. Great Britain 1800–1960,* Oxford 1982

Stettler Niklaus, Haenger Peter, Labhardt Robert, *Baumwolle, Sklaven und Kredite. Die Basler Welthandelsfirma Christoph Burckhardt & Cie. in revolutionärer Zeit, 1789–1815,* Basel 2004

Stettler Niklaus, *Natur erforschen. Perspektiven einer Kulturgeschichte der Biowissenschaft an Schweizer Universitäten 1945–1975,* Zürich 2002

Stoler Ann Laura, *Colonial Archives and the Arts of Governance,* in: Archival Science, Vol. 2, No. 1-2, 2002, pp. 87–109

Stoler Ann Laura, *Rethinking Colonial Categories. European Communities and the Boundaries of Rule,* in: Comparative Studies in Society and History, Vol. 31, No. 1, 1989, pp. 134–161

Strasser Bruno J., *La fabrique d'une nouvelle science. La biologie moléculaire à l'âge atomique,* Florence 2006

Strasser Bruno J., *The Coproduction of Neutral Science and Neutral State in Cold War Europe. Switzerland and International Scientific Cooperation, 1951-69,* in: Osiris, Vol. 24, 2009, pp. 165–187

Straumann Lukas, *Nützliche Schädlinge. Angewandte Entomologie, chemische Industrie und Landwirtschaftspolitik in der Schweiz 1874–1952*, Zürich 2005

Sung Lee, *WHO and the Developing World. The Contest for Ideology*, in: Andrew Cunningham and Bridie Andrews (eds.), Western Medicine as Contested Knowledge, Manchester 1997, pp. 24–45

Swanson Maynard W., *The Sanitation Syndrome. Bubonic Plague and urban Native Policy in the Cape Colony, 1900–1909*, in: Journal of African History, Vol. 18, No. 3, 1977, pp. 387–410

Tilley Helen, *Africa as a Living Laboratory. Empire, Development, and the Problem of Scientific Knowledge, 1870–1950*, Chicago 2011

Tilley Helen, *Global Histories, Vernacular Science, and African Genealogies; or, Is the History of Science Ready for the World?*, in: Isis, Vol. 101, No. 1, 2010, pp. 110–119

Tilly Charles, *Big Structures, Large Processes, Huge Comparisons*, New York 1984

Trachsler Daniel, *Bundesrat Max Petitpierre. Schweizerische Aussenpolitik im Kalten Krieg, 1945–1961*, Zürich 2011

Tripp Aili M., *Changing the Rules. The Politics of Liberalization and the Urban Informal Economy in Tanzania*, Berkeley 1997

Turnbull David, *Local Knowledge and Comparative Scientific Traditions*, in: Knowledge and Policy, Vol. 6, No. 3-4, 1993/94, pp. 29–54

Turshen Meredeth, *Privatizing Health Services in Africa*, New Brunswick, New Jersey 1999

Turshen Meredeth, *The Impact of Colonialism on Health and Health Services in Tanzania*, in: International Journal of Health Services, Vol. 7, No. 1, 1977, pp. 7–35

Turshen Meredeth, *The Political Ecology of Disease in Tanzania*, New Brunswick, New Jersey 1984

Van Laak Dirk, *Kolonien als "Laboratorien der Moderne?,"* in: Sebastian Conrad and Jürgen Osterhammel (eds.), Das Kaiserreich transnational. Deutschland in der Welt, 1871–1914, Göttingen 2004, pp. 257-279

Van de Walle Nicholas, *African Economies and the Politics of Permanent Crisis, 1979–1999*, Cambridge 2001

Vaughan Megan, *Curing their Ills. Colonial Power and African Illness*, Stanford 1991

Verdeaux François, *Du pouvoir des génies au savoir scientifique. Les métamorphoses de la lagune Ebrié (Côte d'Ivoire)*, in: Cahiers d'Etudes Africaines, Vol. 26, No. 1-2, 1986, pp. 145–171

Walsh Julia, Warren Kenneth, *Selective Primary Health Care. An Interim Strategy for Disease Control in Developing Countries*, in: New England Journal of Medicine, Vol. 301, 1979, pp. 967–974

Weber R., *The Beginnings of Developmental Biology in Swiss Universities*, in: International Journal of Developmental Biology, Vol. 46, 2002, pp. 15–22

Wehler Hans-Ulrich, *Transnationale Geschichte – der neue Königsweg historischer Forschung?*, in: Gunilla Budde, Sebastian Conrad, Oliver Janz (eds.), Transnationale Geschichte. Themen, Tendenzen und Theorien, Göttingen 2006, pp. 161–174

Weindling Paul (ed.), *International Health Organizations and Movements, 1918–1939*, Cambridge 1995

Weiskel Timothy C., *Independence and the Longue Durée. The Ivory Coast "Miracle" Reconsidered*, in: William Roger Louis and Prosser Gifford (eds.), Decolonization and African Independence. The Transfers of Power, 1960–1980, New Haven, London 1988, pp. 347–380

Werner Michael, Zimmermann Bénédicte, *Beyond Comparison. Histoire Croisée and the Challenge of Reflexivity*, in: History and Theory, Vol. 45, 2006, pp. 30–50

Werner Michael, Zimmermann Bénédicte, *Vergleich, Transfer, Verflechtung. Der Ansatz der "Histoire croisée" und die Herausforderung des Transnationalen,* in: Geschichte und Gesellschaft, Vol. 28, 2002, pp. 607–636

White Luise, *Speaking with Vampires. Rumor and History in Colonial Africa,* Berkeley, Los Angeles, London 2000

White Luise, Miescher Stephan, Cohen David William, *Introduction. Voices, Words and African History,* in: White, Miescher and Cohen (eds.), African Words, African Voices. Critical Practices in Oral History, Bloomington, Indianapolis 2001, pp. 1–27

Wilhelm Rolf, *Gemeinsam unterwegs. Eine Zeitreise durch 60 Jahre Entwicklungszusammenarbeit Schweiz-Nepal,* Bern 2012

Wilhelm Rolf, *Aus der Anfangszeit der schweizerischen Entwicklungshilfe,* in: Rolf Wilhelm et al. (eds.), August R. Lindt, Patriot und Weltbürger, Bern, Stuttgart, Wien 2002, pp. 127–138

Wirz Albert, *Für eine transnationale Gesellschaftsgeschichte,* in: Geschichte und Gesellschaft, Vol. 27, No. 2, 2001, pp. 489–498

Wirz Albert, *Die humanitäre Schweiz im Spannungsfeld zwischen Philanthropie und Kolonialismus. Gustave Moynier, Afrika und das IKRK,* in: Traverse, No. 2, 1998, pp. 95–110

Worboys Michael, *Science and British Colonial Imperialism, 1895–1940,* PhD Study University of Sussex, Sussex 1979

Worboys Michael, *The Comparative History of Sleeping Sickness in East and Central Africa, 1900–1914,* in: History of Science, Vol. 32, 1994, pp. 89–102

Worboys Michael, *The Discovery of Colonial Malnutrition between the Wars,* in: David Arnold (ed.), Imperial Medicine and Indigenous Societies, Manchester, New York 1988, pp. 208–225

Zangger Andreas, *Koloniale Schweiz. Ein Stück Globalgeschichte zwischen Europa und Südostasien, 1860–1930,* Bielefeld 2011

Zantop Susanne M., *Kolonialphantasien im vorkolonialen Deutschland (1770–1870),* Berlin 1999

Zellmeyer Stephan, *A Place in Space. The History of Swiss Participation in European Space Programmes,* 1960–1987, Basel 2007

Zolberg Aristide, *One-party Government in the Ivory Coast,* Princeton, New Jersey 1969

Zürcher Lukas, *"So fanden wir auf der Karte diesen kleinen Staat." Globale Positionierung und lokale Entwicklungsfantasien der Schweiz in Rwanda in den 1960er Jahren,* in: Hubertus Büschel and Daniel Speich (eds.), Entwicklungswelten. Globalgeschichte der Entwicklungszusammenarbeit, Frankfurt am Main 2009, pp. 275–309

Zürcher Lukas, *Die Schweiz und Ruanda. Mission, Entwicklungshilfe und nationale Selbstbestätigung,* Zürich 2013 (im Druck)

BASLER BEITRÄGE ZUR GESCHICHTSWISSENSCHAFT

Begründet von
E. Bonjour, W. Kaegi und F. Staehelin

Weitergeführt von
F. Graus, K. v. Greyerz, H. R. Guggisberg, H. Haumann,
G. Kreis, H. Lüthy, M. Mattmüller, W. Meyer, J. Mooser,
A. v. Müller, M. Schaffner und R. Wecker

Herausgegeben von
C. Arni, S. Burghartz, L. Burkart, M. Lengwiler,
C. Opitz-Belakhal und F. B. Schenk

Band   1 *Vischer, Christoph.* Die Stellung Basels während des polnischen und österreichischen Erbfolgekrieges 1733–1748. 1938. 160 Seiten. Vergriffen.

Band   2 *Lüthi, Walter.* Die Haltung des Auslandes im zweiten Villmerger Krieg 1712. 1938. 234 Seiten. Vergriffen.

Band   3 *Christ, Salome.* Jacob Burckhardt und die Poesie der Italiener. 1940. 208 Seiten. Vergriffen.

Band   4 *Barth, Dietrich.* Die Protestantisch-Konservative Partei in Genf in den Jahren 1838 bis 1846. 1940. 207 Seiten. Vergriffen.

Band   5 *Grieder, Fritz.* Das Postwesen im helvetischen Einheitsstaat (1798–1803). 1940. 172 Seiten. Vergriffen.

Band   6 *Buxtorf, Peter.* Die lateinischen Grabinschriften in der Stadt Basel. 1940. 224 Seiten. Vergriffen.

Band   7 *Schmid, Hermann Alfred.* Die Entzauberung der Welt in der Schweizer Landeskunde. 1942. 194 Seiten. Vergriffen.

Band   8 *Roth, Paul.* Staatsarchivar. Durchbruch und Festsetzung der Reformation in Basel. Eine Darstellung der Politik der Stadt Basel im Jahre 1529 auf Grund der öffentlichen Akten. 1942. 111 Seiten. Vergriffen.

Band   9 *Fleig, Hans.* Die Schweiz im Schrifttum der deutschen Befreiungszeit (1813 bis 1817). 1942. 254 Seiten. Vergriffen.

Band 10 *Gutzwiller, Hans.* Die Neujahrsrede des Konsuls Claudius Mamertinus vor dem Kaiser Julian. Text, Übersetzung und Kommentar. 1942. 251 Seiten. Vergriffen.

Band 11 *Lötscher, Valentin.* Der deutsche Bauernkrieg in der Darstellung und im Urteil der eidgenössischen Schweizer. 1943. 261 Seiten. Vergriffen.

Band 12 *Bonjour, Edgar.* Englands Anteil an der Lösung des Neuenburger Konflikts 1856/57. 1943. 104 Seiten. Vergriffen.

Band 13 *Niethammer, Adolf.* Das Vormauernsystem an der eidgenössischen Nordgrenze. Ein Beitrag zur Geschichte der schweizerischen Neutralität vom 16. bis 18. Jahrhundert. 1944. 191 Seiten. Vergriffen.

Band 14 *Müller, Georg.* Der amerikanische Sezessionskrieg in der schweizerischen öffentlichen Meinung. 1944. 216 Seiten. Vergriffen.

Band 15 *Bauer, Marianne.* Die italienische Einigung im Spiegel der schweizerischen Öffentlichkeit 1859–1861. 1944. 191 Seiten. Vergriffen.

Band 16 *Gysin, Werner.* Zensur und Pressefreiheit in Basel während der Mediation und Restauration. 1944. 129 Seiten. Vergriffen.

Band 17 *Pieth, Fritz.* Die Entwicklung zum schweizerischen Bundesstaat in der Beleuchtung preussischer Gesandtschaftsberichte aus den Jahren 1819–1833. 1944. 130 Seiten. Vergriffen.

Band 18 *Jacob, Ilse.* Beziehungen Englands zu Russland und zur Türkei in den Jahren 1718–1727. Eine historisch-diplomatische Studie. 1945. 159 Seiten. Vergriffen.

Band 19 *Bächlin, Max.* Das Unterstützungswesen der Helvetik. Staatliche und private Massnahmen zur Linderung der Kriegsnot. 1945. 212 Seiten. Vergriffen.

Band 20 *Rentsch, Hans Ulrich.* Bismarck im Urteil der schweizerischen Presse 1882 bis 1898. 1945. 336 Seiten. Vergriffen.

Band 21 *Meyer, Karl.* Der Neuenburger Konflikt 1856/57 im Spiegel der zeitgenössischen schweizerischen Presse. 1945. 349 Seiten. Vergriffen.

Band 22 *Teuteberg, René.* Prosper de Barante (1782–1866). Ein romantischer Historiker des französischen Liberalismus. 1945. 172 Seiten. Vergriffen.

Band 23 *Bächthold, Rudolf.* Karamzins Weg zur Geschichte. 1946. 103 Seiten. Vergriffen.

Band 24 *Massini, Rudolf.* Das Bistum Basel zur Zeit des Investiturstreites. 1946. 224 Seiten. Vergriffen.

Band 25 *Blumenkranz, Bernhard.* Die Judenpredigt Augustins. Ein Beitrag zur Geschichte der jüdisch-christlichen Beziehungen in den ersten Jahrhunderten. 1946. 218 Seiten. Vergriffen.

Band 26 *Buscher, Hans.* Heinrich Pantaleon und sein Heldenbuch. 1946. 305 Seiten. Vergriffen.

Band 27 *Labhardt, Ricco.* Wilhelm Tell als Patriot und Revolutionär 1700–1800. Wandlungen der Tell-Tradition im Zeitalter des Absolutismus und der Französischen Revolution. 1947. 162 Seiten. Vergriffen.

Band 28 *Lindau, Johann Karl.* Das Medaillenkabinett des Postmeisters Johann Schorndorff zu Basel. Seine Geschichte bis zur Erwerbung durch das Historische Museum Basel. 1947. 246 Seiten. Vergriffen.

Band 29 *Wolf, Kaspar.* Die Lieferungen der Schweiz an die französischen Besetzungstruppen zur Zeit der Helvetik. 1948. 139 Seiten. Vergriffen.

Band 30 *Bütler, Robert.* Nationales und universales Denken im Werke Etienne Pasquiers. 1948. 176 Seiten. Vergriffen.

Band 31 *Ernst, Alfred.* Die Ordnung des militärischen Oberbefehls im schweizerischen Bundesstaat. 1948. 247 Seiten. Vergriffen.

Band 32 *Heitz, Fritz.* Johann Rudolf Iselin, 1705–1779. Ein Beitrag zur Geschichte der schweizerischen Historiographie des 18. Jahrhunderts. 1949. 226 Seiten. Vergriffen.

Band 33 *Gautschy, Heiner.* Die Schweizer Presse um die Mitte des 19. Jahrhunderts – ihre Reaktion auf den Staatsstreich Louis Napoleon Bonapartes. 1949. 211 Seiten. Vergriffen.

Band 34 *Hatze, Margrit.* Die diplomatisch-politischen Beziehungen zwischen England und der Schweiz im Zeitalter der Restauration. 1949. 219 Seiten. Vergriffen.

Band 35 *Haasbauer, Adolphine.* Die historischen Schriften Karl Ludwig von Hallers. 1949. 213 Seiten. Vergriffen.

Band 36 *Schneewind, Wolfgang.* Die diplomatischen Beziehungen Englands mit der alten Eidgenossenschaft zur Zeit Elisabeths, Jakobs I. und Karls I., 1558–1649. 1950. 187 Seiten. Vergriffen.

Band 37 *Walser, Gerold.* Rom, das Reich und die fremden Völker in der Geschichtsschreibung der frühen Kaiserzeit. Studien zur Glaubwürdigkeit des Tacitus. 1951. 179 Seiten. Vergriffen.

Band 38 *Bächthold, Rudolf.* Südwestrussland im Spätmittelalter. Territoriale, wirtschaftliche und soziale Verhältnisse. 1951. 211 Seiten. Vergriffen.

Band 39 *Meyer, Friedrich.* Die Beziehungen zwischen Basel und den Eidgenossen in der Darstellung der Historiographie des 15. und 16. Jahrhunderts. 1951. 211 Seiten. Vergriffen.

Band 40 *Meier, Markus.* Die diplomatische Vertretung Englands in der Schweiz im 18. Jahrhundert (1689–1789). 1952. 157 Seiten. Vergriffen.

Band 41 *Räber, Kuno.* Studien zur Geschichtsbibel Sebastian Francks. 1952. 93 Seiten. Vergriffen.

Band 42 *Vögelin, Hans Adolf.* Die Gründung des schweizerischen Bundesstaates im Urteil der Engländer. 1952. 228 Seiten. Vergriffen.

Band 43 *Staehelin, Andreas.* Peter Ochs als Historiker. 1952. 274 Seiten. Vergriffen.

Band 44 *Vetter, Verena.* Baslerische Italienreisen vom ausgehenden Mittelalter bis in das 17. Jahrhundert. 1952. 218 Seiten. Vergriffen.

Band 45 *Luchsinger, Friedrich.* Der Basler Buchdruck als Vermittler italienischen Geistes 1470–1529. 144 Seiten. Vergriffen.

Band 46 *Sieber, Marc.* Das Nachleben der Alemannen in der schweizerischen Geschichtsschreibung. 1953. 141 Seiten. Vergriffen.

Band 47 *Huber, Paul.* Traditionsfestigkeit und Traditionskritik bei Thomas Morus. 1953. 178 Seiten. Vergriffen.

Band 48 *Schätti, Karl.* Erasmus von Rotterdam und die Römische Kurie. 1954. 169 Seiten. Vergriffen.

Band 49 *Aellig, Johann Jakob.* Die Aufhebung der schweizerischen Söldnerdienste im Meinungskampf des neunzehnten Jahrhunderts. 1954. 255 Seiten. Vergriffen.

Band 50 *Meyer, Rudolf.* Die Flugschriften der Epoche Ludwigs XIV. 1955. 350 Seiten. Vergriffen.

Band 51 *Hanhart, Robert.* Das Bild der Jeanne d'Arc in der französischen Historiographie vom Spätmittelalter bis zur Aufklärung. 1955. 133 Seiten. Vergriffen.

Band 52 *Widmer, Bertha.* Heilsordnung und Zeitgeschehen in der Mystik Hildegards von Bingen. 1955. 286 Seiten. Vergriffen.

Band 53 *Meyer, Paul.* Zeitgenössische Beurteilung und Auswirkung des Siebenjährigen Krieges (1756–1763) in der evangelischen Schweiz. 1955. 174 Seiten. Vergriffen.

Band 54 *Kutter, Markus.* Celio Secondo Curione. Sein Leben und sein Werk (1503 bis 1569). 1955. 310 Seiten. Vergriffen.

Band 55 *Schneider, Elisabeth.* Das Bild der Frau im Werk des Erasmus von Rotterdam. 1955. 133 Seiten. Vergriffen.

Band 56 *Bürck, Gerhart.* Selbstdarstellung und Personenbildnis bei Enea Silvio Piccolomini (Pius II.). 1956. 160 Seiten. Vergriffen.

Band 57 *Guggisberg, Hans Rudolf.* Sebastian Castellio im Urteil seiner Nachwelt vom Späthumanismus bis zur Aufklärung. 1956. 207 Seiten. Vergriffen.

Band 58 *Roth, Dorothea.* Die mittelalterliche Predigttheorie und das Manuale Curatorum des Johann Ulrich Surgant. 1956. 198 Seiten. Vergriffen.

Band 59 *Weis-Müller, Renée.* Die Reform des Klosters Klingental und ihr Personenkreis. 1956. 217 Seiten. Vergriffen.

Band 60 *von Wartburg, Wolfgang.* Zürich und die Französische Revolution. Die Auseinandersetzung einer patriarchalischen Gesellschaft mit den ideellen und politischen Einwirkungen der Französischen Revolution. 1956. 484 Seiten. Vergriffen.

Band 61 *Laube, Bruno.* Joseph Anton Felix Balthasar, 1737–1810. Ein Beitrag zur Geschichte der Aufklärung in Luzern. 1956. 269 Seiten. Vergriffen.

Band 62 *Genner, Lotti.* Die diplomatischen Beziehungen zwischen England und der Schweiz von 1870 bis 1890. Eine Untersuchung der englischen Gesandtschaftsberichte aus Bern. 1956. 227 Seiten. Vergriffen.

Band 63 *Wüthrich, Lukas Heinrich.* Christian von Mechel. Leben und Werk eines Basler Kupferstechers und Kunsthändlers (1737–1817). 1956. 342 Seiten. Vergriffen.

Band 64 *Gelzer, Urs.* Beziehungen Basels zur Innerschweiz während der Regenerationszeit 1830–1848. 1957. 187 Seiten. Vergriffen.

Band 65 *Merkel, Hans Rudolf.* Demokratie und Aristokratie in der schweizerischen Geschichtsschreibung des 18. Jahrhunderts. 1957. 270 Seiten. Vergriffen.

Band 66 *Gessler, Peter.* René Louis d'Argenson, 1694–1757. Seine Ideen über Selbstverwaltung, Einheitsstaat, Wohlfahrt und Freiheit in biographischem Zusammenhang. 1957. 226 Seiten. Vergriffen.

Band 67 *Mattmüller, Markus.* Leonhard Ragaz und der religiöse Sozialismus. Band I: Die Entwicklung der Persönlichkeit und des Werkes bis ins Jahr 1913. 1957. 246 Seiten. Vergriffen.

Band 68 *Sutter, Hans.* Basels Haltung gegenüber dem evangelischen Schirmwerk und dem eidgenössischen Defensionale (1647 und 1668). 1958. 522 Seiten. Vergriffen.

Band 69 *Portmann, Marie-Louise.* Die Darstellung der Frau in der Geschichtsschreibung des früheren Mittelalters. 1958. 147 Seiten. Vergriffen.

Band 70 *Real, Willy.* Von Potsdam nach Basel. Studien zur Geschichte der Beziehungen Preussens zu den europäischen Mächten vom Regierungsantritt Friedrich Wilhelms II. bis zum Abschluss des Friedens von Basel (1786–1795). 1958. 144 Seiten. Vergriffen.

Band 71 *Huber, Max.* Die Staatsphilosophie von Josef de Maistre im Lichte des Thomismus. 1958. 288 Seiten. Vergriffen.

Band 72 *Mommsen, Karl.* Eidgenossen, Kaiser und Reich. Studien zur Stellung der Eidgenossenschaft innerhalb des heiligen römischen Reiches. 1958. 321 Seiten mit 5 Abbildungen. Vergriffen.

Band 73 *Bietenholz, Peter.* Der italienische Humanismus und die Blütezeit des Buchdrucks in Basel. Die Basler Drucke italienischer Autoren von 1530 bis zum Ende des 16. Jahrhunderts. 1959. 171 Seiten. Vergriffen.

Band 74 *Rihm, Werner.* Das Bildungserlebnis der Antike bei Johannes von Müller. 1959. 156 Seiten. Vergriffen.

Band 75 *Wüthrich, Lukas Heinrich.* Das Œuvre des Kupferstechers Christian von Mechel. Vollständiges Verzeichnis der von ihm geschaffenen und verlegten graphischen Arbeiten. 1959. 238 Textseiten und 96 Abbildungen. Vergriffen.

Band 76 *Salathé, René.* Die Anfänge der historischen Fachzeitschrift in der deutschen Schweiz (1694–1813). 1959. 200 Seiten. Vergriffen.

Band 77 *Zaeslin, Peter Leonhard.* Die Schweiz und der lombardische Staat im Revolutionszeitalter (1796–1814). 1960. 179 Seiten. Vergriffen.

Band 78 *Leuenberger, Theodor.* Johannes von Müller und das Christentum. 1960. 85 Seiten. Vergriffen.

Band 79 *Fürstenberger, Markus.* Die Mediationstätigkeit des Basler Bürgermeisters Johann Balthasar Burckhardt (1642–1722). 1960. 178 Seiten. Vergriffen.

Band 80 *Ladner, Pascal.* Das St. Albankloster in Basel und die burgundische Tradition in der Cluniazenserprovinz Alemannia. 1960. 128 Seiten. Vergriffen.

Band 81 *Fromherz, Uta.* Johannes von Segovia als Geschichtsschreiber des Konzils von Basel. 1960. 175 Seiten. Vergriffen.

Band 82 *Stauffer, Paul.* Die Idee des europäischen Gleichgewichts im politischen Denken Johannes von Müllers. 1960. 80 Seiten. Vergriffen.

Band 83 *Uhl, Othmar.* Die diplomatisch-politischen Beziehungen zwischen Grossbritannien und der Schweiz in den Jahrzehnten vor dem Ersten Weltkrieg (1890–1914). 1961. 193 Seiten. Vergriffen.

Band 84 *Wessendorf, Ernst.* Geschichtsschreibung für das Volk und für die Schulen in der alten Eidgenossenschaft. 1962. 223 Seiten. Vergriffen.

Band 85 *Bietenholz, Peter G.* Pietro Della Valle (1586–1652). Studien zur Geschichte der Orientkenntnis und des Orientbildes im Abendlande. 1962. 248 Seiten. Broschiert. Vergriffen.

Band 86 *Schatz, Rudolf.* Der Marquis Clément-Edouard de Moustier und die Schweiz. Seine Gesandtschaft 1823–1825. 1962. 174 Seiten. Vergriffen.

Band 87 *Koprio, Georg.* Basel und die eidgenössische Universität. 1963. 157 Seiten. Vergriffen.

Band 88 *Widmer, Berthe.* Enea Silvio Piccolomini in der sittlichen und politischen Entscheidung. 1963. 180 Seiten. Vergriffen.

Band 89 *Pfaff, Karl.* Kaiser Heinrich II. Sein Nachleben und sein Kult im mittelalterlichen Basel. 1963. 118 Seiten. Vergriffen.

Band 90 *Hartmann, Rudolf.* Das Autobiographische in der Basler Leichenrede. 1963. 194 Seiten. Vergriffen.

Band 91 *Burmeister, Karl-Heinz.* Sebastian Münster. Versuch eines biographischen Gesamtbildes. 2. Auflage 1969. 232 Seiten. Vergriffen.

Band 92 *Guggisberg, Hans Rudolf.* Das europäische Mittelalter im amerikanischen Geschichtsdenken des 19. und des frühen 20. Jahrhunderts. 1964. 190 Seiten. Vergriffen.

Band 93 *Welti, Manfred E.* Der Basler Buchdruck und Britannien. Die Rezeption britischen Gedankenguts in den Basler Pressen von den Anfängen bis zum Beginn des 17. Jahrhunderts. 1964. 304 Seiten. Vergriffen.

Band 94 *Ryser, Heinz.* Johannes von Müller im Urteil seiner schweizerischen und deutschen Zeitgenossen. 1964. 163 Seiten. Vergriffen.

Band 95 *Schmid, Michael.* Staat und Volk im alten Solothurn. Ein Beitrag zur Prosopographie und zum Volkstum des fünfzehnten Jahrhunderts. 1964. 114 Seiten. Vergriffen.

Band 96 *Sieber, Emil.* Basler Trennungswirren und nationale Erneuerung im Meinungsstreit der Schweizer Presse 1830–1833. 1964. 250 Seiten. Vergriffen.

Band 97 *Handschin, Werner.* Francesco Petrarca als Gestalt der Historiographie. Seine Beurteilung in der Geschichtsschreibung vom Frühhumanismus bis zu Jacob Burckhardt. 1964. 192 Seiten. Vergriffen.

Band 98 *Wehrli, Kurt.* Die geistige Entwicklung Johannes von Müllers. Ein historischer Beitrag zum Freiheitsproblem des jungen Idealismus. 1965. 268 Seiten. Vergriffen.

Band 99 *Gugolz, Peter.* Die Schweiz und der Krimkrieg 1853–1856. 1965. 121 Seiten. Vergriffen.

Band 100 *Mattmüller, Hanspeter.* Carl Hilty (1833–1909). 1966. 320 Seiten. Vergriffen.

Band 101 *Wolpert, Paul.* Die diplomatischen Beziehungen zwischen Frankreich und der Eidgenossenschaft 1752–1762. Die Ambassade von A. Th. de Chavigny. 1966. 102 Seiten. Vergriffen.

Band 102 *Dannecker, Rudolf.* Die Schweiz und Österreich-Ungarn. Diplomatische und militärische Beziehungen von 1866 bis zum ersten Weltkrieg. 1966. 312 Seiten. Vergriffen.

Band 103 *Etter, Else-Lilly.* Tacitus in der Geistesgeschichte des 16. und 17. Jahrhunderts. 1966. 245 Seiten mit 9 Abbildungen. Vergriffen.

Band 104 *Burckhardt, Andreas.* Johannes Basilius Herold. Kaiser und Reich im protestantischen Schrifttum des Basler Buchdrucks um die Mitte des 16. Jahrhunderts. 1967. 290 Seiten. Vergriffen.

Band 105 *Steinmann, Martin.* Johannes Oporinus. Ein Basler Buchdrucker um die Mitte des 16. Jahrhunderts. 1967. 160 Seiten. Vergriffen.

Band 106 *Fimpel, Ludwig.* Mino Celsis Traktat gegen die Ketzertötung. Ein Beitrag zum Toleranzproblem des 16. Jahrhunderts. 1967. 100 Seiten. Vergriffen.

Band 107 *Biel, Arnold.* Die Beziehungen zwischen Savoyen und der Eidgenossenschaft zur Zeit Emanuel Philiberts (1559–1580). 1967. 152 Seiten. Vergriffen.

Band 108 *Lacher, Adolf.* Die Schweiz und Frankreich vor dem Ersten Weltkrieg. Diplomatische und politische Beziehungen im Zeichen des deutsch-französischen Gegensatzes 1883–1914. 1967. 465 Seiten. Vergriffen.

Band 109 *Grütter, Thomas.* Johannes von Müllers Begegnung mit England. Ein Beitrag zur Geschichte der Anglophilie im späten 18. Jahrhundert. 1967. 243 Seiten. Vergriffen.

Band 110 *Mattmüller, Markus.* Leonhard Ragaz und der religiöse Sozialismus. Band II: Die Zeit des ersten Weltkriegs und der Revolutionen. 1968. 600 Seiten. Vergriffen.

Band 111 *Gutmann, Elsbeth.* Die Colloquia Familiaria des Erasmus von Rotterdam. 1968. 210 Seiten. Vergriffen.

Band 112 *Ludwig, Marianne.* Der polnische Unabhängigkeitskampf von 1863 und die Schweiz. 1968. 106 Seiten. Vergriffen.

Band 113 *Meyer, Werner.* Die Löwenburg im Berner Jura. Geschichte der Burg, der Herrschaft und ihrer Bewohner. 1968. 291 Seiten mit zwei separaten Karten. Vergriffen.

Band 114 *Jenny, Adrian.* Jean-Baptiste Adolphe Charras und die politische Emigration nach dem Staatsstreich Louis-Napoleon Bonapartes. Gestalten, Ideen und Werke französischer Flüchtlinge. 1969. 314 Seiten. Vergriffen.

Band 115 *Hausmann, Karl Eduard.* Die Armenpflege in der Helvetik. 1969. 108 Seiten. Vergriffen.

Band 116 *Hofer, Viktor.* Die Bedeutung des Berichtes General Guisans über den Aktivdienst 1939–1945 für die Gestaltung des schweizerischen Wehrwesens. 1970. 214 Seiten. Vergriffen.

Band 117 *Bolliger, Markus.* Die Basler Arbeiterbewegung im Zeitalter des Ersten Weltkrieges und der Spaltung der Sozialdemokratischen Partei. Ein Beitrag zur Geschichte der schweizerischen Arbeiterbewegung. 1970. 387 Seiten. Vergriffen.

Band 118 *Trefzger, Marc.* Die nationale Bewegung Ägyptens vor 1928 im Spiegel der schweizerischen Öffentlichkeit. 1970. 422 Seiten. Vergriffen.

Band 119 *Marr-Schelker, Beatrice.* Baslerische Italienreisen vom Beginn des achtzehnten bis in die zweite Hälfte des neunzehnten Jahrhunderts. 1970. 194 Seiten. Vergriffen.

Band 120 *Hunziker, Guido.* Die Schweiz und das Nationalitätsprinzip im 19. Jahrhundert. 1970. 198 Seiten. Vergriffen.

Band 121 *Rytz, Hans Rudolf.* Geistliche des alten Bern zwischen Merkantilismus und Physiokratie. Ein Beitrag zur Schweizer Sozialgeschichte des 18. Jahrhunderts. 1971. 235 Seiten. Vergriffen.

Band 122 *Büttiker, Georges.* Ernest Bovet, 1870–1941. 1971. 180 Seiten. Vergriffen.

Band 123 *Schaffner, Martin.* Die Basler Arbeiterbevölkerung im 19. Jahrhundert. Beiträge zur Geschichte ihrer Lebensformen. 1972. 152 Seiten. Vergriffen.

Band 124 *Isenschmid, Heinz.* Wilhelm Klein, 1825–1887. Ein freisinniger Politiker. 1972. 224 Seiten. Vergriffen.

Band 125 *Renk, Hansjörg.* Bismarcks Konflikt mit der Schweiz. Der Wohlgemuth-Handel von 1889, Vorgeschichte, Hintergründe und Folgen. 432 Seiten. Vergriffen.

Band 126 *Bielmann, Jürg.* Die Lebensverhältnisse im Urnerland während des 18. und zu Beginn des 19. Jahrhunderts. 1972. 247 Seiten. Vergriffen.

Band 127 *Soiron, Rolf.* Der Beitrag der Schweizer Aussenpolitik zum Problem der Friedensorganisation am Ende des Ersten Weltkrieges. 1973. 245 Seiten. Vergriffen.

Band 128 *Germann, Martin.* Johann Jakob Thurneysen der Jüngere, 1754–1803, Verleger, Buchdrucker und Buchhändler in Basel. 1973. 151 Seiten. Vergriffen.

Band 129 *Maurer, Peter.* Die Beurteilung Johannes von Müllers in der Schweiz während der ersten Hälfte des 19. Jahrhunderts. 1973. 220 Seiten. Vergriffen.

Band 130 *Marti, Hans.* Paul Seippel, 1858–1926. 1973. 391 Seiten. Vergriffen.

Band 131 *Scarpatetti, Beat von.* Die Kirche und das Augustiner-Chorherrenstift St. Leonhard in Basel (11./12. Jh.–1525). Ein Beitrag zur Geschichte der Stadt Basel und der späten Devotio Moderna. 1974. 415 Seiten. Vergriffen.

Band 132 *Witzig, Daniel.* Die Vorarlberger Frage. Die Vorarlberger Anschlussbewegung an die Schweiz, territorialer Verzicht und territoriale Ansprüche vor dem Hintergrund der Neugestaltung Europas. 1974. 543 Seiten. Vergriffen.

Band 133 *Plath, Uwe.* Calvin und Basel in den Jahren 1552–1556. 311 Seiten. Vergriffen.

Band 134 *Graus, Frantisek.* Gewalt und Recht im Verständnis des Mittelalters.
          Lüthy, Herbert. Tugend und Menschenrechte.
          Zwei Antrittsvorlesungen. 1974. 60 Seiten. Vergriffen.

Band 135 *Gröbli, Fredy.* Ambassador du Luc und der Trücklibund von 1715. Französische
und   135a Diplomatie und eidgenössisches Gleichgewicht in den letzten Jahren Ludwigs XIV.
          1975. 553 Seiten. Vergriffen.

Band 136 *Neuenschwander-Schindler, Heidi.* Das Gespräch über Calvin – Frankreich 1685
          bis 1870. Historiographische Variationen zu einem interkonfessionellen Thema.
          1975. 264 Seiten. Vergriffen.

Band 137 *Spindler, Katharina.* Die Schweiz und der italienische Faschismus (1922–1930).
          Der Verlauf der diplomatischen Beziehungen und die Beurteilung durch das Bür-
          gertum. 1976. 304 Seiten. Vergriffen.

Band 138 *Marchal, Guy P.* Die frommen Schweden in Schwyz. Das «Herkommen der Schwy-
          zer und Oberhasler» als Quelle zum schwyzerischen Selbstverständnis im 15. und
          16. Jahrhundert. 1977. 109 Seiten. Vergriffen.

Band 139 *Ruesch, Hanspeter.* Lebensverhältnisse in einem frühen schweizerischen Industrie-
und   139a gebiet. Sozialgeschichtliche Studie über die Gemeinden Trogen, Rehetobel, Wald,
          Gais, Speicher und Wolfhalden des Kantons Appenzell Ausserrhoden im 18. und
          frühen 19. Jahrhundert. 1979. 734 Seiten. Vergriffen.

Band 140 *Schär, Max.* Das Nachleben des Origenes im Zeitalter des Humanismus. 1979.
          317 Seiten. Vergriffen.

Band 141 *Wehrle, Kurt.* Analektik und Dialektik der restaurativen Intention. Ein Grund-
          lagenbeitrag zur kontinentaleuropäischen Verhaltensproblematik. 1980. 252 Seiten.
          Vergriffen.

Band 142 *Christ-von Wedel, Christine.* Das Nichtwissen bei Erasmus von Rotterdam. Zum
          philosophischen und theologischen Erkennen in der geistigen Entwicklung eines
          christlichen Humanisten. 1981. 152 Seiten. Vergriffen.

Band 143 *Füglister, Hans.* Handwerksregiment. Untersuchungen und Materialien zur sozialen
          und politischen Struktur der Stadt Basel in der ersten Hälfte des 16. Jahrhunderts.
          1981. 420 Seiten. Vergriffen.

Band 144 *Wirth, Franz.* Johann Jakob Treichler und die soziale Bewegung im Kanton Zürich
          (1845/1846). 1981. 292 Seiten. Vergriffen.

Band 145 *Simon, Christian.* Untertanenverhalten und obrigkeitliche Moralpolitik. Studien
          zum Verhältnis von Stadt und Land im ausgehenden 18. Jahrhundert am Beispiel
          Basels. 1981. 366 Seiten. Vergriffen.

Band 146 *Schaffner, Martin.* Die demokratische Bewegung der 1860er Jahre. Beschreibung
          und Erklärung der Zürcher Volksbewegung von 1867. 1982. 199 Seiten. Vergriffen.

Band 147 *Fink, Paul.* Geschichte der Basler Bandindustrie 1550–1800. 1983. 216 Seiten.
          Vergriffen.

Band 148 *Gasser, Adolf.* Ausgewählte historische Schriften (1933–1983). 1983. 253 Seiten.
          Vergriffen.

Band 149 *Vettori, Arthur.* Finanzhaushalt und Wirtschaftsverwaltung Basels (1689–1789).
          Wirtschafts- und Lebensverhältnisse einer Gesellschaft zwischen Tradition und
          Umbruch. 1984. 454 Seiten. Vergriffen.

Band 150 *Hauser, Benedikt.* Wirtschaftsverbände im frühen schweizerischen Bundesstaat (1848–74). Vom regionalen zum nationalen Einzugsgebiet. 1985. 216 Seiten. Vergriffen.

Band 151 *Gilly, Carlos.* Spanien und der Basler Buchdruck bis 1600. Ein Querschnitt durch die spanische Geistesgeschichte aus der Sicht einer europäischen Buchdruckerstadt. 1985. 574 Seiten. Vergriffen.

Band 152 *Röthlin, Niklaus.* Die Basler Handelspolitik und deren Träger in der zweiten Hälfte des 17. und im 18. Jahrhundert. 1986. 424 Seiten. Vergriffen.

Band 153 *Roeser, Volker.* Politik und religiöse Toleranz vor dem ersten Hugenottenkrieg in Frankreich. 1985. 307 Seiten. Vergriffen.

Band 154 *Mattmüller, Markus.* Bevölkerungsgeschichte der Schweiz I: Die frühe Neuzeit, und 154a 1500–1700. 1987. 757 Seiten.

Band 155 *Wiss-Belleville, Elfriede.* Pierre Coullery und die Anfänge der Arbeiterbewegung in Bern und der Westschweiz. Ein Beitrag zur Geschichte des schweizerischen Frühsozialismus. 1987. 415 Seiten. Vergriffen.

Band 156 *Alioth, Martin.* Gruppen an der Macht. Zünfte und Patriziat in Strassburg im 14. und 15. Jahrhundert. Untersuchungen zu Verfassung, Wirtschaftsgefüge und Sozialstruktur. 1988. 510 Seiten. Vergriffen.

Band 157 *Madurowicz-Urbańska, Helena/Mattmüller, Markus (Hrsg.).* Studia Polono-Helvetica. 1989. 178 Seiten. Vergriffen.

Band 158 *Berner, Hans.* «die gute correspondenz.» Die Politik der Stadt Basel gegenüber dem Fürstbistum Basel in den Jahren 1525–1585. 1989. 260 Seiten.

Band 159 *Rippmann, Dorothee.* Bauern und Städter: Stadt-Land-Beziehungen im 15. Jahrhundert. Das Beispiel Basel, unter besonderer Berücksichtigung der Nahmarktbeziehungen und der sozialen Verhältnisse im Umland. 1990. 382 Seiten. Vergriffen.

Band 160 *Schluchter, André.* Das Gösgeramt im Ancien Régime. Bevölkerung, Wirtschaft und Gesellschaft einer solothurnischen Landvogtei im 17. und 18. Jahrhundert. 1990. 484 Seiten.

Band 161 *Degen, Bernard.* Abschied vom Klassenkampf. Die partielle Integration der schweizerischen Gewerkschaftsbewegung zwischen Landesstreik und Weltwirtschaftskrise 1918–1929. 1991. 326 Seiten.

Band 162 *Winkler, Stephan.* Die Schweiz und das geteilte Italien. Bilaterale Beziehungen in einer Umbruchphase 1943–1945. 1992. 650 Seiten.

Band 163 *Roth, Hans Jakob.* Der britische und französische Agrarmarkt im Jahrhundert vor der Europäischen Gemeinschaft – ein Vergleich. 1993. 210 Seiten.

Band 164 *Guggisberg, Hans R.* Zusammenhänge in historischer Vielfalt: Humanismus, Spanien, Nordamerika. Eine Aufsatzsammlung, herausgegeben unter Mitarbeit von Christian Windler. 1994. 430 Seiten.

Band 165 *Hammer, Urs.* Vom Alpenidyll zum modernen Musterstaat. Der Mythos der Schweiz als «alpine sister republic» in den USA des 19. Jahrhunderts. 1995. 380 Seiten.

Band 166 *Maissen, Thomas.* Von der Legende zum Modell. Das Interesse an Frankreichs Vergangenheit während der italienischen Renaissance. 1994. 492 Seiten.

Band 167 *Weissen, Kurt.* «An der stür ist ganz nütt bezalt». Landesherrschaft, Verwaltung und Wirtschaft in den fürstbischöflichen Ämtern in der Umgebung Basels (1435–1525). 1994. 685 Seiten.

Band 168 *Königs, Diemuth.* Joseph Vogt: Ein Althistoriker in der Weimarer Republik und im Dritten Reich. 1995. 344 Seiten.

Band 169 *Haumann, Heiko/Skowronek, Jerzy (Hrsg.).* «Der letzte Ritter und erste Bürger im Osten Europas». Kościuszko, das aufständische Reformpolen und die Verbundenheit zwischen Polen und der Schweiz. 2. Auflage 2000. 380 Seiten.

Band 170 *Zünd, André.* Gescheiterte Stadt- und Landreformationen des 16. und 17. Jahrhunderts in der Schweiz. 1998. 308 Seiten.

Band 171 *Slanička, Simona (Hrsg.).* Begegnungen mit dem Mittelalter in Basel. Eine Vortragsreihe zur mediävistischen Forschung. 2000. 244 Seiten.

Band 172 *Kaiser, Wolfgang/Sieber-Lehmann, Claudius/Windler, Christian (Hrsg.).* Eidgenössische «Grenzfälle»: Mülhausen und Genf – En marge de la Confédération: Mulhouse et Genève. 2001. 424 Seiten.

Band 173 *Schüpbach-Guggenbühl, Samuel.* Schlüssel zur Macht. Verflechtungen und informelles Verhalten im Kleinen Rat zu Basel, 1570–1600. 2002. 2 Bände, 698 Seiten.

Band 174 *Andrzejewski, Marek.* Schweizer in Polen. Spuren der Geschichte eines Brückenschlages. 2002. 366 Seiten.

Band 175 *Meyer, Werner/von Greyerz, Kaspar (Hrsg.).* Platteriana. Beiträge zum 500. Geburtstag des Thomas Platter (1499?–1582). 2002. 182 Seiten.

Band 176 *Kanyar Becker, Helena (Hrsg.).* Jenische, Sinti und Roma in der Schweiz. 2003. 185 Seiten.

Band 177 *Huber, Katharina.* Felix Platters «Observationes». Studien zum frühneuzeitlichen Gesundheitswesen in Basel. 2003. 397 Seiten.

Band 178 *Leutert, Sebastian.* Geschichten vom Tod. Tod und Sterben in Deutschschweizer und oberdeutschen Selbstzeugnissen des 16. und 17. Jahrhunderts. 2007. 378 Seiten.

Band 179 *Bennewitz, Susanne.* Basler Juden – französische Bürger. Migration und Alltag einer jüdischen Gemeinde im frühen 19. Jahrhundert. 2008. 434 Seiten.

Band 180 *Franc, Andrea.* Wie die Schweiz zur Schokolade kam. Der Kakaohandel der Basler Handelsgesellschaft mit der Kolonie Goldküste (1893–1960). 2008. 297 Seiten.

Band 181 *Opitz-Belakhal, Claudia/Wecker, Regina (Hrsg.).* Vom Nutzen der Geschichte. Nachbardisziplinen im Umgang mit Geschichte. 2009. 119 Seiten.

Band 182 *Kanyar Becker, Helena (Hrsg.).* Vergessene Frauen. Humanitäre Kinderhilfe und offizielle Flüchtlingspolitik 1917–1948. 2010. 282 Seiten.

Band 183 *Montanari Häusler, Beatrice.* Bildung als Auftrag. Die Volkshochschule beider Basel im Wandel ihres Publikums und Programms (1969–2009). 2011. 356 Seiten.

Band 184 *Janner, Sara.* Zwischen Machtanspruch und Autoritätsverlust. Zur Funktion von Religion und Kirchlichkeit in Politik und Selbstverständnis des konservativen alten Bürgertums im Basel des 19. Jahrhunderts. 2012. 595 Seiten.

Band 185 *Florkowska-Frančić, Halina.* «Die Freiheit ist eine grosse Sache». Aktivitäten polnischer Patrioten in der Schweiz während des Ersten Weltkriegs. 2014. 358 Seiten.

Band 186 *Meier, Lukas.* Swiss Science, African Decolonization and the Rise of Global Health, 1940–2010. 2014. 323 Seiten.

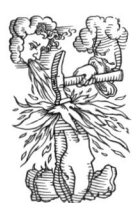

Das Signet des 1488 gegründeten
Druck- und Verlagshauses Schwabe
reicht zurück in die Anfänge der
Buchdruckerkunst und stammt aus
dem Umkreis von Hans Holbein.
Es ist die Druckermarke der Petri;
sie illustriert die Bibelstelle
Jeremia 23,29: «Ist nicht mein Wort
wie Feuer, spricht der Herr,
und wie ein Hammer, der Felsen
zerschmettert?»